NEPHROLOGY NURSING

Concepts and Strategies

NEPHROLOGY NURSING

Concepts and Strategies

Edited by
Beth Tamplet Ulrich, Ed.D., R.N.
Vice President of Patient Services
Southern Baptist Hospital
New Orleans, Louisiana
Past President
American Nephrology Nurses' Association

APPLETON & LANGE
Norwalk, Connecticut/San Mateo, California

0-8385-6699-5

Notice: Our knowledge in clinical sciences is constantly changing. As new information becomes available, changes in treatment and in the use of drugs become necessary. The author(s) and the publisher of this volume have taken care to make certain that the doses of drugs and schedules of treatment are correct and compatible with the standards generally accepted at the time of publication. The reader is advised to consult carefully the instruction and information material included in the package insert of each drug or therapeutic agent before administration. This advice is especially important when using new or infrequently used drugs.

89 90 91 92 93/10 9 8 7 6 5 4 3 2 1

Prentice-Hall International (UK) Limited, *London*
Prentice-Hall of Australia Pty. Limited, *Sydney*
Prentice-Hall Canada, Inc., *Toronto*
Prentice-Hall Hispanoamericana, S.A., *Mexico*
Prentice-Hall of India Private Limited, *New Delhi*
Prentice-Hall of Japan, Inc., *Tokyo*
Simon & Schuster Asia Pte. Ltd., *Singapore*
Editora Prentice-Hall do Brasil Ltda., *Rio de Janeiro*
Prentice-Hall, *Englewood Cliffs, New Jersey*

Library of Congress Cataloging-in-Publication Data

Nephrology nursing: concepts and strategies/Beth Tamplet Ulrich,
    editor.
        p. cm.
    Includes index.
    ISBN 0-8385-6699-5
    1. Kidneys—Diseases—Nursing.   I. Ulrich, Beth Tamplet.
    [DNLM: 1. Kidney Diseases—nursing.   WY 164 N4387]
RC902.N435 1988
610.73'69—dc19
DNLM/DLC   88-14483
for Library of Congress   CIP

Production Editor: Elizabeth C. Ryan
Cover: Michael J. Kelly

PRINTED IN THE UNITED STATES OF AMERICA

Contributors

Betty Irwin Crandall, M.S., R.N.
Clinical Director, Medical-Surgical Nursing
Champlain Valley Physicians Hospital
  Medical Center
Plattsburg, New York

Nancy Fredin, M.S.N., R.N.
Former Administrative Manager, Quality Assurance
Hermann Hospital
Houston, Texas

Karen L. Macheledt, M.S., R.D.
Renal Dietician
Private Practice
Houston, Texas

Marlys E. Nolander, B.S.N., R.N.
Clinical Nurse Specialist
Pediatric Nephrology
University of Minnesota Hospitals
Minneapolis, Minnesota

Janel Parker, M.S.N., R.N.
Nephrology Nurse Consultant
Past President, American Nephrology Nurses' Association
Marietta, Georgia

Sue N. Sauer, M.A., R.N.
Clinical Nurse Specialist
Pediatric Nephrology and Cardiology
University of Minnesota Hospitals
Minneapolis, Minnesota

Beth Tamplet Ulrich, Ed.D., R.N.
Vice President of Patient Services
Southern Baptist Hospital
New Orleans, Louisiana
Past President
American Nephrology Nurses' Association

Reviewers

Dawn T. Brennan, B.S.N.
Research Associate
University of Miami
Diabetes Diagnostic and Treatment Center
Miami, Florida
Past President
American Nephrology Nurses' Association

Janel Parker, M.S.N., R.N.
Nephrology Nurse Consultant
Past President, American Nephrology Nurses' Association
Marietta, Georgia

Contents

Preface

In the early years, before nephrology nursing was recognized as a specialty, the role of the nephrology nurse was to assist the physician in performing hemodialysis. Today, the role of the nephrology nurse has expanded to include all treatment modalities, patients of all ages, many different treatment environments, and a wide range of responsibility.

Nephrology Nursing: Concepts and Strategies is designed to provide valuable information for the nephrology nurse of today regardless of the subspecialty or practice setting. It is based on the philosophy that to be a professional nephrology nurse, one must have a broad knowledge of the specialty as a whole before concentrating on a subspecialty such as dialysis, transplantation, or pediatric nephrology nursing.

This is a pragmatic as well as a theoretical book; and the contributors were selected because of their experience in the field. Betty Crandall is a well-known clinician in the transplant community who, in addition to her role in the field of transplantation, has frequently lectured on acute and chronic renal failure. Karen Macheledt is a renal dietician who worked at the Texas Kidney Institute during the writing of this book, and who is now completing medical school. Janel Parker is an experienced nephrology nurse and past president of the American Nephrology Nurses' Association. In that role, she is best known for having initiated and coordinated the development of a certification examination for professional nephrology nurses that is based on the same philosophy as this book—that professional nephrology nurses must be knowledgeable about all aspects of their specialty.

Sue Sauer and Marlys Nolander practice pediatric nephrology nursing at the University of Minnesota. They have produced an outstanding chapter on the extensive differences in caring for our littlest nephrology patients. Nancy Fredin served as the administrative manager of nursing quality assurance at Hermann Hospital, and is now pursuing her doctorate. All have made valuable contributions to nephrology nursing and to this book.

In developing *Nephrology Nursing: Concepts and Strategies*, we have attempted to provide an educational tool to be used by students and new nephrology nurses as well as a reference text for experienced nephrology nurses and other health-care professionals who work with nephrology patients. We hope that you find it informative and useful.

Beth Tamplet Ulrich, Editor

Acknowledgments

To my colleagues in nephrology who have taught me the art and science of our fine profession.

To my father who long ago taught me that I could do anything I set my mind to do, and my mother who never doubted that I would.

To Walter and Blythe for their inspiration and unlimited support.

1

Renal Anatomy and Physiology

Beth Tamplet Ulrich

OBJECTIVES

After reading this chapter on renal anatomy and physiology, the nurse will be able to:

1. Describe the anatomy of the kidney
2. Trace the blood flow through the kidney
3. Describe the process of urine formation
4. Compare and contrast molecular and fluid transport throughout the nephron
5. Explain the contribution of the renal system in maintaining fluid and electrolyte balance

It is critical that the practicing nephrology nurse have a working knowledge of the normal renal system. By knowing what the kidneys would be doing if they were working properly, it becomes relatively easy to logically determine what the patient with inadequate function needs to establish or maintain fluid and electrolyte balance and duplicate other functions of the kidney.

RENAL SYSTEM ANATOMY

Macrostructure
The main component of the renal system is the kidneys. The kidneys are paired organs located retroperitoneally and lateral to the vertebral column

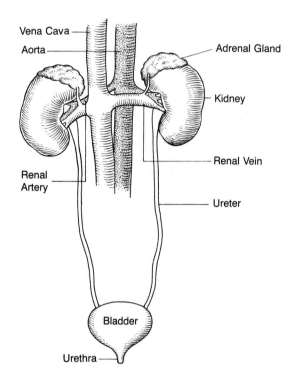

Vena Cava

Aorta

Adrenal Gland

Kidney

Renal Vein

Renal
Artery

Ureter

Bladder

Figure 1-1. Gross anatomy of
the renal system.

Urethra

(Fig. 1-1). The right kidney is situated at the level of the twelfth rib. The left
kidney is slightly higher. An adrenal gland is located atop each kidney. Each
kidney is bean-shaped, measuring approximately 11 cm in length, 5.0 to 7.5
cm in width, and 2.5 cm in thickness. In the adult male, each kidney weighs
125 to 170 grams and, in the adult female, 115 to 155 grams.

A *ureter* connected to each kidney serves to deliver urine to the bladder.
The ureters are 2 to 8 mm in diameter, 25 to 35 cm long, and are profusely in-
nervated. Urine transport is assisted by peristaltic contractions. A ureterovesi-
cal valve, located at the ureter-bladder interface, prevents the backflow of
urine into the ureters.

The *urinary bladder,* composed of muscular elastic tissue, serves as a
collecting reservoir for urine. The inner mucous wall of the bladder has
phagocytic ability to help prevent infection. The bladder is very flexible, with
a capacity of 1000 to 1800 ml. Distention of the bladder stimulates stretch
receptors located in the bladder wall. The stimulated stretch receptors cause
a reflex contraction of the bladder and relaxation of the internal sphincter.
When the external sphincter relaxes, voiding occurs. Parasympathetic nerve
innervation of the bladder coordinates bladder contraction and sphincter
relaxation.

The *urethra* is connected to the bladder and serves primarily as the final
conducting tube for the urine. The female urethra is 3 to 5 cm long. The male

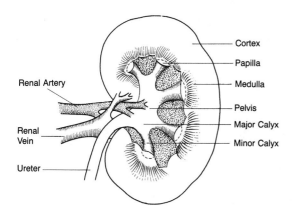

Figure 1-2. Gross anatomy of the kidney.

urethra is about 20 cm long and transports semen as well as urine.

A hard, fibrous capsule surrounds the kidney (Fig. 1-2). The *cortex* is the outermost layer of the kidney and contains all the glomeruli, proximal and distal convoluted tubules, the first portions of the Loops of Henle, and collecting ducts. The inner portion of the kidney, the *medulla,* is composed of conical masses called *pyramids.* The renal artery, renal vein, lymphatics, nerve plexus, and the renal sinus and pelvis are all located at the *hilus.*

Nephrons

The *nephron* is the functional unit of the kidney. Approximately 85 percent of the kidney's one million nephrons originate in glomeruli located in the superficial cortex. These *cortical nephrons* have short Loops of Henle that extend only into the outer medulla (Fig. 1-3).

The remaining 15 percent of the nephrons, the *juxtamedullary nephrons,* originate in glomeruli located in the innermost or juxtamedulary cortex. Juxtamedullary nephrons, in contrast to cortical nephrons, have long Loops of Henle that extend deep into the medulla, where they run parallel to the collecting ducts. This placement contributes to the increased ability of the juxtamedullary nephrons to retain sodium. Each nephron contains Bowman's capsule, a glomerulus, tubules, and renal vasculature (Fig. 1-4).

The *glomerulus* is composed of three layers of cells: the capillary endothelial cell layer, the capillary basement membrane layer, and the urinary epithelial cell layer. These layers form a semipermeable membrane that prevents passage of molecules with a molecular radius greater than 38 to 44 angstroms, but allows easy passage of molecules with a radius of less than 20 angstroms (Brenner & Hostetter, 1981). The presence of anion-rich macromolecular clusters within the glomerular structure further restricts the filtration of negatively charged macromolecules, such as proteins. *Bowman's capsule* is a blind-ended sac that surrounds the glomerulus on its interior side and is open to the first portion of the tubule on its exterior side.

The *proximal convoluted tubule* is composed of a highly coiled portion

4

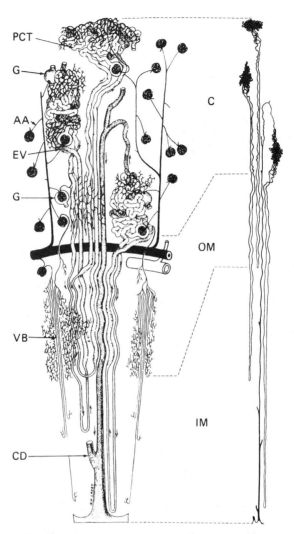

Figure 1–3. Diagram of renal vascular and tubular organization. Only three nephrons (one from each general population) are shown, vascular structures are extensively simplified, and vertical scale is compressed. The same nephrons are shown undistorted to the right. Major zones are: cortex (C), outer medulla (OM), and inner medulla (IM). Afferent arterioles (AA), glomeruli (G), and efferent vessels (EV) are shown together with part of the peritubular capillary network. The proximal convoluted tubules (PCT) and distal convoluted tubules (dark hatching) are generally dissociated from the efferent network arising from their parent glomeruli. Some midcortical efferents directly perfuse Henle loops and collecting ducts in cortical medullary rays. In outer medulla, descending thin limbs of short loops are close to vascular bundles (VB), while thin limbs of long loops are found with thick ascending limbs and collecting ducts (CD) in the interbundle region. Note the relationships of the capillary plexuses (CP) to the vascular bundles. (*Adapted from Beeuwkes, R. III. [1975].* Am J Physiol, 228: *695, with permission.)*

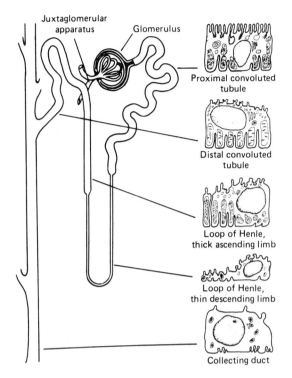

Figure 1-4. The functional nephron. (*From Ganong, W. F. [1985]. Review of medical physiology [13th ed.]. East Norwalk, CT: Appleton & Lange.*)

connected to Bowman's capsule and a straight portion leading to the *Loop of Henle*. The Loop of Henle, a sharp, hairpin loop, leads to the *distal convoluted tubule*. The coiled distal convoluted tubule straightens out to form the *collecting duct*. From the glomerulus to the beginning of the collecting duct, each tubule is separate from its neighbors. At the collecting ducts, the tubules join to form progressively larger ducts that empty into the renal pelvis at the base of each kidney.

Renal Vasculature

Renal blood flow (RBF) is equal to about 25 percent of the cardiac output or approximately 1200 cc per minute. The distribution of the blood flow in the kidney is highest in the superficial cortex and progressively diminishes toward the medulla (Andreoli, Carpenter, Plum, & Smith, 1986). Blood enters the kidney via the *renal artery*, which is located at the hilum next to the ureter. The artery branches, becoming progressively smaller until ultimately about one million *afferent arterioles* result. The branch path is renal artery to interlobar artery to arcuate artery to interlobular artery to afferent arteriole.

Each afferent arteriole leads to a glomerular capillary where filtration occurs. The glomerular capillary bed then merges into the *efferent arteriole*.

The efferent arteriole of cortical nephrons branches into a second capillary bed that lies in the cortex around the proximal and distal tubules. This *peritubular capillary bed* then joins *venules* with the blood finally exiting the kidney via the *renal vein*. Cortical nephrons have high-pressure capillary beds, where filtration occurs and urine is formed, and low-pressure capillary beds that are nutritive, supply blood to the rest of the nephron, and allow for reabsorption from the tubule back into the blood.

Juxtamedullary nephrons have a more complex vasculature (see Fig. 1–3). The efferent arteriole of juxtamedullary nephrons also branches into a second capillary network around the proximal and distal tubules of these nephrons, but this peritubular capillary bed is located in the deep cortex. As with cortical nephrons, blood flows from the peritubular capillary bed to venules and the renal vein.

A series of hairpin loops called *vasa recta* parallel the long Loops of Henle in juxtamedullary nephrons. The vasa recta branch into capillary networks around the ascending limbs of Loops of Henle and the collecting ducts of both types of nephrons. The presence of the vasa recta results in an increased resistance in juxtamedullary nephrons. This resistance leads to a higher filtration rate as well as less blood flow. Vasa recta also act as a counter-current exchanger, preventing the interstitial gradient from being dissipated and thereby contributing significantly to the kidney's ability to concentrate urine.

Juxtaglomerular Apparatus

The *juxtaglomerular apparatus* (JGA) is a combination of specialized tubular and vascular cells located near the glomerulus at the junction of the afferent and efferent arterioles. Juxtaglomerular cells (granular cells) contain granules of inactive renin (Fig. 1–5). The JGA is believed to secrete renin and thus to play a role in both autoregulation of glomerular filtration and renal control of extracellular fluid volume via the renin-angiotension-aldosterone mechanism.

RENAL PHYSIOLOGY

The main purpose of the kidney is to maintain a stable internal environment in which optimal cellular function can occur. This is achieved through a number of specialized renal functions (Table 1–1).

Body Fluids

Body fluids provide an environment for the physical- and chemical-related reactions essential to life. Other functions include cell environment and nutrition, transportation, and acting as a solvent.

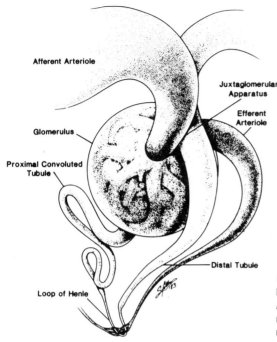

Afferent Arteriole

Juxtaglomerular
Apparatus

Efferent
Arteriole

Glomerulus

Proximal Convoluted
Tubule

Distal Tubule

Loop of Henle

Figure 1-5. The juxtaglomerular apparatus. (*Tauxe, W. N., & Dubovsky, E. [1985].* Nuclear medicine in clinical urology and nephrology. *East Norwalk, CT: Appleton & Lange.*)

Body fluids consist mainly of water and dissolved substances such as salts, minerals, or crystalloids. Body water accounts for about 60 percent of the total weight of adults and about 80 percent of the total weight of infants.

Body fluids are divided into *intracellular fluids* and *extracellular fluids.* Intracellular fluids include fluids located within the cellular structure and account for about two thirds of the total body fluid. Extracellular fluids compose the remaining one-third of the body fluid. Approximately two thirds of the ex-

TABLE 1-1. FUNCTIONS OF THE KIDNEY

1. Regulation of fluid volume and ionic composition of body fluids (homestasis)
2. Excretion of metabolic end products (i.e., urea, creatinine, uric acid)
3. Detoxification and elimination of toxins, drugs, and their metabolites
4. Endocrine regulation of extracellular fluid voume and blood pressure
5. Control of red blood cell mass (erythropoietic principle)
6. Endocrine control of mineral metabolism (formation of 1, 25 dihydroxycholecalciferol or 24, 25 dihydroxycholecalciferol)
7. Degradation and catabolism of peptide hormones (insulin, glucagon, parathyroid hormone)
8. Catabolism of small molecular weight proteins
9. Metabolic interconversions (gluconeogenesis, lipid metabolism)

tracellular fluids are found in the interstitium, and one third in the vascular space. Small amounts of extracellular fluid are found in bones, cerebrospinal fluid, aqueous humor, the respiratory and gastrointestinal tracts, the liver, pancreatic fluids, and serosal cavities. The intracellular and extracellular fluids are separated by cell membranes. These membranes are freely permeable to water, but are not permeable to most solutes. The kidney filters the fluid in the vascular component of the extracellular fluids.

Body Water

Body water is gained through ingestion of liquids, called *sensible gain,* and through ingestion of solid foods and the body's chemical reactions, called *insensible gain.* Body water is lost through the urine termed *sensible loss,* and through the skin, lungs, and stool, termed *insensible loss.* When the kidneys are functioning adequately, the body generally requires 2000 to 2500 cc of water per day to make up for urine and insensible losses. Insensible gains should balance insensible losses and sensible gains should balance sensible losses.

The movement of body fluids from one fluid compartment to another depends on the *permeability* of capillary and cell walls, *osmotic concentrations, colloid osmotic pressure,* and *hydrostatic pressure.* Permeability refers to the size of molecules that can cross a membrane, in this case capillary and cell walls. In order for fluids to move, the membranes must be permeable to the degree that water passage can occur. Osmotic concentration is determined by the amount of solutes in relation to the amount of fluid. Water is pulled from the area of lower osmotic concentration to the area of higher osmotic concentration. Colloid osmotic pressure is the force exerted by nondiffusable particles such as proteins. It appears that the movement of water out of a compartment of relatively high colloid osmotic pressure draws water from an adjacent compartment of lower colloidal osmotic pressure. Hydrostatic pressure is the force of fluid in a compartment. It promotes movement of water from an area of high hydrostatic pressure and into an area of low hydrostatic pressure.

Electrolytes have three major functions: to maintain water distribution, to maintain acid-base balance, and to maintain a balanced degree of neuromuscular excitability. Electrolytes, like body fluid, are divided into those in the extracellular spaces and the intracellular spaces.

The major extracellular electrolytes are sodium (Na^+), chloride (CI^-), bicarbonate (HCO_3^-), and calcium (Ca^{++}). Sodium, chloride, and bicarbonate together account for 90 to 95 percent of the intracellular osmolality.

The body tries to maintain a balance between the number of extracellular and intracellular ions and between the number of positively charged ions (*anions*) and the number of negatively charged ions (*cations*). The body attempts to balance 154 mEq/L of anions with 154 mEq/L of cations, without regard for the composition of anions and cations.

Urine Formation

Urine formation contributes to fluid and electrolyte balance, acid-base balance, and the excretion of metabolic waste products.

Glomerular Filtration

Filtration Pressures. *Starling's hypothesis* clarifies the forces involved in glomerular filtration. According to Starling's hypothesis, the *net filtration pressure* for any capillary is the algebraic sum of the opposing hydrostatic and colloid osmotic pressures that act across the capillary (Vander, 1985). In the glomerular capillaries, the net filtration pressure equals the total of the forces inducing filtration (the glomerular-capillary hydrostatic pressure and the colloid osmotic pressure of fluid in Bowman's capsule) minus the total of the forces opposing filtration (the hydrostatic pressure in Bowman's capsule and the colloid osmotic pressure in glomerular-capillary plasma).

The approximate values for these forces in humans are shown in Figure 1–6. The net filtration pressure declines through the capillary path, finally reaching zero at the efferent end. The result is a mean net filtration pressure of about 5 to 6 mm Hg. Under normal conditions, this pressure is sufficient to force an essentially protein-free plasma filtrate through the glomerular membranes into Bowman's capsule, initiating the formation of urine. Changes in either the hydrostatic pressures in the glomerular capillaries or Bowman's capsule or in the plasma colloid osmotic pressure can alter the net filtration pressure. For example, urethral obstruction can cause a rise in the intratubular pressure in Bowman's capsule, decreasing the net filtration pressure and, therefore, glomerular filtration. An increase in the plasma colloid osmotic pressure, such as that created by the loss of a large quantity of protein-free extracellular fluid with sweating or diarrhea, also reduces the net filtration pressure and the glomerular filtration. In the compromised patient the net filtration pressure may be insufficient or the glomerular membrane may be altered, resulting in the filtration of larger substances such as protein.

Glomerular Filtration Rate. The glomerular filtration rate (GFR) indicates the volume of plasma cleared of a given substance in a specific period of time. The GFR of an individual with adequate renal function and a normal hematocrit is 125 to 140 ml/min or 180 L/day.

To measure GFR accurately, a substance must be utilized that is freely filtered at the glomerulus but is neither secreted or reabsorbed at the tubules. The use of the polysaccharide inulin offers the most accurate measurement of GFR but is inconvenient, because inulin must be given by means of continuous intravenous administration. In clinical situations, creatinine is often used to estimate the GFR. Creatinine is an indigenous substance formed from muscle creatine and released into the blood at a fairly constant rate. Unless

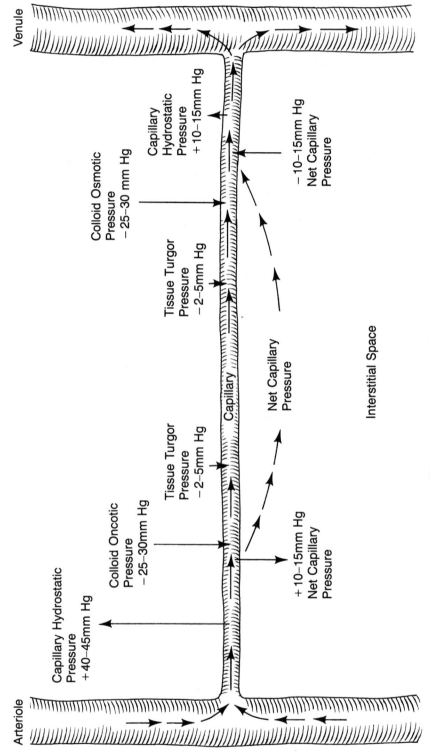

Figure 1-6. Capillary Starling forces.

Arteriole

Venule

Capillary

Interstitial Space

Capillary Hydrostatic Pressure +40–45mm Hg

Colloid Oncotic Pressure –25–30mm Hg

Tissue Turgor Pressure –2–5mm Hg

+10–15mm Hg Net Capillary Pressure

Net Capillary Pressure

Colloid Osmotic Pressure –25–30 mm Hg

Tissue Turgor Pressure –2–5mm Hg

Capillary Hydrostatic Pressure +10–15mm Hg

–10–15mm Hg Net Capillary Pressure

there is dialytic intervention, the creatinine remains stable. The GFR can be estimated by obtaining one serum creatinine level and a 24-hour urine and using the formula

$$\text{GFR} = \frac{(\text{U}_{cr})\ (\text{V})}{\text{P}_{cr}}$$

where U_{cr} = urine creatinine concentration, V = urine volume per time, and P_{cr} = plasma creatinine concentration (Vander, 1985). This method will slightly overestimate the GFR but is quite usable in the clinical setting.

Although the exact mechanisms of GFR determination remain unclear, there is general agreement that the major determinants are the glomerular plasma flow and the hydraulic permeability of the filtration barrier. Either of these determinants can be affected independently by disease conditions, hormones, and drugs. Table 1–2 summarizes the major determinants.

Tubulo-glomerular Balance. The tubulo-glomerular feedback, discussed earlier, primarily functions to regulate GFR (Fig. 1–6), allowing the GFR to re-

TABLE 1–2. SUMMARY OF DIRECT GFR DETERMINANTS AND FACTORS THAT INFLUENCE THEM

Direct determinants of GFR[a] $\text{GFR} = \text{K}_f \cdot (\text{P}_{GC} - \text{P}_{BC} - \pi_{GC})$	Major factors that tend to increase the magnitude of the direct determinant
$\text{K}_f{}^{a}$	↑ Glomerular surface area due to relaxation of glomerular mesangial cells Result: ↑ GFR
$\text{P}_{GC}{}^{a}$	↑ Renal arterial pressure ↓ Afferent arteriolar resistance (afferent dilation) ↑ Efferent arteriolar resistance (efferent constriction) Result: ↑ GFR
$\text{P}_{BC}{}^{a}$	↑ Intratubular pressure due to obstruction of tubule or extrarenal urinary system Result: ↓ GFR
$\pi_{GC}{}^{a}$	↑ Systemic-plasma oncotic pressure (sets π_{GC} at beginnig of glomerular capillaries) ↓ Total renal plasma flow (sets rate of rise of π_{GC} along glomerular capillaries) Result: ↓ GFR

[a]K_f = filtration coefficient; P_{GC} = glomerular-capillary hydraulic pressure; P_{BC} = Bowman's capsule hydraulic pressure; π_{GC} = glomerular-capillary oncotic pressure. A reversal of all arrows in the table will cause a decrease in the magnitudes of K_f, P_{GC}, P_{BC}, and π_{GC}.
From Vander, A. J. (1985). Renal physiology, p 29. New York: McGraw-Hill, with permission.

main constant despite wide fluctuations in blood pressure. In tubulo-glomerular feedback regulation, decreases in the GFR are associated with increases in the flow of tubular fluid through the Loop of Henle (Haberle & von Baeuer, 1983). The decreased GFR results from a reduction in both glomerular capillary blood flow and hydraulic conductivity. Although the tubulo-glomerular feedback regulation can also work to increase the GFR when the tubular flow decreases it is more efficient in its response to increased tubular flow.

Glomerulotubular Balance. In addition to the mechanism of tubulo-glomerular feedback, there is also a phenomenon called glomerulotubular balance. Present evidence indicates that tubular sodium reabsorption is probably more important than GFR in the long-term regulation of sodium balance. Glomerulotubular balance, a completely intrarenal event, accounts for the direct correlation between the GFR and the absolute reabsorption of fluid in the proximal tubules, and possibly the Loops of Henle and distal tubules. If, for example, the GFR decreases by 25 percent, the absolute rate of proximal fluid reabsorption will decrease by almost the same percentage.

The end product of glomerular filtration is an ultrafiltrate containing no formed elements and a lower protein level than the glomerular capillary blood. The differences in protein result in a separation of charges, with anions and cations distributing asymmetrically across the separating membrane. Anion concentration is then higher and cation concentration is lower in the fluid in Bowman's space.

Distribution of Renal Blood Flow. The kidney has the ability to *autoregulate* renal blood flow even with huge changes in the perfusion pressure to the kidney. Over a renal perfusion pressure range of 70 to 180 mm Hg, both renal blood flow and GFR are maintained at relatively constant rates. The exact method for autoregulation is not certain. Internally, the renal blood flow is distributed between the cortex and medulla. The mechanisms controlling this intrarenal distribution are not clearly defined, but may include the sympathetic nervous system, the prostaglandin system, and antidiuretic hormone.

Myogenic Theory. The myogenic theory proposes that the afferent arteriole vasoconstricts in response to an increase in pressure. Thus, the resistance in the afferent arteriole increases, and the blood flow to the kidney remains constant (Fig. 1–7). This mechanism is similar to that found in other autoregulatory vascular beds.

Tubuloglomerular Feedback. Tubuloglomerular feedback is a more complex process. Although its primary function is to regulate glomerular filtration, tubuloglomerular feedback appears to also alter renal blood flow (Fig. 1–8). It has been postulated that this process involves the macula densa feedback mechanism or tubular cells distal to the macula densa, or both, as well as the

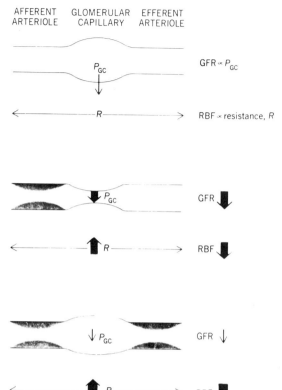

Figure 1-7. *Autoregulation. (From Vander, A. J. [1985].* Renal physiology, *p 78. New York: McGraw-Hill, with permission.)*

generation of a vasoconstrictor chemical. How the macula densa detect changes in rates of fluid flow and which vasoconstrictor is involved remain unclear.

Tubular Function. Tubular function includes the processes of *reabsorption* and *secretion* of substances including electrolytes, waste products, and other substances. Reabsorption is the movement of substances from the filtrate located in the tubular lumen back to the plasma in the peritubular capillaries. This process allows the body to retain necessary substances that have been filtered. Of the 180 L of filtrate that pass to the tubules each day, only approximately one liter is excreted as urine. Virtually all of the filtrate is reabsorbed, most at the proximal tubule. Tubular secretion is the movement of substances from the peritubular capillary plasma into the tubular lumen.

Transport across the tubule requires the movement of the substance across a sequence of membranes (Fig. 1-9). The complex path of substance transport during reabsorption, for example, is from the tubular lumen, across

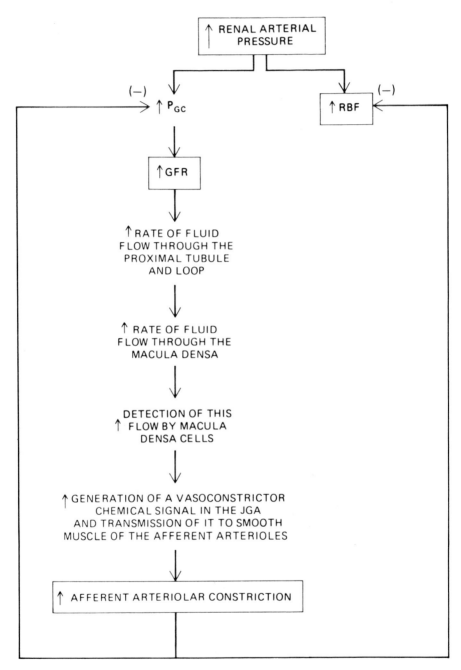

Figure 1-8. Tubulo-glomerular feedback contribution to autoregulation. (*From Vander, A. J. [1985]. Renal physiology, p. 74. New York: McGraw-Hill, with permission.*)

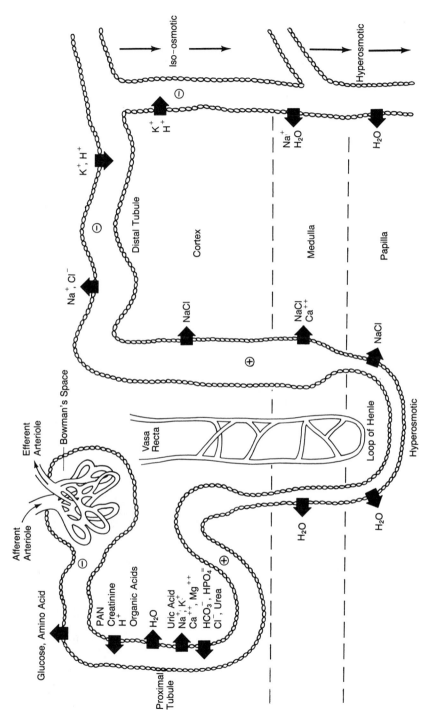

Figure 1-9. Nephron transport.

15

the cell membrane lining the lumen (luminal membrane), into the tubular cell, through the cell's cytoplasm, across the opposite cell membrane, into the interstitial fluid, across the basement membrane and capillary endothelium, and, finally, into the plasma. If one or more of these steps involves the displacing of the substance across a membrane against an electrochemical gradient, then the entire process is called *active transport.* Active transport can be of a primary or secondary nature. *Primary active transport* requires hydrolysis of high-energy compounds, but *secondary active transport* does not (Vander, 1985).

In the case of many substances, the active reabsorption and secretion systems can transport only limited amounts of the substance within a given unit of time. This is referred to as the substance transport maximum or Tm.

Proximal Convoluted Tubule. From Bowman's capsule, the filtrate first moves into the proximal tubule (Fig. 1–10). Most tubular reabsorption occurs at this site. Amino acids, filtered glucose, bicarbonate, and potassium are almost totally reabsorbed. Sixty-five percent of sodium choloride and water reabsorption and a significant amount of phosphate reabsorption take place in the proximal tubule. The fluid leaving the proximal tubule is iso-osmotic to plasma.

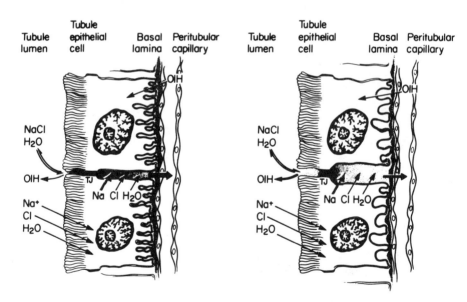

Figure 1–10. A diagrammatic representation of a proximal tubular cell showing its electrical and ion transport properties. (*From Tauxe, W. N., & Dubovsky, E. [1985]. Nuclear medicine in clinical urology and nephrology. East Norwalk, CT: Appleton & Lange.*)

Loop of Henle. The filtrate progresses to the descending limb of the Loop of Henle, which is highly water permeable, but relatively impermeable to electrolytes and solutes. Neither sodium nor chloride is actively transported at this site. Water moves out into the interstitium, as shown in Figure 1–11, and the tubular fluid becomes progressively more concentrated as it equilibrates with the hypertonic interstitium.

The highest solute concentration, 1400 mosm/L, is achieved at the tip of the Loop of Henle (Vander, 1985). As the fluid moves up the ascending limb, almost the reverse of the processes in the descending limb occur. The ascending limb can be divided into the thin ascending limb and the thick ascending limb. Compared to the descending limb, the thin ascending limb has a relatively low water permeability and a higher permeability to sodium and urea. Sodium and chloride are actively transported into the interstitium. As a result, the fluid in the thin ascending limb becomes progressively diluted. The thick ascending limb is virtually impermeable to water. Sodium chloride is removed by secondary active transport, further diluting the tubular fluid. Calcium and magnesium are reabsorbed. By the time the fluid leaves the thick ascending limb, the fluid osmolality is less than that of plasma.

The concentration of urine relies on the success of the Loop of Henle's *countercurrent multiplier system.* As water is reabsorbed, filtrate is progressively concentrated as it flows down the descending limb. With the active transport of sodium and chloride from the tubule into the interstitium, the filtrate is progressively diluted as it flows up the ascending limb. The result, as

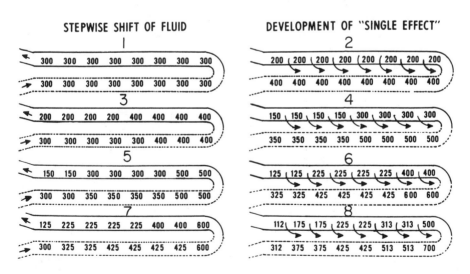

Figure 1-11. The countercurrent multiplier system. (*From Pitts, R. F. [1974]. The physiology of the kidney and body fluids, [3rd ed.]. Chicago: Year Book Medical Publishers, with permission.*)

can be seen in Figure 1-11, is a significant change in the osmotic gradient from the top of the medulla to the bottom. The gradient is said to have been multiplied by the countercurrent flow. The degree to which the hypertonic interstitium is created at the tip of the loop is primarily dependent on the length of the Loop of Henle (the longer the loop, the higher the potential concentration) and the strength of the chloride pump. The development of this hypertonic interstitium is essential for the concentration of urine in the collecting ducts.

Distal Convoluted Tubule. From the ascending limb of the Loop of Henle, the filtrate moves to the distal convoluted tubule. In the presence of aldosterone, sodium is reabsorbed and potassium is secreted at this site. If sufficient potassium to exchange is not present, hydrogen ions are secreted instead. Aldosterone-inhibiting diuretics block sodium reabsorption at this site. While these medications lead to successful diuresis, they may also create potassium imbalances. Calcium and, in the absence of parathyroid hormone, phosphate are reabsorbed. Water permeability remains low and the tubular fluid remains hypotonic.

Collecting Duct. The collecting duct is the site of final concentration or dilution of the urine. Concentration and dilution at this point are totally dependent on the concentration gradient between the filtrate in the duct and the solution in the interstitium (see Fig. 1-11). As previously discussed, a hypertonic interstitium must have been formed if adequate concentration and dilution are to occur. If an adequate concentration gradient is not established, a dilute urine will result. An example of this occurs when Lasix or ethacrynic acid is given to the patient. Both of these medications affect the ascending limb of the Loop of Henle, decreasing sodium and chloride reabsorption. The resulting interstitium is isotonic or hypotonic. Water does not diffuse into the interstitium but rather is eliminated.

Urine. The end result is the daily production of 800 to 1800 cc of light yellow to dark brown urine. The odor of the urine is fresh. The specific gravity varies from 1.005 to 1.025 depending on the concentration, with a pH usually in the range of 4.5 to 7.5. The urine is composed of waste products, excess electrolytes, hormones and their breakdown products, vitamins, drugs, and on occasion, small amounts of sediment. Any alteration in this picture of "normal" urine alerts the nurse to a potential dysfunctional state.

Sodium and Water Balance

The regulation of total body sodium (Na^+) and extracellular volume depends upon a number of systems and interdependent variables (Figs. 1-12 and 1-13). Sodium is the major extracellular cation, with normal serum values ranging from 135 to 145 mEq/L. Approximately 20,000 mEq per day of sodium are filtered by the kidneys, despite the fact that the average healthy in-

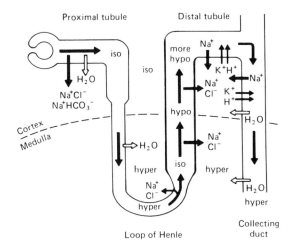

Figure 1-12. Salt and water transport throughout the nephron. (*From Cannon, P. J. [1977]. The kidney in heart failure.* N Engl J Med, 296:26, *with permission.*)

dividual only ingests 50 to 250 mEq in the same time period. If necessary, however, the kidneys have the ability to eliminate a urine that is virtually sodium free. The body's supply of sodium is jealously guarded by the kidney, even at the expense of other electrolytes. The kidneys must also excrete approximately 500 ml/day of water to adequately excrete the obligatory solute load. As could be clearly seen in the previous section on the formation of urine, sodium and water balance are highly interrelated.

Aldosterone. The reabsorption of approximately 2 percent of the total filtered sodium is dependent upon the influence of *aldosterone,* a hormone produced by the zona glomerulosa area of the adrenal cortex. Although 2 percent sounds like a small amount, it is equal to more than the average oral sodium intake.

Aldosterone secretion is controlled by the plasma sodium and potassium concentrations, angiotensin, and, to a minimal degree, adrenocortiotropic hormone (ACTH). Increased plasma sodium results in decreased aldosterone secretion. In contrast, an increased plasma potassium stimulates the adrenal cortex to produce aldosterone, which increases the tubular secretion of potassium and, ultimately, its excretion (Fig. 1-14). Angiotensin is the major controller of aldosterone in sodium regulation reflexes and will be discussed as part of the overall renin-angiotensin system in the following section.

Renin and Angiotensin. Renin is a proteolytic enzyme secreted into the blood by the kidneys, specifically by the specialized area of each nephron known as the juxtaglomerular apparatus (JGA). There are two predominant beliefs regarding the control of renin secretion by the kidneys. The first is that the juxtaglomerular cells function as baroreceptors, sensitive to blood flow through the afferent arteriole. A decrease in arterial pressure stimulates in-

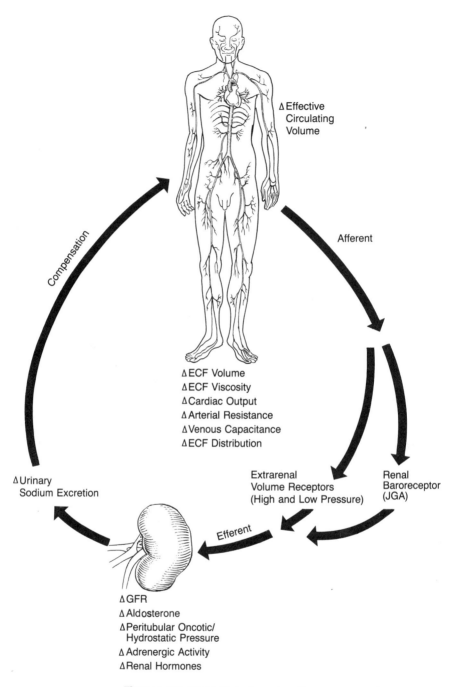

ΔEffective
Circulating
Volume

Afferent

Compensation

ΔECF Volume
ΔECF Viscosity
ΔCardiac Output
ΔArterial Resistance
ΔVenous Capacitance
ΔECF Distribution

ΔUrinary
Sodium Excretion

Extrarenal
Volume Receptors
(High and Low Pressure)

Renal
Baroreceptor
(JGA)

Efferent

ΔGFR
ΔAldosterone
ΔPeritubular Oncotic/
  Hydrostatic Pressure
ΔAdrenergic Activity
ΔRenal Hormones

Figure 1–13. Regulation of renal sodium.

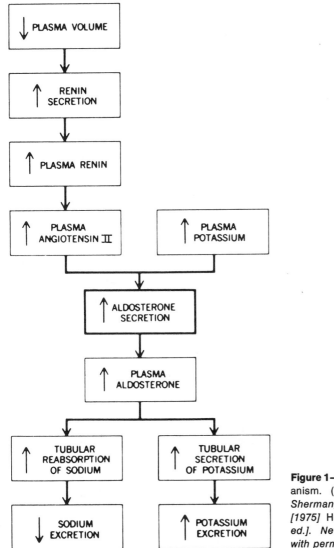

Figure 1-14. Aldosterone mechanism. (*From Vander, A. J., Sherman, J. H., & Luciano, D. [1975] Human physiology [2nd ed.]. New York: McGraw-Hill, with permission.*)

creased granularity of the juxtaglomerular cells and increases renal secretion (Fig. 1-15). The second alternative holds that the macula densa cells of the distal tubule act as chemoreceptors, sensitive to the sodium concentration of the tubular fluid. These chemoreceptors stimulate the juxtaglomerular cells to increase renin output. In addition to these two alternatives, there is also some evidence that the sympathetic nervous system and catecholamines also influence renin secretion (Vander, 1985).

Regardless of the process, a low plasma volume results in a decreased

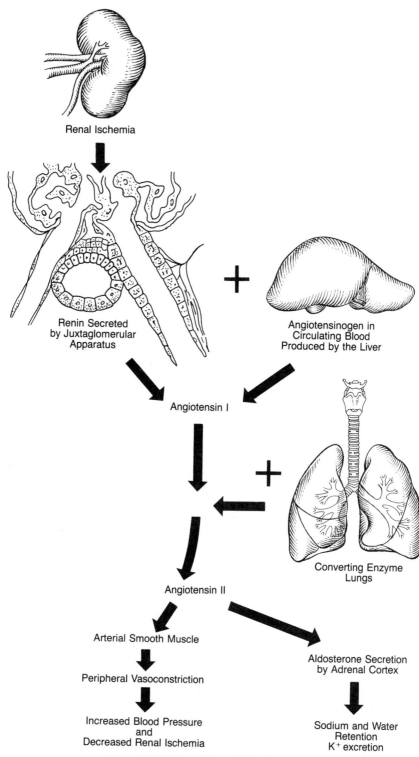

Renal Ischemia

Renin Secreted
by Juxtaglomerular
Apparatus

Angiotensinogen in
Circulating Blood
Produced by the Liver

+

Angiotensin I

+

Converting Enzyme
Lungs

Angiotensin II

Arterial Smooth Muscle

Peripheral Vasoconstriction

Increased Blood Pressure
and
Decreased Renal Ischemia

Aldosterone Secretion
by Adrenal Cortex

Sodium and Water
Retention
K^+ excretion

Figure 1–15. The renin-angiotensin system.

glomerular filtration rate. This leads to a low intratubular sodium load. Juxtaglomerular cells then secrete renin. Figure 1–15 illustrates the progression of the events that follow renin secretion.

The combination of the secreted renin with angiotensinogin in the blood yields angiotensin I, which is then converted to angiotensin II. The presence of angiotensin II causes peripheral vasoconstriction, which is evidenced by an increased blood pressure and decreased renal ischemia. Angiotensin II stimulates the release of aldosterone by the adrenal cortex and the activation of the thirst mechanism (Fig. 1–16).

Antidiuretic Hormone. The ability for water to follow when sodium is reabsorbed depends on *antidiuretic hormone* (ADH). ADH is an octopeptide produced by the hypothalamus and secreted in the blood by the posterior pituary gland. Vascular baroreceptors, especially those in the left atrium, are stimulated by changes in atrial blood pressure. Afferent nerves transmit this information to the hypothalamus where ADH production is appropriately inhibited or increased (Fig. 1–17).

Pure water deficits or gains also influence ADH secretion through changes in body fluid osmolarity. Osmoreceptors, located in the hypothalamus, detect water osmolarity changes and, through neural input, alert the hypothalamus cells that secrete ADH. In the situation where the hypothalamus cells receive conflicting input from the baroreceptors and osmoreceptors, the stronger input prevails.

In addition to the major regulators of ADH secretion, hypothalamus cells are also subject to short-term influences like pain, fear, and alcohol, and long-term influences such as diabetes insipidus.

Potassium Balance

Potassium (K^+) is the major intracellular cation and is responsible for the regulation of resting membrane potentials that control cell excitability. The intracellular concentration of 150 mEq/L is far beyond the extracellular concentration of 3 to 5 mEq/L. Even a small change in the cellular transport of potassium can result in a large change in the extracellular concentration. Although the kidneys do not have the ability to compose a potassium-free urine, they can respond successfully to a wide range of potassium levels.

Potassium is freely filtered at the glomerulus with 85 to 90 percent of the filtered potassium being reabsorbed by the time the filtrate reaches the distal tubule. Under most conditions, potassium reabsorption prior to the distal tubule appears to occur without regard to body potassium. This does not appear to be the case in the distal tubule and collecting ducts where potassium is both reabsorbed and secreted.

Potassium secretion is influenced by potassium concentration of the distal-tubular cells, aldosterone secretion, sodium changes, and certain medications. Changes in the potassium concentration of the distal tubular cells result in a corresponding balancing change in potassium secretion. Aldo-

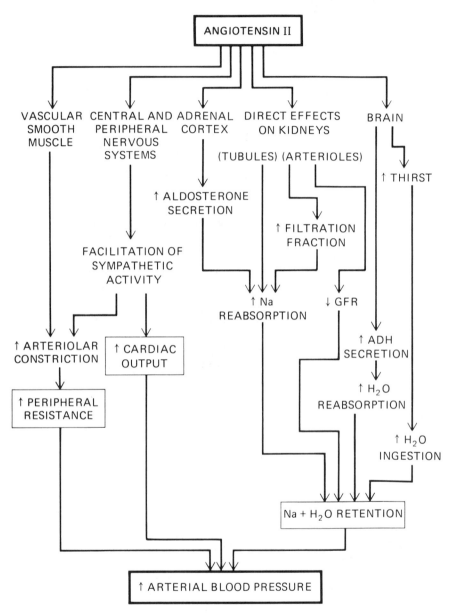

Figure 1-16. Detailed effects of angiotensin II. (*From Vander, A. J. [1985]. Renal physiology, p 130. New York: McGraw-Hill, with permission.*)

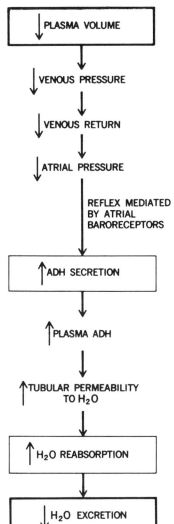

Figure 1-17. ADH response to plasma volume decrease. (*From Vander, A. J., Sherman, J. H., & Luciano, D. [1975]. Human physiology,* (2nd Ed.). New York: McGraw-Hill, with permission.)

sterone, previously discussed, enhances potassium secretion. In response to an alteration in potassium concentration, the adrenal cortex secretes or withholds aldosterone to balance body potassium.

Potassium secretion also appears to be related to sodium excretion, but the mechanisms of this relationship remain unclear. Medications such as diuretics can also be responsible for altering potassium excretion.

Acid-base Balance
The body is an acid-producing organism. Some acid is excreted by the lungs as carbon dioxide. Fixed acids cannot be excreted by the lungs and must be ex-

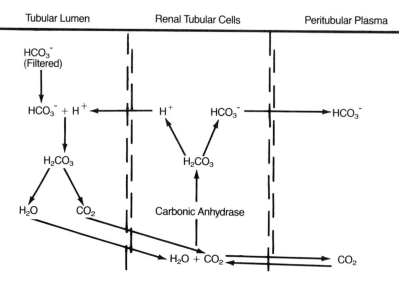

Figure 1-18. Bicarbonate reabsorption.

creted by the kidneys. The lungs are generally seen as the first line of defense when acid-base imbalances occur; they attempt to quickly rectify the situation. The kidneys are the second line of defense and offer a more long-term solution through the reabsorption of bicarbonate filtered at the glomerulus (Fig. 1-18) and the addition of new bicarbonate to renal plasma (Fig. 1-19).

Bicarbonate. Bicarbonate (HCO_3^-) is freely filtered at the glomerulus. The normal serum bicarbonate is 24 to 26 mEq/L. With a normal GFR, about 4500 mEq of bicarbonate is filtered each day. Ninety percent of the filtered bicarbonate is reabsorbed at the proximal tubule and the remaining bicarbonate is reabsorbed by the Loop of Henle and the distal tubule. Bicarbonate is actively transported and has a transport maximum, beyond which the excess is excreted.

Filtered bicarbonate cannot be reabsorbed directly. It must first be converted to carbonic acid by combining with hydrogen ions secreted into the tubule. This process is detailed in Figure 1-18.

The kidneys also contribute new bicarbonate to plasma through tubular acid secretion, a process fundamentally the same as that for bicarbonate reabsorption. In bicarbonate generation, illustrated in Figure 1-19, the secreted acid combines with other buffers in the tubular lumen or remains free in solution and is excreted.

Ammonia and phosphate are the major urinary buffers. This bicarbonate generation process contrasts to the bicarbonate reabsorption process in which the secreted acid combines with the filtered bicarbonate and is reabsorbed as water. The net result of the bicarbonate generation process is that

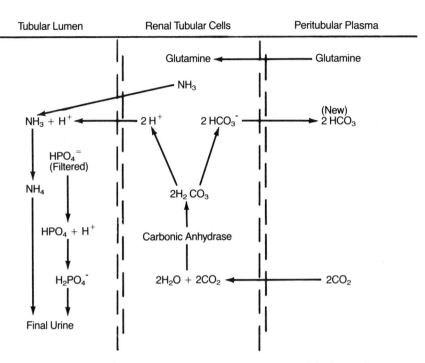

Figure 1-19. Bicarbonate generation and renal regulation of hydrogen-ion balance.

new bicarbonate is added to the plasma and an equivalent amount of acid is excreted.

Acid Secretion. The kidney also regulates acid-base balance by tubular acid secretion. An important regulatory mechanism is the ability of the kidney to vary hydrogen secretion with the GFR. The main stimulus for acid secretion is the P_{CO_2} of the arterial blood, which causes an equivalent P_{CO_2} increase in the tubular cells. Increased formation of carbonic acid results and leads to an elevated intracellular hydrogen-ion concentration (decreased pH).

   Acid secretion mechanisms can be altered in the presence of salt depletion, which stimulates sodium reabsorption and hydrogen-ion secretion such that virtually all of the filtered bicarbonate is reabsorbed. This reduces the ability of the kidneys to compensate for established metabolic alkalosis. Potassium also influences the ability of the kidney to secrete acid.

Calcium and Phosphate

Calcium (Ca^{++}) is the main element in the bone, and is necessary for muscle contraction, neurotransmission, and clotting. The normal serum calcium ranges from 8.7 to 10.7 mg/dl. About 98 percent of the filtered calcium is reabsorbed through many of the same pathways used by sodium. The majority of reabsorption (65 to 70 percent) occurs at the proximal tubule, with the remainder occurring at the Loop of Henle (20 to 25 percent) and the distal tubule (10 percent). The amount of calcium reabsorption is primarily determined by parathyroid hormone (PTH) and vitamin D. The effect of PTH is shown in Figure 1–20.

In order to stimulate the reabsorption of calcium, vitamin D must be in its active form. Vitamin D_3 is hydroxylated first by the liver (in the 25 position) and then by the kidneys (in the 1 position). The end result is 1, 25 dihydroxy vitamin D_3 (1, 25 $(OH)_2D_3$), the active form of vitamin D.

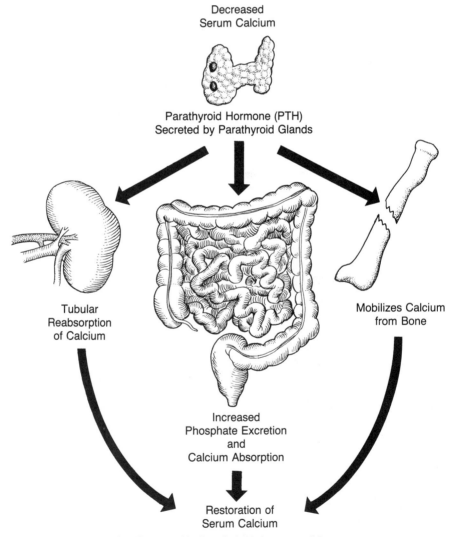

Decreased
Serum Calcium

Parathyroid Hormone (PTH)
Secreted by Parathyroid Glands

Tubular
Reabsorption
of Calcium

Mobilizes Calcium
from Bone

Increased
Phosphate Excretion
and
Calcium Absorption

Restoration of
Serum Calcium

Figure 1–20. Regulation of serum calcium.

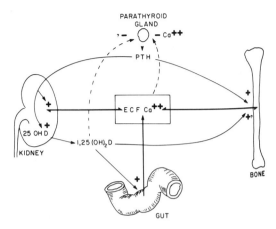

Figure 1-21. Interrelationship of calcium, phosphate, and vitamin D. (*From Nissenson, A. R., Fine, R. N., & Gentile, D. E. [1984]. Clinical dialysis. East Norwalk, CT: Appleton & Lange.*)

Phosphate (PO_4^-) is actively reabsorbed in the proximal tubule in the presence of sodium. Phosphorus balance is inversely related to calcium balance. Normal serum phosphorus levels range from 2.5 to 4.5 mg/dl. Phosphate, calcium, PTH, and vitamin D are intimately related (Fig. 1-21).

SUMMARY

A complete understanding of normal renal anatomy and physiology is necessary before proceeding to the study of abnormal or dysfunctional states. It is recommended that the nephrology practitioner also become quite familiar with general anatomy and physiology and the interrelationships with the renal system.

REFERENCES

Andreoli, T. E., Carpenter, C. C. J., Plum, F., & Smith, L. H., Jr. (1986). *Cecil essentials of medicine.* Philadelphia: Saunders.

Brenner, B. M., & Hostetter, T. H. (1981). Mechanisms of glomerular barrier function. *Contrib Nephrol, 26,* 9-16.

Cannon, P. J. (1977). The kidney in heart failure. *N Engl J Med, 269,* 26.

Ganong, W. F. (1985). *Review of medical physiology* (13th ed.). East Norwalk, CT: Appleton & Lange.

Haberle, D. A., & von Baeuer, H. (1983). Characteristics of glomerulo-tubular balance. *Am. J Phys, 244,* 355-366.

Vander, A. J. (1985). *Renal physiology.* New York: McGraw-Hill.

Nissenson, A. R., Fine, R. N. & Gentile, D. E. (1984). *Clinical dialysis.* East Norwalk, CT: Appleton & Lange.

Pitts, R. F. (1974). *The physiology of the kidney and body fluids* (3rd ed.). Chicago: Yearbook Medical Publishers.

Tauxe, W. N., & Dubovsky, E. (1985). Nuclear medicine in clinical urology and nephrology. East Norwalk, CT: Appleton & Lange.

Vander, A. J., Sherman, J. H., & Luciano, D. (1975). *Human physiology.* (2nd ed.). New York: McGraw-Hill.

2

Diagnosing Renal System Failure

Beth Tamplet Ulrich

OBJECTIVES

After reading this chapter on diagnostic tests associated with renal disease, the nurse will be able to:

1. Evaluate the results of urine studies in relation to adequate renal function
2. Determine the clearance of a substance, given the necessary laboratory data
3. Describe the radiographic studies used to diagnose the cause of renal dysfunction
4. Care for the patient undergoing renal arteriography studies or a renal biopsy

Diagnosing failure of the renal system requires first that the diagnostician be intimately familiar with the normal or adequately functioning renal system. Fortner (1978) has suggested that in order to effectively diagnose and manage renal function, the nephrology professional must "think like a tubule." A wide variety of renal function tests are available to provide valuable information to health care personnel working with the nephrology patient. These tests range from the very simple urinalysis to complicated radionucleotide studies.

INITIAL ASSESSMENT

The *initial patient history* is very important in diagnosing failure of the renal system, especially in the complex situation of the patient with multisystem failure. Some patients will present with only mild, nonspecific signs and symptoms, while others will be in overt failure. The order and speed in which various indicators of the declining renal function occurred can assist the nephrology professional in determining whether the primary cause of the decline was renal-related or was initiated as a result of other organ failures.

It is necessary to know the adequacy of renal function prior to the onset of the presenting problem. Is there a history of dysuria, nocturia, or polyuria? If the patient is hospitalized, what is the relationship of intake to output? Has the patient experienced flank pain or passed a renal stone? Has hematuria ever been observed?

Family history should be investigated. Is there a history of polycystic kidney disease, renal calculi, or hereditary nephritis?

Does the patient have one of several systemic diseases that are known to contribute to the development of renal failure, such as diabetes mellitus, systemic lupus erythematosus, hypertension, or sickle cell anemia? Has the patient been exposed to any nephrotoxic agents? Nephrotoxic agents include certain drugs, chemical agents, and radiographic contrast materials.

Has the patient had any of the more subtle signs of impending renal failure like weight loss, fatigue, itchy skin, edema, anorexia, or nausea and vomiting?

PHYSICAL EXAMINATION

Because the kidney is interrelated with virtually every other body system, the physical examination must be extensive and thorough, covering every system. The diagnostician must be especially observant for signs of volume depletion or volume excess.

URINE STUDIES

Urinalysis
One of the most informative, but often overlooked, renal function tests is the *urinalysis*. The specimen for a routine urinalysis may be collected at any time, but the first voided specimen in the morning provides the most information. Once the specimen is collected, it should be examined within the hour (Table 2-1). Beyond that time, the accuracy of the test results is questionable, because bacteria multiply, red blood cells hemolyze, and casts disintegrate.

With normal renal function, the urine will be very light yellow to dark brown, depending on the concentration of urochrome pigment. A reddish

TABLE 2-1. MICROSCOPIC EXAMINATION OF THE URINE

	Finding	Associations
Casts	Red blood cell	Glomerulonephritis, vasculitis
	White blood cell	Interstitial nephritis, pyelonephritis
	Epithelial cell	Acute tubular necrosis, interstitial nephritis, glomerulonephritis
	Granular	Renal parenchymal disease (nonspecific)
	Waxy, broad	Advanced renal failure
	Hyaline	Normal finding in concentrated urine
	Fatty	Heavy proteinuria
Cells	Red blood cell	Urinary tract infection, urinary tract inflammation
	White blood cell	Urinary tract infection, urinary tract inflammation
	Eosinophil	Drug-induced interstitial nephritis
	(Squamous) epithelial cell	Contaminants
Crystals	Uric acid	Acid urine, acute uric acid nephropathy, hyperuricosuria
	Calcium phosphate	Alkaline urine
	Calcium oxalate	Acid urine, hyperoxaluria, ethylene glycol poisoning
	Cystine	Cystinuria
	Sulfur	Sulfadiazine antibiotics

From Andreoli, T. E. et al. (1986). Cecil essentials of medicine, p. 2 0 7. Philadelphia: Saunders, with permission.

urine indicates the presence of red blood cells, and a cloudy urine may result from the presence of white blood cells (Table 2-2).

The odor is fresh. The specific gravity varies from 1.005 to 1.025, with a pH in the range of 4.5 to 7.5. An alteration in the urine pH may distort urinalysis results. The urine is composed of waste products such as urea and creatinine, excess electrolytes, hormones and their breakdown products, vitamins, drugs, and, occasionally, sediment. The microscopic portion of the urinalysis will identify the presence and absence of waste products and cellular elements. *Urine osmolality* is also an important diagnostic tool, indicating the concentration of the urine. In adults, osmolality may vary from 75 to 1200 mOsm/kg (Smith, 1987).

The urinalysis may be requested as a routine, a clean catch (midstream), or a sample collected sterilely. For the routine urinalysis or a bedside determination of specific gravity or pH, the patient merely voids into a nonsterile urine cup. A clean catch or midstream urinalysis requires that the patient begin voiding, urinate into a sterile urine container to fill the container, and complete the voiding into the toilet or bedpan. The sterile collection of urine for a urinalysis requires that the patient be catheterized if a catheter is not already in place. The catheter is inserted, the urine flow is allowed to begin,

TABLE 2-2. URINE COLORS

Color	Association
Colorless	Dilute urine, diabetes mellitus, diabetes insipidus
Yellow	Normal, riboflavin, quinacrine
Amber	Concentrated urine, Pyridium, sulfasalizine
Blue, blue-green	biliverdin, methylene blue, amitriptyline, triamterene
Red	Hematuria, hemoglobinuria, myoglobinuria, phenytoin, phenolphthalein, rifampin, adriamycin, anthrocyanin (pigment in beets and blackberries)
Red-brown	Porphyria, urobilinogen, bilirubin, nitrofurantoin, primaquine, chloroquine, metronidazole
Brown-black	Acidification of hemoglobin pigment, melanin, alkaptonuria, senna, cascara, rhubarb
Milky white	Chyluria, pyuria

From Andreoli, T. E. et al. (1986). Cecil essentials of medicine, p 207. Philadelphia: Saunders, with permission.

and the specimen is collected. The catheter is then removed unless an indwelling catheter has been ordered.

Urine Specimen for Culture and Sensitivity
A urine sample for culture and sensitivity, often referred to as a urine C&S, is collected when the specific contaminating organism must be identified. The urine for culture and sensitivity requires a sterile collection of the urine specimen by means of the catheterization procedure just described.

Timed Urine Collections
Urine may also be collected over extended periods of time, usually for 12 to 24 hours. Examples are urine studies for catecholamines and creatinine. For example, renal excretion of protein may be significantly increased in patients with glomerular or tubular disorders. Normal protein excretion is less than 150 mg in a 24-hour period. In cases of glomerular disease, protein excretion may be in excess of 2 to 3 g in the same time period.

To collect an extended specimen, the nurse instructs the patient to void. This first specimen is discarded and the time is noted (start time). All urine voided is then collected until the preestablished completion time. At the completion time, the patient is asked to void a final time. This last specimen is added to the total specimen which is sent to the laboratory. Different extended urine study tests require special containers, preservatives, and refrigeration. Directions for the specific study ordered should be clarified before beginning the study.

TABLE 2-3. SERUM ANALYSIS

Test	Normal Serum Level
Serum urea nitrogen	8 to 24 mg/dl
Creatinine	0.5 to 1.5 mg/dl
Sodium	135 to 145 mEq/L
Chloride	96 to 106 mEq/L
Potassium	3.5 to 5.0 mEq/L
Calcium	8.7 to 10.7 mg/dl
Phosphate	2.5 to 4.5 mg/dl
Magnesium	1.5 to 2.5 mEq/L
Hematocrit	40 to 48% men
	38 to 46% women
Ferritin	30 to 300 mg/ml
Alkaline phosphates	25 to 100 U/ml
Serum glutamic pyurevic acid (SGPT)	5 to 35 U/ml
Serum protein	6.0 to 8.4 gm/dl
Albumin	3.5 to 5.1 gm/dl
Parathyroid hormone	40 to 150 NLEO/ml

SERUM ANALYSIS

Serum Creatinine
Serum creatine and serum urea nitrogen are the two blood chemistries most closely associated with renal function (Table 2–3). Creatinine is a metabolite of the muscle protein creatine. The production of creatinine is determined by an individual's skeletal muscle mass and is fairly constant. Normal creatinine values range 0.85 to 1.5 mg/dl in males and 0.70 to 1.25 mg/dl in females. Because serum creatinine varies with muscle mass, the serum creatinine must not be used as the sole indicator of renal function, but rather must be considered in combination with other diagnostic indices.

Serum Urea Nitrogen
Urea is the major end product of protein metabolism. The serum urea level (BUN) reflects the dietary intake of protein as well as the protein catabolic rate. Like creatinine, urea is freely filtered at the glomerulus; but unlike creatinine, urea is reabsorbed throughout the renal tubule, especially when the kidney is attempting to conserve salt and water. As a result, serum urea levels are affected by extracellular fluid volume. Normal serum urea nitrogen levels range from 5 to 25 mg/dl.

Serum Creatinine: Urea Nitrogen Ratio
Perhaps more important than either of the serum levels alone is the ratio of serum urea nitrogen to serum creatinine (Table 2-4). A deviation from the

TABLE 2-4. CAUSES OF ALTERED UREA NITROGEN-TO-CREATININE RATIO

Increased Ratio (> 10:1)
Increased urea input
  Increased dietary protein intake
  Gastrointestinal hemorrhage
  Hemolysis
  Sepsis/catabolic states
  Drugs that inhibit anabolism
    Corticosteroids
    Tetracyclines
Decreased effective circulating volume
  Volume depletion
  Congestive heart failure
  Cirrhosis/ascites
  Nephrotic syndrome
Obstructive uropathy
Decreased Ratio (<10:1)
Decreased urea input
  Starvation
  Liver disease
Increased creatinine production
  Rhabdomyolysis
Volume expansion
  SIADH
  Iatrogenic
Chronic renal failure with dialysis

From Andreoli, T. E. et al. (1986). Cecil essentials of medicine, p 2 0 8 . Philadelphia: Saunders, with permission.

normal 10:1 ratio can be very useful diagnostically. A urea-to-creatinine ratio greater than 10:1 may indicate increased urea input from increased protein intake, hemolysis, septic states, or drugs that inhibit anabolism; decreased creatinine production; or decreased effective circulation volume resulting from volume depletion, congestive heart failure, or ascites. A urea-to-creatinine ratio less than 10:1 may indicate decreased urea input as a result of decreased protein intake or liver disease, increased creatinine production, overhydration, or end-stage renal disease with dialysis (Table 2–3).

Serum Electrolytes
A primary function of the kidney is the regulation of electrolytes in the body. Ongoing serum electrolyte determination is critical to the successful treatment in the patient with acute renal failure or the unstable chronic dialysis patient. It is less time critical, but still important, in the stable chronic dialysis patient and the post-transplant patient. The serum electrolytes usually measured are sodium, potassium, calcium, phosphorus, and bicarbonate.

RENAL FUNCTION STUDIES

Renal function studies combine urine and serum analyses to assess the glomerular and tubular functional capacity of the kidneys.

Fractional Excretion Studies

Fractional excretion of solutes is another measure of filtration. The urinary excretion of a solute is measured relative to the urinary excretion of creatinine. The formula for fractional excretion is:

$$FE_x = \frac{(U_x)\ (P_{cr})}{(R_{cr})\ (P_x)}$$

where FE_x = fraction (percent) of the solute in plasma that is excreted, U_x = amount of solute excreted, P_{cr} = plasma creatinine, U_{cr} = urine creatinine, and P_x = amount of solute in plasma.

Fractional excretion of sodium is useful in the differential diagnosis of acute renal insufficiency. A fractional sodium excretion of less than 1 percent indicates prerenal causative factors, early obstruction, or acute glomerulonephritis. A fractional sodium excretion of more than 1 percent indicates acute tubular necrosis, toxic nephropathy, or acute interstitial nephritis (Andreoli, Carpenter, Plum, & Smith, 1986). Figure 2–1 illustrates the decision tree for acute renal insufficiency using fractional sodium excretion as a key diagnostic element. Fractional excretion values for calcium, phosphate, amino acids, and uric acid contribute to the diagnosis of tubular problems.

Clearance Studies

Clearance is closely related to glomerular filtration rate (GFR) and is defined as the volume of plasma from which a substance is completely cleared in a given period of time. Each substance in the blood has a clearance value. The basic formula for determining the clearance of a substance is:

$$C_x\ (ml/min) = \frac{[\text{urine concentration} \times (U_x)]\ [\text{urine flow rate } (V)]}{\text{plasma concentration} \times (P_x)}$$

The accuracy of the clearance study depends on the use of a substance that is freely filtered and that undergoes neither tubular reabsorption nor secretion. Inulin remains the standard to which all other substances are measured. It is not, however, pragmatic in the general clinical setting.

Creatinine has been shown to be an adequate substitute. *Creatinine* is an amino acid, normally present in plasma as a result of muscle metabolism, with fairly constant production and a proportional relationship to body muscle mass and surface area. Normal creatinine clearance values are 100 to 150 ml/min for males and 85 to 125 ml/min for females. When normalized to body surface area, normal creatinine clearance is 95 to 105 ml/min per 1.73 m^2 of body surface.

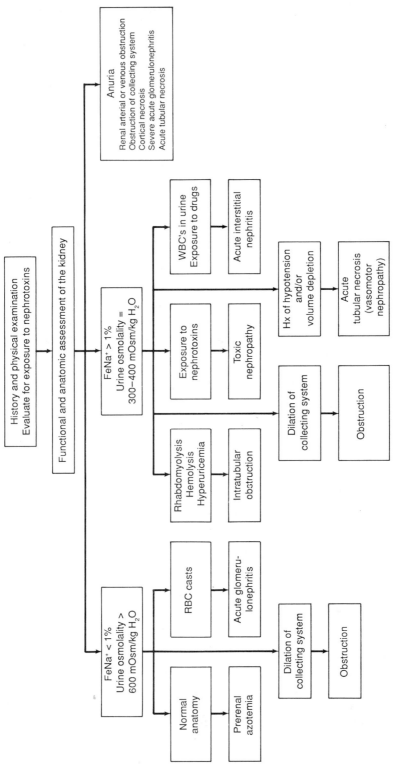

Figure 2-1. Diagnostic plan in a patient with acute renal insufficiency. (*From Andreoli, T. E. et al. [1986]. Cecil essentials of medicine, p 216. Philadelphia: Saunders, with permission.*)

CYSTOSCOPY

Cystoscopy allows direct visualization of the interior of the bladder using a lighted cystoscope. The cystoscope can also be used to insert ureteral catheters, obtain biopsies, and remove calculi.

Fluids are usually forced prior to the procedure to ensure an adequate urine flow. Cystoscopy can be painful due to spasms and contractions that occur in the bladder sphincters. The procedure may be performed under sedation or general anesthesia. If general anesthesia is not used (and it usually is not unless the patient is a child, or other operative procedures are anticipated), the nurse should assist the patient in relaxing as much as possible.

The patient is placed in the lithotomy position. A local anesthetic is instilled into the urethra, and the cystoscope is inserted. The bladder is distended with saline to allow better visualization. The patient will have to resist the urge to void.

Immediately after the cystoscopy, the patient may experience postural hypotension due to the prolonged time in the lithotomy position. The patient may also experience urinary frequency, burning on urination, and mild hematuria. Frank bleeding should be reported to the physician immediately. Potential complications of the cystoscopy procedure include bladder perforation, urinary tract hemorrhage, urinary retention, and urinary or bladder infection.

RADIOLOGICAL STUDIES

Abdominal X-Ray

X-ray of the abdomen, often called a *kidney-ureter-bladder (KUB) film,* offers a one-dimensional view of the entire renal system. Evaluating the size of the kidneys can aid in the initial diagnosis. Small kidneys, for example, are suggestive of a chronic disease process. Large kidneys can indicate obstructive, inflammatory, infiltrative, or cystic disease. Occasionally, renal calculi can be visualized on the abdominal x-ray, as can blockages or constrictions of the urinary tract.

Intravenous Pyelogram

An *intravenous pyelogram* (IVP) allows accurate visualization of the entire renal system. An iodinated radiographic contrast medium is administered intravenously. Within a few minutes of the administration, the medium is concentrated in the tubules and a nephrogram image is seen. The medium progresses through the filtrate tract, and sequential films allow for visualization of each portion of the tract. Cysts, tumors, calculi, and obstructions are easily observed.

Preparation of the patient involves assessment of past allergic reactions to iodinated radiographic contrast mediums, iodine, or seafood; administration of cathartics or enemas the evening before; and educating the patient concerning the warm to hot flushing that may occur when the medium is administered. Usually, fluids will be withheld for 8 hours prior to testing to allow for better concentration of the medium. Fluid restriction should not be a part of the preparation of patients with known renal dysfunction; multiple myeloma, where the contrast medium can potentiate precipitation of myeloma protein in the kidney; diabetes mellitus; sickle cell anemia, since elevation in renal tissue oncotic pressure can promote sickling and infarction of renal tissue; and congestive heart failure, due to the acute osmotic effect of the contrast medium which can further compromise heart failure. The chance for contrast medium-induced nephrotoxicity is the major drawback of this test and others using similar contrast mediums.

Retrograde Pyelogram

A *retrograde pyelogram*, like an IVP, allows for evaluation of the renal system. The radiographic contrast medium is injected directly into the ureters by means of a ureteral catheter introduced through a cystoscope. A retrograde pyelogram allows for visualization of the ureters when this has not been possible with an IVP. It is very useful for observing obstructions which can, in fact, often be removed or bypassed by the placement of the ureteral catheter during the retrograde pyelogram procedure. Risks associated with the retrograde pyelogram include ureteral trauma, bleeding, and infection. Since these risks are significant, especially in the already compromised patient, Brezis, Rosen, and Epstein (1986) recommend only performing the procedure on one side if the patient has two normal-sized kidneys and obstruction has been ruled out as a cause of the renal failure.

Renal Arteriography

Renal arteriograms allow the accurate evaluation of the renal vasculature and are especially useful in patients with suspected renal artery stenosis or thrombois, in patients with a renal mass, and in the performance of pretransplant donor workups. The renal arteriogram is a more invasive procedure and as such carries with it more danger than minimally invasive or noninvasive techniques. The risk must be weighed against the need for additional information.

Initial preparation of the patient is similar to that for an IVP. In addition, the patient will be given a sedative prior to the procedure. A contrast medium is injected through a catheter which is inserted into the femoral artery up the aorta to the renal arteries (Fig. 2-2). Sequential x-rays are taken as the dye moves through the renal system. As with the IVP, the patient may experience a warm to hot flush as the dye is injected. After the procedure is completed, the femoral catheter is removed. A pressure dressing is placed over the site and left in place. The patient remains on bed rest for 12 to 24 hours. The site is checked for bleeding, and peripheral pulses in the legs are taken every 30

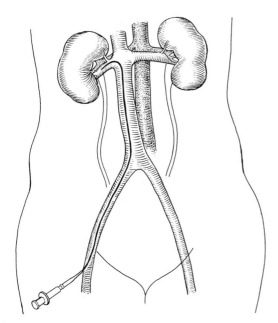

Figure 2-2. Catheter insertion for renal arteriography.

minutes initially and then every hour. Potential complications of renal arteriograms include thrombosis, embolis, excessive bleeding, and infection.

ULTRASONOGRAPHY

A more accurate noninvasive determination of kidney size and shape can be made using *renal ultrasonography*. A small external ultrasound probe is moved back and forth over the renal area, which has been covered with conductive gel. Sound waves from the probe reflect back to the probe from body structures. The ultrasound computer interprets the soundwaves and creates a picture. Cortical thinning or edema can sometimes be visualized clearly enough to suggest chronic parenchymal disease or acute inflammation, respectively. Hydronephrosis appears as an enlargement of the echo-free pelvis and dilated calyces (Brezis, Rosen, & Epstein, 1986). Ultrasonography is beneficial in ruling out the possibility of an obstruction, having been shown to be almost as reliable as the more traumatic intravenous pyelogram (Ellenbogen, Scheible, Talner, & Leopold, 1978). Masses and cysts can also be diagnosed in this manner.

RADIONUCLIDE IMAGING

Radionuclide imaging of the kidneys, often called a *renal scan*, involves the intravenous administration of radioactive isotopes that are excreted by the kidney. External radiation detector probes are placed over the kidney to measure the appearance and disappearance of the radioactive material in the kidney. Uptake and excretion of the material are calculated. The most comonly used radionuclide for renal vascular imaging is technetium-99-labeled diethylene triamine pentacetic acid (^{99m}Tc DTPA). Hippuran ^{131}I, a compound excreted by tubular secretion, is used to assess renal tubular function.

A normal scan reveals symmetric vascularization and function of the kidneys. In addition to diagnosing renal problems, the scan is also useful in determining perfusion and function of a transplanted kidney.

Preparation of the patient is usually minimal. The patient lies quietly during the test and should not experience any pain or discomfort. Since only a tracer dose of radioactive material is used, no special precautions are necessary.

COMPUTED TOMOGRAPHY

Closely akin to the IVP is the *computed tomograph (CT) scan* of the kidneys. As in the IVP, a contrast medium is administered intravenously and its course through the renal system is scanned. The CT scan uses tissue contrast produced by the density of the tissue under examination to differentiate solid from cystic lesions.

MAGNETIC RESONANCE IMAGING

Magnetic resonance imaging (MRI) is a rapidly evolving technology that offers considerable promise in the field of nephrology. Magnetic resonance describes the property of subatomic particles (electrons and nuclei) to absorb and emit (resonate) radiofrequency energy when placed in a magnetic field (Weiner, 1986). The resonance frequency of a nucleus depends on the magnetic field strength and the physical characteristics of, and the electrical environment around, the nucleus under study. The range of contrast available by MRI greatly surpasses that of other imaging methods.

MRI involves the use of a powerful magnet, radiofrequency coil, radiofrequency transmitter, radiofrequency receiver, and computer to operate the equipment and process the data. The tissue to be examined must be placed between the transmitter and the receiver. This may necessitate the use of a very large instrument if the whole body is involved, or smaller instruments for a portion of the body that can be isolated.

There are two problems with MRI. Because of its relative slowness (5 to 10 minutes to obtain an image), distorted images can occur due to motion of the targeted tissue. The other problem is safety and inconvenience. Pacemakers, watches, and even credit cards may be made inoperative by exposure to the MRI equipment. Nothing made of metal can be near the magnet. The MRI magnet is capable of attracting a pair of hemostats from across the room! After a few initial "flying hemostat" incidents, MRI facilities have installed metal detectors to prevent the presence of any metal near the magnet.

Although these problems sound major, the sight of one magnetic resonance image is enough to convince most practitioners that the problems can and should be overcome. Comparing the MRI to the x-ray or CT scan is like comparing a fine color television to an inexpensive black and white set. The potential appears unlimited.

RENAL BIOPSY

A *renal biopsy* is used to diagnose the existence, extent, or origin of a renal disease process. Open biopsies, which require a surgical procedure and anesthesia, are rarely done. A closed biopsy using a percutaneous needle is much more common.

An IVP or ultrasound is performed prior to the biopsy to determine the exact location of the kidneys. The patient lies in the prone position with a pillow or sandbag used to elevate the midbody area. After the administration of a local anesthetic, the biopsy needle is inserted. Once the biopsy is obtained, the needle is removed and a pressure dressing is applied.

Preparation of the patient includes assessment of the patient's coagulation ability and status, and explanation of the procedure and postprocedure care. The patient will remain in the prone position for 30 to 60 minutes and on bed rest for 24 hours. The biopsy dressing should be checked for bleeding and vital signs should be taken every 10 minutes the first hour and, based on the findings, progressively decreased once every hour. All urine should be observed for hematuria. Potential complications of a renal biopsy include hematoma, excessive bleeding, and infection.

SUMMARY

The patient with renal failure presents a complicated diagnostic challenge. Although nephrology nurses are generally not responsible for making the diagnosis, they are responsible for gathering critical data, instructing the patient and family in what certain diagnostic procedures can contribute to the diagnostic process and what the patient can expect during the procedure, assisting the physician during the procedure, and caring for the patient before and after the procedure. Information concerning diagnostic testing is therefore an integral part of the knowledge base of a professional nephrology nurse.

REFERENCES

Andreoli, T. E., Carpenter, C. C. J., Plum, F., & Smith, L. H., Jr. (1986). *Cecil essentials of medicine.* Philadelphia: Saunders.

Brezis, M., Rosen, S., & Epstein, F. H. (1986). Acute renal failure. In B. M. Brenner & F. J. Rector, Jr. (Eds.), *The kidney* (3rd ed., pp. 735–799). Philadelphia: Saunders.

Ellenbogen, P. H., Scheible, F. W., Talner, L. B., & Leopold, G. R. (1978). Sensitivity of grey scale ultrasound in detecting urinary tract obstruction. *Am J Roent, 130,* 731.

Fortner, R. W. (1978, May). *Pathophysiology: Acute renal failure.* Paper presented at Advanced Concepts of Care, San Francisco.

Smith, E. K. M. (1987). *Renal disease: A conceptual approach.* New York: Churchill Livingstone.

Weiner, M. W. (1986). Magnetic resonance imaging and spectroscopy of the kidney. In H. C. Gonick (Ed.), *Current nephrology.* Chicago: Year Book Medical Publishers.

3

Acute Renal Failure

Betty Irwin Crandall

OBJECTIVES

After reading this chapter on acute renal failure, the nurse will be able to:

1. Define acute renal failure
2. State and define the three categories of acute renal failure and give at least two examples of each
3. Using the five phases, describe a typical patient's clinical course after developing acute renal failure
4. Identify the clinical signs and symptoms and laboratory findings that can be used to differentiate prerenal azotemia from acute tubular necrosis
5. State at least five principles that guide medical and nursing practice in caring for the patient with acute renal failure
6. State at least three factors to consider in deciding which treatment modality to use with a patient experiencing acute renal failure

Acute renal failure (ARF) is defined as a sudden impairment or decline in renal function associated with an increase in the serum concentrations of urea (azotemia) and creatinine. It is frequently, but not always, associated with oliguria ($\leqslant$ 400 cc urine/24 hr), hyperkalemia, and sodium retention. Acute renal failure is often reversible, but prolonged episodes may lead to irreversible renal failure and the need for chronic dialysis or renal transplantation.

Acute renal failure rarely occurs in isolation. Patients who develop acute renal failure are often critically ill individuals with multisystem failure.

ETIOLOGY

The causes of acute renal failure are numerous. To facilitate making a diagnosis and establishing a treatment plan, clinicians have organized them into three categories depending on the physiological location of the insult: prerenal, postrenal, and intrarenal.

Prerenal Acute Renal Failure

Causes of *prerenal acute renal failure* are events that result in hypoperfusion or a decrease in the amount of blood supplied to the kidneys. The function of the kidneys themselves is normal in a prerenal state of ARF, but the kidneys are unable to adequately filter blood because of a reduction in renal blood flow. Conditions that result in decreased cardiac output, vasodilitation, or decreased effective circulating blood volume can result in decreased blood flow to the kidneys and thus in prerenal acute renal failure. Cardiogenic shock, arrhythmias, severe congestive heart failure, pericardial tamponade, and acute pulmonary embolism may all reduce cardiac output to such a degree as to result in prerenal ARF. Sepsis and anaphylaxis are examples of conditions that result in vasodilation and may cause hypoperfusion of the kidneys. The effective circulating blood volume may be decreased to a critical level by conditions such as hemorrhage, dehydration, burns, diarrhea, vomiting, third spacing, cirrhosis, peritonitis, and nephrotic syndrome. Vascular disorders such as renal artery or vein thrombosis or stenosis and renal infarction may also reduce renal blood suppply sufficiently to cause ARF.

Because the kidneys themselves remain functionally normal, prerenal acute renal failure can often be reversed by improving myocardial function, expanding the effective circulating blood volume, promoting vasoconstriction, or correcting a vascular problem. If the decreased perfusion to the kidneys is allowed to continue for too long, irreversible ischemia may result, and the prerenal acute renal failure may become intrarenal. By definition, an episode of acute renal failure is prerenal only if it is reversed when the underlying cause of hypoperfusion is corrected.

Postrenal Acute Renal Failure

Obstruction to the flow of urine anywhere from the calyces to the urethral meatus may result in *postrenal acute renal failure*. For renal failure to develop, the obstruction must be bilateral, be below the level of the bladder, or be unilateral in the individual with only one functioning kidney. A unilateral obstruction above the bladder in someone with two normal kidneys will result in problems such as infection, but will not result in ARF because the unobstructed kidney will hypertrophy and excrete the nitrogenous wastes.

Causes of postrenal or obstructive acute renal failure may be thought of as either mechanical or functional. Mechanical causes include calculi, tumors, urethral strictures, prostatic hypertrophy, blood clots, and sloughed necrotic papillae. Obstruction of an indwelling catheter, bladder neck obstruction, and congenital malformations of the urinary tract may also be mechanical causes of obstruction. A neurogenic bladder resulting from spinal cord injury, diabetic neuropathy, or medications such as ganglionic blocking agents may be a functional cause of obstruction.

As with prerenal causes of azotemia, postrenal acute renal failure is very often reversible. However, prolonged obstruction may result in intrarenal damage and potentially irreversible renal failure.

Intrarenal Acute Renal Failure

Damage to the renal tissue itself that results in a sudden deterioration of kidney function and the development of ARF is known as *intrarenal acute renal failure*. The damage may be to the glomerulus, as occurs in acute poststreptococcal glomerulonephritis and systemic lupus erythematosis. Other causes of intrarenal failure are papillary necrosis, interstitial nephritis, and vascular diseases such as polyarteritis nodosa. Damage to the tubular portion of the nephron is, however, the most common cause of intrarenal failure and in fact the most common form of acute renal failure itself (Stark, 1982).

Acute Tubular Necrosis (ATN). Acute tubular necrosis (ATN) is the name given to acute renal failure that results from tubular damage. ATN results from either ischemia or nephrotoxicity.

Ischemia. Ischemic injury to the kidney should be anticipated when perfusion to the kidneys is obliterated or reduced below a mean systematic arterial pressure of 60 to 70 mm Hg in the afferent arteriole (Mars & Treloar, 1984). Below this critical level, the ability of the afferent and efferent arterioles to maintain glomerular filtration due to the property of autoregulation is lost and the glomerular filtration rate decreases. Ischemia is also likely whenever circulation to the kidneys is interrupted for longer than 30 minutes, as occurs during vascular surgery when the aorta is cross-clamped above the renal arteries or with the procurement of cadaver kidneys for transplantation.

Prolonged or severe prerenal acute renal failure is a very common cause of ATN. In such cases, prerenal causes of azotemia are not corrected and progress to intrarenal damage due to ischemia of the tubules.

Ischemic injuries damage not only tubular epithelial cells but also cells of the basement membrane. The basement membrane cells, unlike epithelial cells, are not able to regenerate (Stark, 1982). Thus, ATN resulting from ischemia may cause areas of the nephron to be irreparably damaged.

Nephrotoxicity. A wide variety of substances may cause injury to the renal tubules and are thus potential nephrotoxins. Heavy metals and ions such as mercuric chloride, copper sulfate, and gold may damage the kidney, as may organic solvents such as carbon tetrachloride and ethylene glycol. The most common nephrotoxic agents are, however, medications, especially antibiotics. Aminoglycosides such as gentamicin, tobramycin, kanamycin, and amikacin are particular offenders. They appear to bind to the cells of the proximal tubule, where they have a very prolonged half-life; damage to the tubule then causes acute renal failure. Other antibiotics or antimicrobials that are frequently nephrotoxic are vancomycin, amphotericin-B, methicillin, tetracycline, and some cephalosporins. Phenacetin, acetaminophen, and nonsteroidal anti-inflammatory agents such as ibuprofen, are other medications that are known nephrotoxins. Finally, of great clinical importance are radiologic contrast media. The iodine-based dyes used for intravenous pyelography, angiography, cardiac catheterization, and CT scanning may cause tubular damage. Patients with underlying renal disease, the elderly, those with volume deficits, and those receiving other nephrotoxic agents are at greatest risk. Adequate hydration and close monitoring will reduce the number of complications seen when such dye studies are necessary.

Nephrotoxic injuries usually damage the epithelial cells of the tubule but not the cells of the basement membrane. For that reason, the chances of the ATN being reversible are good.

Some instances of ATN involve both ischemia and nephrotoxicity. Many nephrotoxins also cause ischemia. At times it may not be possible to clearly determine the cause of ATN. When one has eliminated both prerenal and postrenal causes of acute renal failure as well as causes of acute glomerular injury, it is generally safe to assume that the acute renal failure is a result of ATN.

Pathogenesis of ATN. Despite extensive research, the mechanisms causing the decreased renal function in acute tubular necrosis are not well understood. Several theories exist, including decreased glomerular capillary pressure related to the renin-angiotensin system, glomerular endothelial cell swelling, decreased glomerular permeability, intratubular obstruction, and the backleak of glomerular filtrate (Van Stone, 1983). On pathological examination, histological findings have included patchy areas of necrosis involving the tubular epithelial cells and possibly the tubular basement membrane. Both the proximal and distal tubules may be involved.

CLINICAL COURSE

A patient with acute renal failure proceeds through several fairly well-defined stages: onset, oliguric-anuric, early diuretic, late diuretic or recovery, and convalescent. Nursing and medical care will vary depending on the phase in which the patient is at any given time.

Onset

This is the period of time from the precipitating event until oliguria or anuria develops. *Oliguria* is defined as a urine output of less than 400 ml in 24 hours, with 400 ml being the amount of urine output required for solute removal. *Anuria* is a urine output of less than 50 ml in 24 hours. Occasionally, patients with acute renal failure do not develop oliguria. In such cases, the period of onset would be that time from the precipitating event until *azotemia,* the accumulation of toxic levels of nitrogenous wastes in the blood, develops. The period of onset in acute renal failure is quite different from the progressive loss of nephrons and slow decline in function often seen in those who develop chronic renal failure. There is no time for adaptation and patients often present quite ill and in need of aggressive therapy. Medical and nursing care during this phase center on determining the precipitating event and correcting any conditions that might contribute to worsening of the renal failure. Patients are often placed on a restricted diet to control uremia, hyperkalemia, and excessive salt and water retention. Blood pressure is controlled with diuretics, antihypertensives, and salt and fluid restrictions.

Oliguric-anuric Phase

This is the period of time during which urine output is less than 400 ml/24 hr. It usually lasts 1 to 2 weeks. If the oliguric-anuric phase is prolonged beyond 2 weeks, the prognosis for recovery is not as good. Controlling life-threatening hyperkalemia with dietary restrictions, medications, and dialysis if necessary is one priority of both medical and nursing care during the oliguric-anuric phase. Other priorities include managing fluid overload and hypertension with fluid and dietary restrictions, medications, and dialysis. Finally, uremia may become so severe as to also require dialysis to prevent adverse effects on multiple body systems.

Early Diuretic Phase

This phase begins when the 24-hour urine volume exceeds 400 ml and ends when the blood urea nitrogen (BUN) and serum creatinine levels stop rising. Frequently, the BUN and creatinine will continue to rise for several days after the diuretic phase begins. Once they begin to fall, the early diuretic phase ends and recovery begins. During the early diuretic phase, fluid and electrolyte balance is often difficult to maintain. Urine volumes may exceed several liters daily due to the defect in concentrating ability and to the osmotic diuretic effect of the high BUN level. Prevention of dehydration becomes a challenge. Assessing the patient's fluid status and maintaining fluid and electrolyte balance are the priorities of care during this phase.

Late Diuretic or Recovery Phase

Once the BUN and serum creatinine levels begin to fall, the late diuretic or recovery phase begins. This stage ends when these levels stabilize or return to the normal range. During this period, fluid and electrolyte balance must be closely monitored. Potential nephrotoxins should be avoided. Some drugs may require dose modification.

Convalescent Phase

The convalescent period begins when the BUN level stabilizes and continues until the patient resumes previous activities. This phase may extend as long as 12 months. The patient's renal function must be monitored at regular intervals. Fluids and dietary intake may be restricted. Some patients may have irreversible acute renal failure and require dialysis permanently. Patient and family education and careful follow-up are the priorities of care.

ASSESSMENT

When an individual suddenly develops an acute deterioration of renal function, assessment should begin with compiling a careful patient history to identify potential causative factors. The patient, family, previous care givers, and the medical record may be sources of information. Preexisting medical conditions should be enumerated with particular attention to cardiac conditions, vascular disease, diseases of the kidneys or urinary tract, and systemic diseases (such as diabetes mellitus and systemic lupus erythematosus) known to affect renal function. Exposure to potential nephrotoxins should be evaluated. Inquiries should be made about recent surgeries or acute illnesses. If the patient has been recently hospitalized, the medical record should be carefully reviewed to elicit risk factors such as hypotensive episodes, cardiac arrests, sepsis, or anaphylaxis.

Excluding Postrenal and Prerenal Causes of ARF

Early recognition of a potentially reversible cause of acute renal failure is mandatory. This demands exclusion of postrenal and prerenal causes of ARF. The goal is to prevent damage to the kidney tissue itself—to prevent intrarenal acute renal failure from occurring due to untreated prerenal or postrenal causes.

To exclude postrenal causes, patency of the urinary tract must be assured. Successful insertion of an indwelling catheter into the bladder will confirm that neither a urethral or bladder neck obstruction, nor a nonfunctional, overdistended bladder, is the cause of the renal failure. Sonography is a helpful, noninvasive tool to exclude obstruction of the ureters or calyceal system as causes of azotemia. An intravenous pyelogram (IVP) may be done to visualize the urinary tract but the risks of nephrotoxicity from the contrast material must be carefully considered prior to performing this test. It should also be remembered that an IVP will not visualize in a patient who is significantly uremic.

Once postrenal or obstructive causes have been excluded, attention should be directed to evaluating renal perfusion. Assessment of the patient's hydration status should include daily weights; frequent measurements of urine output, pulse, and blood pressure; evaluation of skin turgor and the condition of mucous membranes; assessment of the degree of edema; and evaluation of distention of the neck veins. Decreased weights, hypotension, tachycardia, low volumes of concentrated urine, poor skin turgor, and flat neck veins suggest volume depletion. Edema, distended neck veins, hypertension, and increases in weight in the face of oliguria and azotemia are suggestive of an intrarenal disorder. In critically ill patients, lines for invasive monitoring will be present and central venous pressure (CVP), pulmonary capillary wedge pressure (PCWP), mean arterial pressure, and cardiac output can be easily determined. Fluid gains or losses should be carefully calculated and recorded. Myocardial function and the degree of systemic vasodilitation must be estimated. Sepsis and anaphylaxis should be excluded as possible causes. Finally, vascular diseases such as renal artery or vein stenosis or thrombosis and aortic aneurysm must be investigated if clinical examination or findings from the history are suggestive.

One of the most difficult tasks is to differentiate between prerenal ARF and ATN. This differentiation is critical because the patient with a prerenal disorder needs aggressive volume replacement. If a patient in ATN is treated with large amounts of fluid, overload with congestive failure or pulmonary edema may result. Several laboratory tests may be helpful. In prerenal ARF, the serum urea level is disproportionally elevated from the serum creatinine level. In addition, high urine osmolality, low urine sodium concentration, and high urine to plasma urea or creatinine ratios suggest volume depletion. Conversely, in ATN the ability to concentrate urine is lost, resulting in urine with a low specific gravity and low osmolality. Urine electrolyte concentration (Na^+ and Cl^-) is inappropriately high in ATN. Table 3-1 lists laboratory findings that are helpful in differentiating decreased renal function secondary to volume depletion from that caused by tubular damage.

Clinical Manifestations

The person with acute renal failure presents with signs of rapid deterioration of kidney function. Most commonly oliguria develops, but some patients

TABLE 3-1. LABORATORY FINDINGS IN ACUTE RENAL FAILURE DUE TO VOLUME DEPLETION AND TUBULAR DAMAGE

Test	Prerenal ARF		ATN	
Serum urea: creatinine ratio	High	(>20:1)	Low	(<15:1)
Urine osmolality (mOsm/L)	High	(>500)	Low	(<350)
Urine sodium concentration (mEq/L)	Low	(<20)	High	(>40)
Urine specific gravity	High	(>1.015)	Low	(<1.010)
Urine creatinine: plasma creatinine ratio	High	(>40:1)	Low	(<20:1)

become anuric while others maintain a normal urine volume. Azotemia, the accumulation of nitrogenous waste products, invariably occurs. Laboratory testing shows elevated BUN and creatinine levels. Electrolyte abnormalities are likely but not necessarily present. Fluid retention, edema, and hypertension are common clinical findings in oliguric patients. As renal failure progresses, its effect on multiple body systems begins to become evident.

Genitourinary System. Findings in acute renal failure that are related to the urinary system include decreased volume (in most cases) and a rise in serum levels of urea nitrogen and creatinine. Alterations in urine osmolality, specific gravity, and electrolyte concentrations may occur, as discussed previously. Urinalysis may show proteinuria, cellular debris, and even casts. Renal excretion of medications may be seriously altered and dose adjustments are frequently necessary.

Cardiovascular System. Changes in blood pressure are frequently seen in acute renal failure. Prerenal azotemia is often associated with hypotension and tachycardia. Intrarenal acute renal failure, particularily if associated with oliguria, often results in hypertension, volume overload, and even congestive heart failure. Arrhythmias may develop from alterations in electrolyte balance, especially potassium, calcium, and hydrogen ion (acid-base disorders). Pericarditis can develop in patients who become profoundly uremic.

Respiratory System. Acute renal failure can severely hinder the body's attempts to rid itself of hydrogen ions, resulting in a metabolic acidosis. The respiratory system will attempt to compensate by expiring carbon dioxide through hyperventilation. Sputum becomes thick and tenacious and the cough reflex is depressed, both of which predispose to pneumonia. The other major effect of acute renal failure on the respiratory system is volume overload resulting in pulmonary edema.

Gastrointestinal System. As uremia progresses, anorexia, nausea, and vomiting frequently develop. Stomatitis may further reduce the ability to take in adequate calories. The dietary and fluid restrictions necessary for management of the renal failure may make food less appealing. Constipation is frequently seen as a result of fluid restrictions, low-fiber diets, inactivity, and antacids used to control phosphate levels.

Hematopoietic System. When renal tissue is damaged, its ability to secrete erythropoietin decreases, resulting in anemia. Laboratory studies show a fall in hemoglobin and hematocrit levels, indicative of a normochromic, normocytic anemia. Uremia interferes with platelet adhesiveness, predisposing the patient to bleeding. Response to infection is altered as a nonspecific interference with cellular immunity occurs. Patients with renal failure are more susceptible to infection. In fact, infection is said to be the leading cause of death in acute renal failure, accounting for 60 to 75 percent of total mortality (Van Stone, 1983).

Neurological System. The accumulation of urea, creatinine, and other toxins may result in alterations of mental state. Drowsiness, disorientation, delirium, coma, and psychosis have all been reported in patients with acute renal failure. Convulsions may occur as a result of electrolyte imbalances or a too rapid urea clearance by dialysis.

Integumentary System. Dryness and itching of the skin may result from the accumulation of uremic wastes or from calcium and phosphate imbalances. Platelet abnormalities make bruising and purpura common findings. There is often a disruption in skin integrity.

MANAGEMENT OF ACUTE RENAL FAILURE

Determine the Cause and Correct When Possible

The first step in the treatment of acute renal failure is to determine the reason for the deterioration of renal function. It is at this time that prerenal, post-renal, and intrarenal causes must be identified and differentiated. Previous sections of this chapter describe the observations, tests, and procedures that can assist in identifying the etiology of the renal failure. Conditions that can be corrected must be in order to prevent further damage to the renal parenchyma. Obstruction must be relieved. Adequate renal perfusion must be restored. Nephrotoxic agents should be discontinued unless necessary to treat life-threatening conditions.

Assess Volume Status and Correct Fluid Excess or Deficit

Altered renal function frequently has a great effect on volume status. Prerenal acute renal failure, the postobstructive diuretic phase of postrenal acute renal failure, nonoliguric ATN, and the diuretic phase of oliguric ATN may all be associated with volume deficits. To prevent further intrarenal damage, fluid replacement, based upon a thorough assessment of the patient's hydration status, is essential.

Fluid excess or overload can also compromise renal function by causing hypertension and by decreasing myocardial efficiency. Both can cause further deterioration of renal function. In addition, overhydration can pre-cipitate life-threatening complications such as congestive heart failure and pulmonary edema. Excess fluid can be removed by potent diuretics if there is sufficient residual renal function to respond. Dialysis or continuous hemo-filtration may be required to remove excess fluid. Strict adherence to fluid restrictions will help prevent reaccumulation.

Treat Hyperkalemia and Prevent Cardiac Arrhythmias

Hyperkalemia is the most important sudden hazard in oliguric acute renal failure because of its relationship to life-threatening cardiac arrhythmias. Serum potassium levels must be closely monitored and hyperkalemia aggressively treated. Treatment options include the administration of hypertonic glucose, insulin, and sodium bicarbonate; the oral or rectal administration of cation exchange resins; and dialysis.

The intravenous administration of hypertonic glucose, insulin, and sodium bicarbonate works to treat hyperkalemia by shifting potassium into the intracellular compartment where it will not affect myocardial contractility. It is a temporalizing measure, however, because within a few hours, the potassium will move back into the extracellular compartment. Correcting the acidosis associated with renal failure and administering calcium gluconate intravenously also help to reduce myocardial irritability.

Cation exchange resins remove potassium from the serum quite effectively. They act by exchanging sodium for potassium, binding potassium in the gut, and excreting it in the stool. They significantly add to the total body sodium, and so must be used with caution in patients with renal failure.

Dialysis will usually be required in the patient with oliguric acute renal failure who is hyperkalemic, especially if he or she is also fluid overloaded and acidotic. Diets should also be restricted in potassium.

Restore or Maintain Normal Blood Pressure

Both hypotension and hypertension can result in further deterioration of renal function. Hypotension can most often be treated with volume replacement and correction of the underlying problem, although vasopressors may occasionally be necessary. Hypertension may respond to control of fluid overload or may require the use of antihypertensive agents. Adequate control of hypertension is essential not only to prevent further deterioration of renal function but to prevent vascular complications such as myocardial infarctions and cerebrovascular accidents. Dietary restrictions of sodium will assist in the management of hypertension.

Correct Uremia

The accumulation of nitrogenous wastes is the hallmark of renal failure. Uremia has adverse effects on many body systems including the neurological, cardiovascular, and hematopoietic systems. To control uremia, diets must be restricted in protein while still providing adequate calories to prevent catabolism (see "Maintain Adequate Nutrition and Prevent Catabolism" later in this chapter for details about how this is done). Dialysis is indicated in patients with overt uremic symptoms and generally in those with a BUN level over 100 or a creatine level greater than 12 (Van Stone, 1983).

Correct Metabolic Acidosis

Acute renal failure results in a metabolic acidosis because of the inability of the kidneys to secrete hydrogen ions and generate bicarbonate. Profound acidosis is incompatible with life. Acidosis may be treated by administering sodium bicarbonate. Because of the high sodium content, prolonged administration may not be possible in someone with renal failure. Severe acidosis is an indication for dialysis.

Maintain Adequate Nutrition and Prevent Catabolism

Nutrition plays a very important role in the patient with acute renal failure. Quite often these are critically ill patients with multiple medical problems. Many are postsurgical. Infection is the major cause of mortality in this patient population. The prevention of infection, wound healing, and recovery from multiple medical problems demand a good nutritional state.

Providing adequate calories to prevent catabolism is no easy feat in someone whose intake of protein, potassium, sodium, and fluid must be restricted. Supplementation with essential amino acids, the use of fats, and high carbohydrate diets are methods of providing the necessary calories and nutrients. If oral feeding is not possible or if adequate caloric intake cannot be achieved, hyperalimentation is recommended. Feeding tubes are preferred to intravenous hyperalimentation because of the risk of infections. If hyperalimentation is used, electrolytes must be closely monitored.

Prevent and Treat Infection

As previously stated, infection is the leading cause of death in acute renal failure. These patients are particularly susceptible to infection for several reasons. They are immunocompromised due to their uremic state. Many are critically ill, with large surgical incisions and invasive lines. Their sputum is thick and tenacious and their cough reflex depressed. Many are catabolic or in poor nutritional states. Skin integrity may be interrupted and wound healing is delayed.

Nursing care must be directed to preventing infection. Patients should be ambulatory if possible, and those who cannot be should be turned and encouraged to cough and deep breathe frequently. Meticulous care must be given to wounds, incisions, and invasive lines using aseptic techniques. Good skin care should be given and the patient turned frequently to maintain skin integrity and prevent decubiti. The use of an indwelling urinary catheter should be avoided. The nurse must be alert to signs of infection such as fever; local redness, swelling, heat, or drainage; and an elevated white blood cell count.

When infections do develop they must be treated appropriately. If antibotics are administered, care must be taken to adjust the dosage for the degree of renal impairment.

Provide Supportive Care to Patient and Family

In patients with so many physical problems it is easy to overlook the needs for emotional support and education; however, these patients and their families are in great need of this aspect of nursing care. They are often overwhelmed by the acute onset of physical illness and its associated emotional stresses. Time for patient and family education has been limited and their readiness to learn is not optimal due to the acute nature of the illness, the multiple physical derangements, and the many distractions. Brief, uncomplicated explanations are needed and repetition is important. The use of written materials will enhance learning.

Patients and families will also need emotional support. They face an acute illness, the possible need for dialysis, the potential for permanent kidney failure, a significant change in their life style, and possibly death. Any one of these is frightening and a crisis. Together, they are often overwhelming. Nurses must express concern and understanding of the patient's and family's reactions and provide support during this difficult time.

DIALYSIS IN ACUTE RENAL FAILURE

Dialysis is often indicated in the treatment of acute renal failure, especially in those patients who are oliguric or anuric. Indications for dialysis include fluid overload, hyperkalemia refractory to treatment with dietary restrictions and medications, overt uremia, and in most patients, a BUN level greater than 100 or creatinine level greater than 12. Severe acidosis unresponsive to medical treatment may also require dialysis for adequate treatment. Delaying dialysis in patients with such clinical indications may place them in danger of life-threatening complications such as cardiac arrhythmias, congestive heart failure, pulmonary edema, or uremic encephalopathy. Dialysis will also allow a more reasonable diet and thus improve the patient's nutritional status.

Either hemodialysis or peritoneal dialysis may be used to treat acute renal failure. Comparisons have not demonstrated a clear advantage of one type of dialysis over the other. Individual patient considerations should dictate whether hemodialysis or peritoneal dialysis will be prescribed. Consideration must also be given to the resources available in the institution for dialysis and to the expertise of the medical and nursing personnel.

Subsequent chapters will address both hemodialysis and peritoneal dialysis and the care of patients undergoing those treatments in some detail. The discussion in the present chapter will therefore be limited to the factors that must be taken into consideration in deciding which modality will be employed in the patient with acute renal failure.

Hemodialysis Versus Peritoneal Dialysis: Patient Considerations

Hemodialysis is more efficient than peritoneal dialysis and allows a more rapid clearance of wastes. Therefore, it may be the modality of choice for those patients whose rate of urea generation is high, such as severely catabolic patients. Likewise, hemodialysis is preferred in the severely hyperkalemic patient who is demonstrating ECG changes and in whom life-threatening cardiac arrhythmias are likely. Care must be taken in profoundly uremic patients not to lower the urea level too rapidly because disequilibrium syndrome may occur.

Patients with cardiovascular instability may not tolerate hemodialysis as well as peritoneal dialysis. Hemodialysis requires that blood be passed through an extracorporeal circuit. This reduces effective intracorporeal circulating blood volume. In patients with volume depletion, poor myocardial function, or vasodilatation, this small reduction in intravascular blood volume may be sufficient to reduce cardiac output to a critical level. Such individuals may be candidates for treatment with peritoneal dialysis. This same principle holds true for small children in whom the extracorporeal volume may represent an abnormally high proportion of total cardiac output. They too may better tolerate peritoneal dialysis.

Patients with recent abdominal surgery, especially if drains remain in place, may not be able to retain peritoneal dialysate in the cavity for a sufficient period of time to achieve adequate clearances to make peritoneal dialysis feasible. In addition, leakage of peritoneal dialysate through incisions may delay wound healing. Multiple abdominal surgeries or multiple episodes of peritonitis may result in adhesions in the peritoneal cavity that interfere with clearance. A current episode of peritonitis is not a contraindication to peritoneal dialysis. In fact, peritoneal dialysis with the addition of appropriate antibiotics to the dialysate is an accepted treatment for peritonitis.

Hemodialysis requires heparinization to prevent clotting of blood in the extracorporeal circuit. For some patients, heparinization presents a significant risk. Such patients include those with recent cerebral bleeds, pericardial effusions that may become bloody, gastrointestinal bleeding, or significant blood dyscrasias. Peritoneal dialysis does not require heparinization and offers a safer alternative for such patients.

Access for dialysis must also be taken into consideration. Hemodialysis requires vascular access which, with recent developments in catheters, is relatively easily established in most patients. Peritoneal dialysis requires the insertion of a catheter into the peritoneal cavity either surgically or by paracentesis. Access rarely dictates the choice of modality, because most patients can have access for either hemodialysis or peritoneal dialysis established without significant difficulty.

The final patient consideration is certainly not the least important. Patient and family wishes should be ascertained after the options, the advantages and disadvantages of each, and the recommendations of the health care team have been made known to them. In some instances, other considerations such as the patient's medical condition or resource availability will dictate the modality. However, if there is no clear advantage to one type of dialysis over another, patient and family wishes should be determined and followed.

Resource Considerations: Equipment and Personnel

Hemodialysis is a complex procedure that requires very specialized equipment and a highly skilled staff. In addition, water treatment, electrical requirements, and drain facilities must be considered. Although the procedure itself is relatively short (3 to 4 hours), the intensity of nursing care needed is quite high (often one nurse to one patient in those with acute renal failure). Many community hospitals do not have the resources to offer hemodialysis. They must either transfer the patient or contract with another facility to provide the necessary personnel and equipment.

In contrast, peritoneal dialysis is a relatively simple procedure that does not require complex equipment, water treatment, special electrical requirements, or drain facilities. The time required for the treatment is longer (often as long as 24 to 36 hours) but the intensity of nursing care is much less. Nursing staff can be adequately trained to perform peritoneal dialysis safely in a short period of time. Most hospitals have the resources to be able to perform peritoneal dialysis either in an intensive care or medical surgical unit. Table 3–2 summarizes the factors to be taken into consideration when choosing a dialysis therapy for a patient with acute renal failure.

TABLE 3-2. CONSIDERATIONS IN CHOOSING A DIALYSIS THERAPY FOR THE PATIENT WITH ACUTE RENAL FAILURE

	Hemodialysis	Peritoneal Dialysis
Efficiency	Much more efficient	Less efficient waste clearance
Equipment	Complex	Simple
Facility considerations	Water treatment Electrical requirements Drain facilities	Not necessarily required
Personnel	Highly specialized staff Long period of training	Skilled nurses Short period of training
Treatment time	3–4 hours	May be as long as 24–36 hours
Patient considerations	Caution in patients with cardiovascular instability May be difficult in small children Heparinization may present risks for some patients	Recent abdominal surgery, adhesions may reduce clearance May not allow rapid enough clearance of urea or potassium in some patients
Access	Requires vascular access	Requires insertion of peritoneal catheter
Complications	Hemodynamic instability Hemorrhage Air embolus Disequilibrium syndrome Membrane sensitivity Vascular access problems (stenosis, infection, clotting, hematoma) Pyrogen reactions	Hyperglycemia Peritonitis Catheter problems (infection, obstruction) Hypernatremia Protein loss Decreased diaphragmatic excursion (decreased ventilation) Bowel perforation

Nurses are very appropriately included in the decision-making process about the type of dialysis to be instituted. Nursing roles include patient assessment and the presentation of findings that could influence the decision. Experienced nephrology nurses often recommend a treatment modality to the physician. Once the decision has been made, nurses should understand the rationale for the decision and support it. At this time patient and family education must be continued. A great deal of fear and apprehension accompany the beginning of dialytic therapy.

CONCLUSION

The patient with acute renal failure represents a great nursing challenge. Such patients often have involvement of multiple body systems and require intensive nursing care. Ongoing patient assessment and revision of the plan of care to meet the patient's changing needs are essential. The development of acute renal failure is an event for which patients and families are unprepared. They are presented with a disease that may require frightening treatments such as dialysis and that may result in a chronic condition. In some patients, acute renal failure may be fatal. During this stressful time, education and emotional support must be an integral part of the nursing care provided.

REFERENCES

Mars, D. R., & Treloar, D. (1984). Acute tubular necrosis—pathophysiology and treatment. *Heart & Lung 13*(2), 194–202.

Stark, J. L. (1982). How to succeed against acute renal failure. *Nursing 82, 12*(7), 26–33.

Van Stone, J. C. (1983). *Dialysis and the treatment of renal insufficiency.* New York: Grune & Stratton.

4

Chronic Renal Failure

Betty Irwin Crandall

OBJECTIVES

After reading this chapter on chronic renal failure, the nurse will be able to:

1. Name and describe the clinical findings of the four stages along the continuum from diminished renal reserve to end stage renal disease
2. Describe the changes in the integumentary system that commonly occur in renal failure
3. Name three major disorders of the cardiovascular system that commonly occur in renal failure and identify at least two implications for nursing care related to each
4. Name three nursing interventions that are appropriate due to the hematological abnormalities frequently seen in chronic renal failure
5. Describe the medical and nursing interventions necessary to help prevent the development of hyperparathyroidism and renal osteodystrophy
6. Name three effects of renal failure on the nervous system and describe appropriate nursing interventions to provide care to a patient who demonstrates those effects

Chronic renal failure may be defined as a state in which the kidneys no longer function adequately to rid the body of wastes and maintain homeostasis. The hallmark of renal failure is azotemia. Chronic renal failure may develop rather rapidly (over only a few weeks) or may occur more slowly over a period of months or years. It is an irreversible condition.

As renal failure progresses, it results in uremia or the uremic syndrome, a term originally defined as "urine in the blood." *Uremia* refers to the clinical syndrome of toxicity that results from the retention of those products normally excreted in the urine. The uremic syndrome is manifested by fluid and electrolyte abnormalities, altered regulatory functions of the kidneys, and the physiological changes and alterations of function on many organ systems caused by the accumulation of toxins usually excreted by the kidney.

Renal disease may be viewed as progressing along a continuum from diminished renal reserve to *end stage renal disease* (ESRD). At first, the process is a subclinical one involving the loss of functioning nephrons without clinical symptoms. The loss of renal reserve in this stage can only be detected by laboratory testing. In fact, the most often measured parameters of renal function (BUN and creatinine) will remain normal until over 50 percent of renal function has been lost. In this stage of diminished renal reserve, creatinine clearance may be the only indicator of dysfunction.

The stage of diminished renal reserve will progress to renal insufficiency as more nephrons cease to function. During this stage, the function of the kidneys is obviously abnormal but the individual may not demonstrate physical limitations in daily activities. Detectable abnormalities may include azotemia, anemia, and a loss of the ability to concentrate urine. This is a precarious state because the kidneys have lost the ability to adjust their function when challenged with conditions such as dehydration, heart failure, or salt depletion. Such conditions may rapidly tip the patient with renal insufficiency into renal failure.

Renal insufficiency progresses to renal failure. In this stage the patient begins to show limitations in performing daily activities. Anemia, hypertension, metabolic acidosis, azotemia, hypocalcemia, and other metabolic derangements are seen. Eventually, the patient shows evidence of uremia, a syndrome that encompasses all of the overt signs and symptoms of renal failure. If not already instituted, dialysis is begun and it relieves many of the symptoms of uremia. The patient has reached end stage disease.

ESRD is defined as irreversible renal failure that necessitates dialysis or transplantation for survival. It is the final stage along the continuum that begins with diminished renal reserve.

It is beyond the scope of this chapter to discuss the numerous causes of chronic renal failure and the pathology of each disease process. Common causes include pyelonephritis, glomerulonephritis, hypertensive nephropathy, diabetic nephropathy, obstructive nephropathy, and congenital and hereditary disorders. Many other less common disease states may result in chronic renal failure. In addition, irreversible acute renal failure may result in ESRD. The reader is referred to the many good texts available if specific information about the pathology of various disease states is desired.

The purpose of this chapter is to review the pathophysiology of chronic renal failure. Renal disease causes pathological changes in almost all body systems. The changes discussed in this chapter occur when renal function deteriorates to 20 to 25 percent of normal. Patients can often be managed without dialysis or transplantation still longer, often until the glomerular filtration rate (GFR) is only 10 to 15 percent of normal. Understanding the alterations in the functioning of major body systems caused by the development of chronic renal failure provides the basis of knowledge necessary to understand the medical regimen and to assess, plan, implement, and evaluate nursing care for this group of patients.

CHANGES IN THE INTEGUMENTARY SYSTEM

Persons who are uremic have a characteristic grayish-bronze tone to the skin. Some individuals exhibit a yellowish hue to the skin even without evidence of liver dysfunction. This discoloration is a result of retained pigments that are normally excreted by the kidneys. Because of the anemia that commonly accompanies renal failure, these persons also have an underlying pallor. Decreased activity of the oil glands and reductions in the size of sweat glands result in dryness of the skin and decreased perspiration. Skin dryness and the deposition of urea and phosphate crystals cause severe itching.

Uremic Frost
Uremic frost is a condition rarely seen today due to the early initiation of dialysis to treat azotemia. It is a white dust-like material usually seen on the face, nose, forehead, and sometimes the upper trunk. It results when severely azotemic individuals excrete urea crystals via the sweat glands.

Abnormal blood clotting activity and increased capillary fragility associated with uremia combine with the itching and scratching to cause excoriations, purpura, and ecchymoses on the skin. Even relatively minor trauma can result in severe bruising. Areas of excoriation, bruising, or scratches may become infected. Edema may reduce circulation and make infection an even greater possibility.

Nails are thin, brittle, and break easily. They may have a whitened proximal section with a much darker brown distal edge. Ridges are commonly seen on the nails. Hair is dry and tends to fall out easily.

Nursing Care Implications. The uremic manifestations in the integumentary system present some of the most uncomfortable symptoms patients experience. The constant itching and scratching make patients irritable, restless, and frustrated. In addition, they add greatly to the risk of infection.

Nursing care is directed to maintain skin integrity and relieve the symptoms. Patients must be taught the importance of good hygiene and assisted if they are unable to perform their own care. The use of soap should be avoided when possible because soaps may cause further drying of the skin.

Bath oils and lotions should be applied liberally. Nails should be trimmed and kept short to prevent excoriations from scratching. Hair should be kept clean and moisturized. Shampooing too frequently should be avoided to prevent drying. Antipruritic medications may be used during intense periods of itching. Control of phosphate levels and dialysis to lower urea levels will assist in the control of itching.

Particular care must be taken to maintain skin integrity in hospitalized or nonambulatory patients. Frequent turning, proper positioning, and massage of pressure areas will help prevent decubitus formation. Eggcrate mattresses or flotation pads may also be used. Early ambulation should be encouraged. Range of motion exercises not only prevent contractures but also improve circulation.

Patients will often become frustrated and irritable because of failure to control these symptoms. An understanding, sympathetic attitude on the part of the nurse and a willingness to try new approaches will do much to convey concern and support to a patient who is quite distressed.

DISORDERS OF FLUIDS, ELECTROLYTES, AND ACID-BASE BALANCE

Disturbances in body water, many electrolytes, and acid-base balance occur often in patients with ESRD.

Body Water Disturbances
Patients with renal failure may be either dehydrated or fluid overloaded, depending on the underlying disease process and the degree of renal impairment. Large urinary losses may occur early in renal failure due to a loss of the ability of the renal tubules to concentrate urine. In some disease states such as polycystic kidney disease, excessive losses of body water may continue even once end stage disease is reached. Most often, however, once GFR falls below 4 to 5 ml/min, volume overload is the major problem (Lancaster, 1984). Volume overload results from severe renal impairment that prevents the kidney from filtering water at the glomerulus.

It should be remembered that in addition to causing other complications, both dehydration and fluid overload can cause further deterioration of renal function. Maintaining the patient in an euvolemic state will optimize his or her residual renal function.

Metabolic Acidosis
The kidneys serve as the final pathway for excreting the hydrogen ions produced in the body during metabolism. They control the acid-base balance of the body by secreting excessive hydrogen ions in the urine, by reabsorbing filtered bicarbonate, and by regenerating bicarbonate in the renal tubules. In addition, the kidneys excrete other acid end products of protein metabolism.

When the kidneys fail, they are unable to perform these functions. Other acid end products of protein metabolism are also retained, and consume available blood buffers. All of these processes result in a metabolic acidosis, indicated by a low arterial blood pH and a low serum bicarbonate level.

The respiratory system attempts to compensate for the metabolic acidosis by increasing the rate and depth of breathing to excrete carbon dioxide. This is a normal compensatory mechanism known as Kussmaul respiration, which allows the body to maintain a normal pH for a time despite the renal impairment. This pattern of hyperventilation may be the only clinical sign of the acid-base imbalance.

Nursing Care Implications. Management of fluid balance is usually achieved by carefully matching intake to fluid losses. Most patients with chronic renal failure will require fluid restriction to prevent volume overload. Intake of fluids in all forms (oral and intravenous) is usually restricted to the total urine output for the previous 24 hours plus an allowance of 500 to 600 ml daily for insensible water losses. This figure represents customary losses for an adult under normal metabolic conditions. Allowances must be made for febrile states, the patient who is vomiting or has diarrhea, and other conditions that cause increased fluid losses.

Nursing responsibilities include careful monitoring and recording of intake and output as well as patient and family education about the need for fluid restriction and the dietary sources of fluid. Patients should be taught that all foods that are liquid at room temperature must be counted as fluids. Thirst may be controlled by having the patient suck on hard candy or a lemon.

In the early stages of renal failure, diuretic therapy may be useful to control fluid balance. As renal failure progresses, diuretics are ineffective. Dialysis may become necessary for fluid removal.

Control of the metabolic acidosis that results from chronic renal failure eventually requires the administration of alkalizing agents such as Shohl's solution, Bicitra, or sodium bicarbonate, or the institution of dialysis. Dialysis corrects the acidosis by removing hydrogen ions and by adding either acetate or bicarbonate to serve as buffers.

DISORDERS OF THE CARDIOVASCULAR SYSTEM

A large percentage of individuals with chronic renal failure have cardiovascular disease of one kind or another. Among those patients undergoing maintenance dialysis, cardiovascular events are the leading cause of mortality (Young, Krothapalli, & Ayues, 1984). Patients with ESRD exhibit a 10 to 30 times greater risk of cardiovascular mortality than the U.S. population at large (Cummings & Klahr, 1985). Four major cardiovascular conditions will be discussed in this section: hypertension, accelerated atherosclerosis, myocardial dysfunction, and pericarditis. Hyperkalemia is also discussed as a cardiovascular complication of chronic renal failure because the primary effect of high serum potassium levels is on cardiac functioning.

Hypertension

The most frequent cardiovascular complication of renal failure is hypertension. It results primarily from sodium and water retention and from malfunction of the renin-angiotensin mechanism.

Sodium and water retention occur when the kidneys lose their ability to filter and excrete salt and water. This results in expansion of the extracellular fluid volume and hypertension. An elevated blood pressure caused by the retention of sodium and water usually responds to dietary and fluid restrictions and dialysis.

The second major cause of hypertension in patients with renal failure is malfunction of the renin-angiotensin system. (Refer to Chapter 1 for a discussion of the normal mechanism.) Patients in renal failure often produce excessive amounts of renin. Renin is converted to angiotensin II, a potent vasoconstrictor and a substance that stimulates aldosterone secretion. Both aldosterone secretion and peripheral vasoconstriction serve to raise blood pressure. Normally, an increase in blood pressure reduces renin production. In patients with renal failure, renin is often produced even in the face of an elevated blood pressure. Antihypertensives such as captopril, which block aspects of the renin-angiotensin system, may be used successfully to control blood pressure. In severe cases of renin-induced hypertension, bilateral nephrectomy may be indicated for hypertension control.

Uncontrolled hypertension has many potentially lethal effects. It accelerates the process of atherosclerosis by causing further vascular damage. This results in an increased risk of myocardial infarction and cerebrovascular accidents as well as worsening renal function by increasing renal ischemia. Hypertensive encephalopathy may result in increased intracranial pressure, seizures, coma, and even death. Left ventricular hypertrophy and congestive heart failure may result from the extra work load on the heart caused by uncontrolled hypertension.

Nursing Care Implications. Many patients with renal failure will have antihypertensive medication prescribed. Nurses may be responsible for administering medications in the hospital or dialysis unit as well as assuring that patients and their families are educated about the medications, the importance of taking them as prescribed, and the actions and adverse effects of the antihypertensive drugs. Because patients may not "feel bad" when hypertensive and because the adverse effects of these medications may make patients feel worse, adherence to the prescribed regimen is often a problem. Nurses must assess patients' responses to the medications and work collaboratively with patients and physicians to achieve a reasonable regimen. Care must be taken in administering antihypertensives prior to hemodialysis because they may alter the cardiovascular response to fluid removal and precipitate shock.

In general, antihypertensives should not be given immediately prior to or during hemodialysis.

Controlling extracellular fluid volume through dietary restrictions of sodium and fluid is an important aspect of the management of hypertension. The goal is to reduce blood return to the heart (preload) and thus reduce cardiac output, reducing blood pressure. Nurses must assure that patients understand the need for sodium and fluid restriction and know the dietary sources of sodium.

Accelerated Atherosclerosis

Patients with chronic renal failure have an increased incidence of atherosclerotic disease when compared to age-matched controls. The reasons for this are not completely understood. Certainly, these patients have an increased incidence of risk factors for atherosclerosis. The most significant risk factor experienced by ESRD patients is hypertension. Hyperlipidemia is another cardiovascular risk factor frequently seen in this patient population. It has been suggested that if the incidence of these risk factors is taken into consideration, the incidence of atherosclerotic disease and therefore of mortality from cardiovascular causes may not be higher in patients with renal failure than in age-matched controls (Van Stone, 1983). However, patients with ESRD do demonstrate an increased incidence if one looks only at the development of atherosclerotic disease and its lethal complications such as myocardial infarction and cerebrovascular accidents. Atherosclerotic disease remains a significant problem in the management of these patients.

Nursing Care Implications. Nursing interventions to reduce morbidity and mortality from accelerated atherosclerosis center around patient education. Patients and their families must be instructed in the importance of controlling blood pressure and the regimen prescribed for doing this, as described earlier. Control of serum cholesterol and triglyceride levels will also reduce the risk of atherosclerotic disease. Control is usually achieved by dietary restrictions. Patient education is important for compliance.

Another important aspect of nursing care is assessment for evidence of atherosclerotic disease. Detecting early signs of cerebral or myocardial ischemia may allow medical or surgical intervention to prevent significant morbidity or even mortality.

Myocardial Dysfunction

Hypertension, atherosclerosis, and the anemia that frequently accompanies chronic renal failure result in an increased work load on the heart. Hypertrophy of the left ventricular musculature often results (left ventricular hypertrophy or LVH). Reports indicate that 25 to 40 percent of chronic dialysis patients have evidence of left ventricular hypertrophy (Van Stone, 1983). Excessive myocardial hypertrophy reduces myocardial function probably because there is insufficient blood supply for the increased muscle mass. In addition, the stress of extracellular volume excess (fluid overload) may precipitate congestive failure in a patient whose myocardial function is already compromised.

Clinically, the first sign of depressed cardiac function may be congestive heart failure with dyspnea on exertion, orthopnea, paroxysmal nocturnal dyspnea, and the accumulation of peripheral edema. Anginal attacks may indicate insufficient perfusion of an enlarged myocardium. Chest radiography may show an enlarged heart shadow. Echocardiography may demonstrate a dilated and less than optimally functioning left ventricle. Cardiac function as measured by ejection fraction is frequently decreased.

Nursing Care Implications. Hypertension is thought to be the primary factor in the development of left ventricular hypertrophy. Nursing interventions to assist in blood pressure control have previously been discussed. Adequate transfusion as well as interventions to reduce blood loss from laboratory testing and loss during hemodialysis will assist in controlling anemia and thus also reduce the work load on the heart.

Patient assessment is an important aspect of nursing care. Nurses may evaluate myocardial function by watching for the signs of congestive failure and myocardial ischemia. Review of testing requested by the physician may provide early clues to the development of left ventricular hypertrophy. Patients must be taught to be alert to the signs of myocardial dysfunction and to report them to the physicians and nurses caring for them. Dialysis may improve myocardial function by removing excess fluid, controlling hypertension, and removing substances that may themselves be toxic to the myocardium.

Hyperkalemia

Hyperkalemia is a life-threatening complication of renal failure that almost always occurs once urine outputs fall below 500 ml for 24 hours. Until the output drops below that level, normal serum potassium levels (3.5 to 5.0 mEq/L) are usually maintained despite potassium ingestion because of the ability of the kidneys to both filter and secrete potassium. Once GFR falls sufficiently to reduce daily urine output to 500 ml, serum potassium levels rise rapidly. In patients with chronic renal failure, few signs of hyperkalemia are evident until potassium levels exceed 6.5 mEq/L, when electrocardiographic changes may indicate potentially lethal cardiac arrhythmias that can result in cardiac arrest and death. If the patient is not monitored, these changes may not be seen until the patient arrests.

High serum potassium levels alter the balance between intracellular and extracellular potassium. This alters the membrane potential and thus the electrical activity of the heart. The result is the potentially lethal cardiac arrhythmias seen in hyperkalemia. Ultimately, interference with contraction of the myocardium may result. Acidosis and hypocalcemia may increase serum potassium levels and increase myocardial irritability.

The single most important indications of elevated serum potassium levels are the classic electrocardiogram (ECG) changes. In fact, no clinical evidence of hyperkalemia may be present. Tall, tented T waves are most often the first change seen. Other changes include a prolonged PR interval, ST segment depression, and a widened QRS complex. Eventually, the P wave is lost and ventricular fibrillation and cardiac standstill result.

Nursing Care Implications. Hyperkalemia must be treated as an emergency life-threatening condition when it occurs. In severe hyperkalemia, medical treatment often includes the administration of hypertonic glucose and short-acting (regular) insulin intravenously to lower serum potassium levels by moving potassium into the cells. Intravenous sodium bicarbonate is used to correct acidosis and to assist in the movement of potassium intracellularly. Calcium gluconate antagonizes the effect of elevated potassium on the heart. When potassium levels are less dangerously elevated and ECG changes are not evident, cation exchange resins such as polystyrene sulfonate (Kayexalate) may be administered orally or as a retention enema. Kayexalate reduces serum potassium levels by exchanging sodium for potassium in the intestine. Potassium is then excreted in the stool. Finally, dialysis may be used to definitively treat hyperkalemia by removing potassium ions from the plasma. A low potassium dialysate may be used to speed potassium removal.

Nursing responsibilities in the treatment of hyperkalemia include, of course, the administration of the medications ordered and performing dialysis. It must always be remembered that treatment by administering glucose and insulin is only a temporary measure because once the glucose is metabolized in the cell, potassium again moves into the plasma, resulting in hyperkalemia. When giving a patient Kayexalate, care must be taken not to administer excessive amounts of sodium to a patient who can easily become volume overloaded.

Prevention of hyperkalemia is an important aspect of nursing care for the chronic renal failure patient. Causes of hyperkalemia include excessive dietary intake of potassium, ingestion of potassium in medications, blood transfusions, bleeding, and a catabolic state. Nurses can have the greatest impact in helping to assure dietary compliance. Patients must be taught the sources of dietary potassium and the significance of excessive potassium levels. They must be encouraged to maintain an adequate caloric intake to prevent catabolism. Medications high in potassium should be avoided. For example, sodium penicillin, rather than potassium penicillin, should be used. Blood transfusions should be administered during dialysis when possible so that the potassium present in stored blood can be removed.

Assessment is an obvious component of the nursing care of patients with renal failure. Laboratory monitoring of patients' serum potassium levels must be performed as indicated. In a recently diagnosed patient, one who is acutely ill, recovering from surgery, bleeding, or severely catabolic, serum potassium levels must be checked at least daily, often as frequently as every few hours.

In a stable, chronic patient, potassium levels may only be monitored weekly or even monthly. These results should be shared with the patient and used to reinforce teaching and adherence to the prescribed regimen. An ECG should be done whenever a patient is known to be profoundly hyperkalemic. Continuous monitoring is recommended in an acutely ill patient or one who has shown ECG changes.

Pericarditis, Pericardial Effusion, Tamponade

Pericarditis is a frequent cardiovascular complication of chronic renal failure, occurring in approximately 30 to 50 percent of patients (Lancaster, 1984). Many of these patients are asymptomatic and may, in fact, be undiagnosed. Two types of pericarditis are commonly seen in chronic renal failure: uremic pericarditis and dialysis-associated pericarditis.

Uremic pericarditis occurs prior to the onset of dialysis, is usually associated with other signs and symptoms of uremia, and responds to dialysis (Van Stone, 1983). Fever and chest pain are frequently not seen. Cardiac tamponade is rare in uremic pericarditis. This type of pericarditis is thought to be caused by an irritating effect of uremic toxins on the pericardium. Initiation of dialysis is usually all that is needed to treat the condition.

The etiology of dialysis-associated pericarditis is not clear. No definite correlation is seen with serum urea or creatinine levels or other common indicators of the control of uremia. Chronic fluid overload may be a factor. Infection, particularly viral infection, may be the cause in some patients. Often no positive cultures are reported but viral agents are known to be difficult to culture. Dialysis-associated pericarditis is frequently associated with fever and chest pain. Cardiac tamponade is not uncommon. Dialysis may not improve the condition.

The clinical signs and symptoms of pericarditis are related to the underlying pathology. In nondisease states, a few milliliters of fluid are present between the visceral and parietal layers of the pericardium. During cardiac contraction the two layers are able to glide over each other because of this lubrication. With the inflammation seen in pericarditis, the layers no longer glide but rather rub together harshly. This produces a pericardial friction rub heard on auscultation of the chest. Other clinical signs may include fever, hypotension and chest pain that may be relieved when the patient sits up and leans forward.

The inflammatory process of pericarditis may cause the effusion of fluid and bleeding into the pericardial space. This is known as a *pericardial effusion.* Clinically, one may note the disappearance of a friction rub that previously existed as the fluid accumulation again allows the two layers to glide over each other. A marked decrease in systolic blood pressure on inspiration (paradoxical pulse) is frequently cited as specific evidence of a pericardial effusion (Lancaster, 1984). This is an exaggeration of a normal event since blood pressure falls as much as 10 mm Hg on inspiration. Paradoxical pulse is caused by the restriction of cardiac filling caused by the effusion. Chest roentgenograms and echocardiograms are useful diagnostic studies to detect pericardial effusions.

Cardiac tamponade may develop despite attempts to reduce the effusion. This usually results from bleeding into the pericardial space and is more common in dialysis-associated pericarditis than in uremic pericarditis. Large amounts of fluid in the pericardial sac prevent adequate filling of the heart and reduce cardiac output. Signs and symptoms include hypotension, muffled heart sounds, bulging neck veins, narrowing pulse pressure, and weak peripheral pulses. Tamponade is a life-threatening complication. Pericardiocentesis or surgery to create a pericardial window or perform pericardiectomy must be performed to maintain cardiac output and prevent death.

Nursing Care Implications. Therapy for uremic pericarditis is usually the initiation of dialysis. Symptoms usually resolve once dialysis is begun. Dialysis-associated pericarditis is usually treated by increasing the time and frequency of dialysis. Control of fluid overload may also be beneficial. Some physicians may use steroids or indomethicin, although controlled clinical trials do not prove their usefulness.

Assessment for evidence of pericarditis in patients with chronic renal failure is an important nursing function. Auscultation of the chest may detect a friction rub. Blood pressure should be closely monitored, as should other indicators of cardiac output. Minimizing the amount of heparin used during hemodialysis and controlling bleeding times may help prevent bleeding into the pericardial sac. Detection and early treatment of infections may prevent infective pericarditis.

DISORDERS OF THE PULMONARY SYSTEM

Pulmonary problems of chronic renal failure include pulmonary edema, pneumonia, pleuritis, and pleural effusions. In addition, the respiratory system attempts to control the body's acid-base balance by expiring carbon dioxide to compensate for the inability of the kidneys to secrete hydrogen ions and reabsorb bicarbonate. This results in the Kussmaul respirations often seen in metabolic acidosis. The breath of patients with chronic renal failure may have a characteristic uremic odor.

The sputum in individuals with renal failure is thick and tenacious. The cough reflex is depressed. These factors, combined with the altered immunologic state and decreased pulmonary macrophage activity seen in this patient population, produce an increased risk of pulmonary infection. Infection is the most common adverse pulmonary consequence of renal failure (Bernard & Brigham, 1984). Bacterial pneumonia is the most frequent pulmonary infection seen, although viral and fungal infections do occur. The incidence of tuberculosis in patients with chronic renal failure is 6 to 16 times that of the general population (Bernard & Brigham, 1984).

Pleuritis and pleural effusions may develop in patients with renal failure. The etiology and treatment are not fully understood. Undoubtedly, as with pericarditis and pericardial effusions, the etiology is multifactorial. An irritating effect of uremic toxins on the pleural membrane is believed to be one factor. Effusions increase in size with fluid overload. Hemorrhagic effusions may result from heparinization during hemodialysis. Large pleural effusions may compromise pulmonary function.

Fluid overload and congestive heart failure may result in pulmonary edema. Low serum oncotic pressure due to low levels of serum proteins and changes in pulmonary microvascular permeability undoubtedly add to the tendency for fluid accumulation in the lungs. Pulmonary edema is most frequently seen in inadequately dialyzed patients or those who do not adhere to fluid and sodium restrictions. It is a life-threatening complication but usually responds well to dialysis and fluid removal.

Nursing Care Implications. Interventions to prevent and treat fluid overload are extremely important in avoiding the pulmonary complications of renal failure. Fluid and sodium restrictions and adequate dialysis will help maintain the patient in an euvolemic state. Patient education about the necessity for preventing fluid overload and the ways to do so is an important aspect of nursing care. Patient assessment for the signs of extracellular volume excess may allow for early intervention and prevention of pulmonary complications.

Prevention, detection, and treatment of pulmonary infections is vitally important. Patients who are hospitalized or not fully ambulatory must be encouraged to cough, deep breathe, and use incentive spirometers to achieve full lung expansion and prevent atelectasis and infection. Frequent auscultation of the chest should be a routine part of the assessment of all patients with chronic renal failure. Chest roentgenograms are indicated whenever abnormal sounds are heard on auscultation and in all cases of unexplained febrile episodes. Early treatment of pulmonary infections with appropriate antibiotics is important. Pleuritis and pleural effusions may be detected by chest auscultation or may be evident on chest x-rays. Patients may complain of pain in the chest which is most severe on inspiration. Compromise of pulmonary function is a late finding in pleural effusions.

HEMATOLOGIC ABNORMALITIES

Three major hematologic abnormalities are seen in patients with chronic renal failure: anemia, abnormal platelet functioning, and changes in immune and granulocyte function. These three abnormalities may produce significant problems and complications for patients and demand careful attention by health professionals.

Anemia

Anemia is the primary hematologic abnormality found in patients with chronic renal failure. Most dialysis patients demonstrate a significant anemia with a hemoglobin concentration averaging between 6 and 8 g/dl (Van Stone, 1983) and a hematocrit of about 20 percent. The anemia of renal failure, if uncomplicated, is normochromic and normocytic. In general, the severity of the anemia is not correlated with the etiology of the renal failure. One exception is the patient with polycystic kidney disease who, because of an increased renal mass, usually develops anemia more slowly than those without polycystic kidney disease.

The cause of the anemia of renal failure is multifactorial. A major factor is the decreased production of erythropoietin, a hormone normally produced by the kidney that stimulates the bone marrow to produce red blood cells. Even the diseased kidney is still capable of producing some erythropoietin and bilateral nephrectomy uniformly decreases plasma erythropoietin concentrations, increasing the severity of the anemia (Van Stone, 1983). Other organs, such as the liver and possibly the salivary glands, do produce small amounts of erythropoietin, so that even the anephric patient will often have some detectable level of plasma erythropoietin.

Although decreased erythropoietin production is the major factor in the development of anemia in patients with renal failure, toxins present in the serum of these patients also inhibit erythropoiesis and cause an accelerated rate of red blood cell destruction. These toxins are not well defined but at least some of them are believed to be dialyzable molecules, as suggested by the fact that one often sees a slight improvement in the anemia in the first few months after dialysis is initiated. The decrease in red blood cell survival is relatively small, from a normal time of 115 days to 73 days (Van Stone, 1983), but probably contributes significantly to the anemia. It has been shown that red blood cells from patients with chronic renal failure survive normally when transfused into normal individuals. This finding supports the view that the decreased red blood cell survival time is a result of circulating toxins in the plasma of uremic individuals rather than an inherent defect in the cells themselves.

Blood loss in patients with renal failure also contributes to the anemia. Blood loss may occur from excessive laboratory testing, bleeding from the gastrointestinal mucosa, and as a result of leaks, rupture, or residual blood remaining in the dialyzer after hemodialysis. It has also been suggested that severe secondary hyperparathyroidism may increase bone marrow fibrosis and thus inhibit erythropoiesis. Well-controlled studies have not been published that substantiate the role of hyperparathyroidism in the anemia of chronic renal failure. Finally, deficiencies of both iron and folic acid may contribute to the anemia.

It is difficult to quantitate the clinical significance of this anemia in patients with renal failure. The pallor is usually quite evident. Fatigue is prevalent and activity tolerance is usually reduced. Anemia can contribute to the left ventrical hypertrophy, congestive heart failure, and angina, which frequently complicate the management of these patients.

Abnormal Platelet Function

There may be a small reduction in the platelet count in chronic renal failure but it usually remains within the limits of normal. Of much greater significance are the abnormalities of platelet function seen in these patients. There is a reduction in both platelet adhesiveness and platelet aggregation. This results in a prolonged bleeding time and abnormalities of hemostasis. Patients with renal failure are prone to prolonged bleeding from venipuncture sites and to difficulties maintaining hemostasis after surgery. Bruising and purpura may be evident. Bleeding from mucous membranes or body orifices may occur.

Changes in Immune and Granulocyte Function

Infection is reported to account for 10 percent of all deaths in patients with chronic renal failure (Anagnostou & Fried, 1984). This increased rate of life-threatening infection results from abnormalities in both granulocyte function and immune response.

The total white blood cell count is usually normal or slightly increased, but the total peripheral lymphocyte counts are commonly below normal. the number of both T and B lymphocytes is decreased. The percentage of T cells is normal, but there is a decrease in the percentage of B cells. Both cellular and humoral immunity are impaired in renal failure. Cellular immune deficiencies have been demonstrated through cutaneous anergy testing. Anergy seems to improve slightly immediately after dialysis is initiated but then seems to worsen if dialysis therapy is necessary longer than one year. Antibody production is frequently not normal when the patient is stimulated with an antigen. Despite diminished antibody production in response to antigen stimulation, vaccination may still be effective.

There are also abnormalities in both the mobility and chemotaxis of granulocytes in chronic renal failure. The effect of renal failure on phagocytic activity has not yet been fully determined. Some studies show normal phagocytic activity and a few show diminished activity (Van Stone, 1983).

Hemodialysis itself is known to have a significant effect on the circulating granulocyte count. Early in the dialysis treatment, there is a severe, sudden granulocytopenia. This apparently results from the activation of complement compounds by the dialyzer membrane, resulting in the sequestration of granulocytes in the pulmonary vascular bed. This is believed to be one of the causes of the hypoxia seen during hemodialysis. The severity of the granulocytopenia varies with different dialyzer membranes and is reduced when reprocessed dialyzers are used.

Nursing Care Implications. Prevention of complications that may result from the hematologic abnormalities occurring in renal failure is a significant part of the nursing care required for these patients. Nurses must assist other health professionals in avoiding excess blood loss for unnecessary laboratory testing and from clotting, leaks, rupture, or inadequate rinsing of the dialyzer during hemodialysis. Applying adequate pressure to venipuncture sites will prevent excessive blood loss there. Antacid therapy and prevention of trauma to mucous membranes will help prevent ulceration and subsequent bleeding. Appropriate use of aseptic technique and avoidance of contact with persons who are infected will do much to prevent these susceptible individuals from contracting infections. Infections of the pulmonary system and of the vascular access or peritoneal catheter are likely sites of infection. Careful attention to skin care and prevention of trauma will help prevent bruising, purpura, and excessive bleeding.

Anemia itself may be treated with blood transfusions. The risks of transmitting viral infections through blood transfusions must be weighed against the potential complications of anemia, particularly on the cardiovascular system. Nurses are usually responsible for monitoring the degree of anemia and its effect on the patient's daily activities.

Iron and folic acid supplements may also be administered. Oral iron supplements may cause gastric irritation. Customarily, these supplements are given with meals, but in patients with renal failure the supplements cannot be given with meals because of the need to administer phosphate-binding medications at that time. The absorption of iron is severely reduced as a large part of the iron is bound to the antacid. In patients receiving large numbers of blood transfusions, iron overload may occur. Serum ferritin levels must be closely monitored in such patients. Iron overload may be treated with desferrioxamine, an iron chelating agent that binds iron and permits its elimination during dialysis. Folic acid supplements are often administered to patients with renal failure. Because they are water soluble and dialyzable, they should be administered following hemodialysis.

Androgens (male hormones) have been used with some success to raise the hematocrit levels of patients with chronic renal failure. Commonly, androgens such as testosterone or nandrolone decanoate (Deca-Durabolin) are administered at weekly intervals. They appear to increase the renal production of erythropoietin and may also improve the response of the bone marrow to erythropoietin. The potential advantages of androgen therapy must be weighed against such disadvantages as hirsuitism in female patients, acne, hair loss, cost, and injection site hematomas. Most physicians recommend long-term androgen treatment only for those patients who show significant improvement in the anemia after a six-month trial without evidence of major adverse effects. Nurses are involved in administering androgens as well as in monitoring their effectiveness and adverse reactions.

An optional treatment currently under investigation is synthetic erythropoietin. This drug should significantly reduce the need for transfusions.

One major aspect of nursing care for all of these hematologic abnormalities is assuring adequate dialysis of the patient. Dialysis itself improves many of these abnormalities by removing the uremic toxins that are in part responsible for the problems.

EFFECTS ON THE GASTROINTESTINAL SYSTEM

Chronic renal failure is associated with changes throughout the entire gastrointestinal tract from the mouth to the anus. General gastrointestinal symptoms such an anorexia, nausea, vomiting, and a metallic or ammonia-like taste in the mouth are commonly seen. Gastritis, ulceration, and lesions in the intestine may present more serious problems. The etiology of the gastrointestinal complications associated with chronic renal failure is not fully understood, but uremic toxins are believed to play a major role.

Anorexia, especially for high-protein foods, is a frequently seen early symptom of uremia. As renal failure progresses nausea and vomiting may develop, interfering with adequate nutrition. The nausea and vomiting of uremia typically occur in the early morning and often resemble the morning sickness of early pregnancy. The cause of this early morning nausea and vomiting is not entirely clear. Elevated serum levels of uremic wastes produce some of the symptomatology but the degree of azstemia does not always correlate with the amount of nausea and vomiting exhibited. The role that lesions in the GI tract play in producing these symptoms has not yet been fully evaluated. The symptoms often improve with the initiation of dialysis.

Oral Cavity

Stomatitis, characterized by painful ulcerations of the buccal mucosa, a coated tongue, and a metallic taste in the mouth, is seen in many patients with severe renal failure. There is frequently a characteristic odor to the breath that is sometimes described as "ammoniacal" or "fishy." This odor is referred to as *fetor uremicus,* translated as the smell of urine and ammonia on the breath. Patients with renal failure often suffer bleeding from the gums or from ulcerated areas. The bleeding and pain inhibit good oral hygiene. These patients become susceptible to infections such as candida and herpes and to tooth decay. The compromised immune status of individuals with renal failure makes them even more susceptible to infections in the mouth.

Many of the symptoms described above are believed to be due to ammonia. Urea concentration in the saliva is approximately three fourths that in the serum. Bacteria in the mouth produce urease, an enzyme that converts the excessive salivary urea to ammonia. The high ammonia concentrations are believed to be the cause of the fetor uremicus, gum ulceration, bleeding, metallic taste, and stomatitis seen in renal failure (Lancaster, 1984).

Esophagus, Stomach, Intestine

Uremia may cause mucosal alterations in all segments of the gastrointestinal tract. The changes include mild edema, submucosal hemorrhage, mucosal ulceration, and necrosis. Hemorrhagic lesions are more likely to occur in the esophagus, stomach, and proximal colon, whereas ulceration is more common in the ileum and colon. The accumulation of uremic toxins seems to be the cause of these lesions. Bleeding may occur from these lesions (Van Stone, 1983).

Gastric acid secretion may be variably affected by chronic renal failure. Patients with advanced renal failure who have not yet begun dialysis have markedly impaired gastric acid secretion whereas those treated with hemodialysis have an increased secretion of gastric acid. Gastrin, a hormone secreted by the small intestine, stimulates acid secretion in the stomach. Serum gastrin concentrations increase with progressive renal failure. Thus, one would expect increased gastric acid secretion in all patients with renal failure. In the undialyzed uremic patient, both structural mucosal changes that allow leakage of acid out of the stomach, and local conversion of some of the acid secreted, may mask the true hypersecretion of acid (Van Stone, 1983). Despite this increase in gastric acid secretion, studies have not demonstrated an increased incidence of peptic ulcer disease (Gilbert & Goyal, 1984).

Constipation

Constipation is a very common problem in patients with renal failure. The causes are many and include a diet low in fiber, fluid restriction, inactivity, and the administration of phosphate-binding antacids. Care must be taken to prevent fecal impaction, which can lead to bowel obstruction, mucosal ulceration, bleeding, and even perforation.

Liver

Patients with renal failure frequently exhibit abnormalities in liver function. The most common cause of liver dysfunction in this patient population is viral hepatitis. Prior to the availability of a test to screen for the hepatitis B antigen, that was the most common agent causing viral hepatitis; transmission by means of blood transfusions or from patient to patient in a dialysis unit was common. Now that patients, staff, and blood donors can be screened for the presence of the hepatitis B virus and those without antibody can be vaccinated, hepatitis B is becoming less of a problem. Infection with non-A, non-B hepatitis is increasingly problematic.

Frequently, patients with renal failure develop hepatitis without clinical symptoms. In such patients, elevation of liver enzymes may be the only indication that the patient is infected. Some patients will develop mild clinical illness with fever, nausea, and jaundice. A few will develop fulminating hepatitis with profound elevation of the bilirubin and enzymes, bleeding dyscrasias, and clinical liver failure. Some patients may develop chronic active hepatitis and show progressive liver failure over a period of years.

Nursing Care Implications. Management of the symptoms of the gastrointestinal problems associated with renal failure and the prevention of complications are major aspects of nursing responsibility. Patients who are anorexic or suffering from nausea and vomiting need encouragement to maintain adequate nutrition. Good oral hygiene including brushing gently with a soft toothbrush several times daily will help kill bacteria that contribute to the ammonia-like taste and smell many suffer. Mouthwash, sour balls, or lemon may help improve taste and alleviate thirst. Bland, soft foods in small amounts are usually better tolerated than spicy foods or large meals. Eating later in the morning or in the afternoon rather than immediately upon arising may be advisable due to the early morning nausea. Preventive dentistry is to be encouraged to prevent cavity formation or to ensure early treatment. Nurses should regularly examine the oral cavities of patients with renal failure to detect ulceration, tooth decay, bleeding, or infection.

Reflux and increased gastric acidity may produce symptoms of gastritis or esophagitis. Patients should be questioned routinely to ascertain problems. Small feedings, eaten slowly, with the patient in an upright position may help resolve symptoms. Antacids or H-2 blockers such as cimetidine or ranitidine may help.

Constipation should be avoided by encouraging a higher fiber intake in the diet and by using stool softeners. Activity should be increased to tolerance. Laxatives not containing magnesium should be used to prevent severe constipation and impaction.

All patients with renal failure should be screened routinely for evidence of liver disease. Nurses should be alert to the physical findings associated with liver disease, and should also review laboratory reports for evidence of enzyme or bilirubin elevation. Patients at high risk, such as those on hemodialysis, should be screened for antibody to the hepatitis B virus. Those without the antibody should be vaccinated.

METABOLIC PROBLEMS

Chronic renal failure and uremia result in numerous metabolic problems. Carbohydrate intolerance, hyperlipidemia, and alterations in protein metabolism are particularly significant.

Carbohydrate Intolerance

Patients with renal failure demonstrate an abnormal clearance of a load of either oral or intravenous glucose. During a glucose tolerance test, the maximum level of serum glucose is not extremely high, but the clearance phase is prolonged. Additionally, the initial insulin response to a glucose infusion is excessive and the decline of circulating insulin is prolonged (Kelly & Mitch, 1984). Peripheral tissues become insensitive to the action of insulin. Thus, although the circulating level of insulin is higher than normal in those with renal failure, its effectiveness is decreased due to tissue resistance to its action.

These abnormalities in carbohydrate metabolism do not usually result in hyperglycemia or ketoacidosis. There is usually sufficient insulin released to prevent such clinical manifestations. Regular dialysis will most often improve insulin and glucose metabolism, but they do not normalize. Other conditions such as obesity or the use of steroids may produce clinical hyperglycemia.

Hyperlipidemia

Abnormalities of lipid metabolism are common in renal failure. Except for those with nephrotic syndrome, hypertriglyceridemia is the most common abnormality encountered. The cause is multifactorial. Hyperinsulinemia results in an increase in triglyceride synthesis due to increased hepatic output of glycerides. Triglyceride clearance is impaired in renal failure. In those treated with continuous ambulatory peritoneal dialysis (CAPD), the continuous glucose load in the dialysate probably contributes to triglyceride synthesis. The result is an elevated triglyceride level.

There is a well-documented relationship between hyperlipoproteinemia (especially Type IV) and atherosclerotic cardiovascular disease (Lancaster, (1984). Uremic patients are at significant risk of developing vascular disease for many reasons including hypertriglyceridemia.

Protein Metabolism

With decreased renal function, there is an accumulation of the end products of protein metabolism. Control of the uremic syndrome necessitates restricting protein intake, which may result in inadequate intake of the essential amino acids. Hormone produciton, enzyme activity, and many other body functions dependent on protein synthesis may be affected.

Nursing Care Implications. Assuring adequate nutrition despite multiple restrictions is no easy task for nurses and dieticians caring for patients with chronic renal failure. One must be certain that as many sources of high biologic value protein-containing essential amino acids are included as possible. Protein sources with low biologic value should be avoided, because they contain few essential amino acids and actually worsen uremia by producing large amounts of unusable end products. Ongoing nutritional assessment is important to prevent catabolism and muscle wasting.

Carbohydrate excess in the diet should be avoided to prevent hyperglycemia. Weight control is important to avoid obesity and its potential for worsening the carbohydrate intolerance. Nurses can assist patients in dietary planning and provide positive reinforcement for appropriate weight control. Blood glucose levels should be monitored to detect a tendency toward hyperglycemia.

Dietary control of hyperlipidemia may be important in preventing cardiovascular disease. Nurses should monitor triglyceride and cholesterol levels and provide appropriate patient and family education. Dietary restrictions may be necessary.

CHANGES IN THE NEUROLOGICAL SYSTEM

Neurological function is altered to some degree in nearly all uremic patients. Disturbances may minimally affect functioning or may be so severe as to disable the individual. Any of the three parts of the nervous system—central, peripheral, or autonomic—may be affected. Dysfunction of the nervous system may lead to abnormal functioning of the muscles themselves.

Many neurological disorders are related to the effect of uremic toxins on the nervous system. The effects of electrolyte disturbances and hormonal and hemodynamic problems must also be considered. Additionally, neurological problems may reflect altered drug metabolism and excretion or the effects of certain disease process on the nervous system. This discussion will be limited to those neurological changes that appear to be a primary manifestation of renal failure itself.

Central Nervous System

Changes in mentation and behavioral changes frequently accompany renal failure. They are often among the earliest symptoms of uremia. Patients may exhibit a shortened attention span, shortened memory, confusion, and an inability to think as clearly as they were able to prior to becoming ill. They may develop a flat affect, be difficult to engage, and appear depressed. At the same time they may be irritable, emotionally labile, difficult to deal with, and demanding. Less frequently seen are delusions and psychoses. Decreased or absent libido is not uncommon.

These changes in mentation and behavior are believed to be a result of a metabolic encephalopathy secondary to uremia. Electroencephalographic changes are indicative of metabolic encephalopathy and are characterized by disturbances of cortical background rhythm and replacement of normal alpha waves by a low irregular rhythm. This is often read as a diffuse slowing of cerebral activity.

Untreated, this metabolic encephalopathy may progress to stupor, coma, and death. The initiation of dialysis and the control of uremia usually improve these symptoms.

Seizures may develop in patients with renal failure. Frequently, they are related to rapid changes in electrolytes, acid-base balance, or urea levels or to hypertension. Focal seizure activity is unusual and usually reflects underlying focal cerebral pathology such as bleeding or a mass lesion (Tyler & Tyler, 1984).

Peripheral Nervous System

The effect of uremia on the peripheral nervous system is the development of a peripheral neuropathy. It is usually confined to the lower extremities, although in severe cases it may affect the upper extremities. Most commonly it begins as a sensory loss in the feet. The paresthesia may be accompanied by pricking, tingling, or painful sensations.

With progression, weakness of the feet and atrophy of leg muscles develop. One of the earliest symptoms may be a "restless leg syndrome," a condition described by patients as a feeling in the leg, not painful or paresthetic, that is relieved by movement. At this point, objective neurologic changes may not be present, but motor nerve conduction usually shows minor slowing (Tyler & Tyler, 1984).

A second problem is known as the "burning feet" syndrome. There is swelling, redness, and exquisite tenderness of the soles and dorsum of the feet. Patients with poor nutrition may be more susceptible to this problem, and an improved nutritional status may relieve some of the symptoms (Tyler & Tyler, 1984).

The changes associated with uremic peripheral neuropathy are symmetrical and begin distally before progressing proximally. Motor involvement can lead to foot drop and a debilitating loss of function of the lower extremities.

Pathologically, uremic peripheral neuropathy is manifested by axonal atrophy and demyelination of nerve fibers. It is believed that the loss of myelin results from axonal destruction. High levels of uremic toxins, especially the so-called middle molecules, have been implicated in the axonal damage, although this has not been proven. It is likely that malnutrition may also play a role (Van Stone, 1983).

Autonomic Nervous System

The effects of uremia on the autonomic nervous system are most classically seen in the decreased responsiveness of the baroreceptors. Patients so affected are not able to compensate for a drop in blood pressure with reflex tachycardia nor to correct for an increase in blood pressure with bradycardia. The depressed cough reflex seen in patients with renal failure may also be a reflection of autonomic dysfunction.

Nursing Care Implications. Nursing assessment of the functioning of all aspects of the neurological system is an important part of the care delivered to patients with renal failure. Careful assessment and accurate documentation of findings will allow for the comparison of findings and an evaluation of therapeutic interventions. Serial electroencephalograms, cortical function tests, and nerve conduction studies should be reviewed for they provide objective evidence of improvement, deterioration, or stabilization of neurological function.

Assuring adequate nutrition appears to be important, especially in controlling peripheral neuropathy. Providing adequate dialysis also appears to be important in controlling symptoms. In order to achieve these two goals, patient cooperation is essential. Nurses must educate patients and their families about the importance of adequate nutrition and adherence to the prescribed dialysis regimen.

The development of neurological symptoms can be very frightening and disturbing to patients and their families. Patients may be unable to control their behavior. Their independence may be compromised. A supporting attitude on the part of all members of the health care team, as well as education about the reasons for the changes, will assist both patient and family to adjust. Assistance with activities of daily living may be required and a referral for home care may become necessary.

During dialysis, the effects on the autonomic nervous system must be remembered. When the blood pressure falls due to fluid removal, patients may become unresponsive due to a decrease in cardiac output that occurs because there is no reflex tachycardia. Close monitoring with this in mind is important, as is immediate action when the problem arises.

ABNORMALITIES OF CALCIUM, PHOSPHORUS, AND VITAMIN D; HYPERPARATHYROIDISM; SKELETAL PROBLEMS

Normally, calcium, phosphorus, vitamin D, the parathyroid glands, the skeletal system, and the kidneys exist in an intricate and carefully balanced interrelationship. The development of renal failure inevitably disrupts this balance. As a result, individuals with renal failure will demonstrate one or more of the following problems: hyperphosphatemia, hypocalcemia, hyperparathyroidism, inadequate vitamin D metabolism, osteodystrophies, or metastatic calcifications. Abnormalities of calcium, phosphorus, or vitamin D metabolism are important because they are among the earliest changes to occur with progressive loss of renal function and because they are treatable. Early recognition and treatment can be successful in preventing the significant morbidity and mortality that can result from these disorders.

Three primary abnormalities cause the problems related to calcium, phosphorus, and vitamin D metabolism that occur in renal failure. These are phosphorus retention due to a decrease in phosphate excretion, decreased calcium absorption due to abnormal vitamin D metabolism, and resistance to the action of parathyroid hormone.

Phosphorus Retention
The normal diet contains 1500 to 2000 mg of phosphorus, of which approximately 1000 mg is absorbed from the gastrointestinal tract. The kidneys pro-

vide the primary method of excreting phosphorus from the body. To maintain a normal level of phosphorus, the average person must excrete one gram of phosphorus in the urine each day. Plasma phosphorus is freely filtered at the glomerulus. The amount reabsorbed in the tubules, and thus the amount excreted in the urine, is controlled by the circulating concentration of parathyroid hormone. As the levels of parathyroid hormone increase, the reabsorption of phosphorus by the tubules decreases, resulting in increased excretion of phosphorus (Van Stone, 1983).

As renal failure progresses, the ability of the kidneys to filter phosphorus decreases. Serum concentrations of phosphorus rise. Because serum phosphorus and ionized calcium are in dynamic equilibrium, this results in a fall in the level of ionized calcium. A low calcium level stimulates the secretion of parathyroid hormone, which results in decreased tubular reabsorption of phosphorus and increased urinary excretion of phosphorus. In the early stages of renal failure, this mechanism allows plasma calcium and phosphorus levels to remain within normal limits. However, this is accomplished with high levels of circulating parathyroid hormone levels that have deleterious effects on the bones and other organs of patients with renal failure. The constant stimulation of the parathyroid gland eventually results in hypertrophy of the gland, making secondary hyperparathyroidism more difficult to control later in the course of the disease.

Eventually, glomerular filtration rate deteriorates so significantly that phosphate excretion essentially ceases. Serum phosphate levels rise despite very high levels of parathyroid hormone. Plasma levels of ionized calcium continue to fall. At this point, only dietary restrictions and the administration of phosphate-binding antacids will control plasma phosphate levels.

Abnormal Vitamin D Metabolism

Vitamin D is a steroid compound normally obtained in the diet and synthesized from cholesterol in the skin after exposure to ultraviolet radiation from the sun. This parent vitamin D compound is essentially inactive until it is hydroxylated once by the liver and subsequently by the kidney. The major action of this active form of vitamin D ($1, 25 (OH)_2D_3$ or 1, 25 dihydroxycholecalciferol) is to increase calcium absorption in the small intestine. In the absence of $1, 25 (OH)_2D_3$, less than 25 percent of dietary calcium may be absorbed. With high levels of the hormone, greater than 75 percent is absorbed (Van Stone, 1983).

$1, 25 (OH)_2D_3$ may rightly be considered a hormone rather than a vitamin since it is produced in one organ (the kidney), secreted into the blood stream, and affects other organ systems. Its production by the kidney is regulated on the basis of the body's need for calcium. The primary function of $1, 25 (OH)_2D_3$ is to maintain the plasma calcium concentration within normal limits. Vitamin D affects muscle metabolism and may also help regulate parathyroid hormone secretion.

Renal insufficiency greatly reduces the synthesis of 1, 25 $(OH)_2D_3$. Plasma concentrations fall when glomerular filtration rates decrease to 25 cc/min, and it is not detectable in patients who have undergone bilateral nephrectomies. Serum calcium concentrations fall as a result of low levels of vitamin D. This too stimulates the parathyroid gland.

Parathyroid Hormone Resistance
Finally, patients with renal failure demonstrate a skeletal resistance to the calcemic action of parathyroid hormone (Massry, 1984). Similar doses of parathyroid hormone result in smaller elevations of serum calcium in patients with renal insufficiency than in normal controls (Van Stone, 1983). The cause of this resistance is not fully understood.

Hyperparathyroidism
Hyperplasia of the parathyroid glands is seen in nearly all patients with renal failure, but the increase in volume and mass varies among patients. The glands may increase to 10 to 50 times normal (Massry, 1984). Marked elevations in the blood levels of parathyroid hormone (PTH) are frequently seen in patients with renal failure.

Hypocalcemia is the primary stimulus for PTH secretion. If phosphorus and calcium levels are controlled early in the disease, secondary hyperparathyroidism can be prevented. The spontaneous development of hypercalcemia in a patient with renal failure or the development of renal osteodystrophy should alert one to the possibility of hyperparathyroidism. Surgery to remove part of the hypertrophied gland (3½ of 4 lobes) may be necessary to prevent debilitating bone disease.

Renal Osteodystrophy and Metastatic Calcification
The term *renal osteodystrophy* is a general term used to describe the bone abnormalities that occur with chronic renal failure. It is really a combination of three to five different processes: osteomalacia, osteitis fibrosa cystica, osteosclerosis, osteoporosis, and subchrondal resorption. Often these disorders occur simultaneously, but usually one or two predominate (Van Stone, 1983). All result from the abnormalities of calcium, phosphorus, and vitamin D metabolism, and from hyperparathyroidism.

Clinically, these disorders cause the demineralization of bone with pain, fractures, and abnormal body alignment. The bone disease can be debilitating and can lead to the inability to support the body's weight in an erect position. Patients may become wheelchair-bound or bedridden.

If the hyperparathyroidism continues unchecked, the product of serum calcium and phosphorus may become so high that metastatic calcifications occur. Soft tissues and the vascular system are frequently involved. Metastatic calcifications may occur in the brain, eyes, gums, joints, lungs, myocardium, heart valves, blood vessels, and skin. Some of these present life-threatening complications.

Medical Therapy

Controlling serum phosphate levels by restricting dietary phosphorus intake and by administering phosphate-binding antacids is the single most important step in preventing and treating renal osteodystrophy and hyperparathyroidism. Once phosphate levels are controlled, vitamin D supplements may be administered to enhance intestinal absorption of calcium. Vitamin D is now available as dihydrotachysterol or as calcitriol, the active metabolite $1, 25 (OH)_2D_3$. Oral calcium can also be administered to increase serum calcium levels. It can be given as calcium lactate or as calcium carbonate.

As previously stated, subtotal parathyroidectomy may be necessary if hyperparathyroidism persists despite adequate control of calcium and phosphate levels. Remineralization of bone begins soon after the surgery. Structural changes and bone deformities may not be reversible, however.

Nursing Care Implications. Skeletal abnormalities, bone disease, and hyperparathyroidism are preventable and treatable complications of renal failure. Nurses must focus on early patient education to prevent these disorders. Patients must be taught the reasons for taking the phosphate-binding antacids and and adhering to dietary restrictions. They must be kept informed (to the ability they are able to understand) of their calcium and phosphate levels and the results of bone surveys. Positive reinforcement for adhering to the prescribed regimen is essential.

Nurses must follow the results of calcium, phosphorus, and PTH levels. They should review the reports of bone surveys. Physical assessment should include monitoring for bone pain, fractures, or malalignment of the skeletal system. Abnormal findings should be discussed with the patient and the physician so that appropriate changes may be made in the medical regimen.

Once the GFR falls below 10 percent of normal, regular maintenance dialysis is necessary. Dialysis assists in controlling metabolic acidosis, maintaining electrolyte balance, and removing uremic toxins, all of which may contribute to renal osteodystrophy. Nurses administer dialytic therapy, monitor its effectiveness, and educate patients about the prescribed regimen.

CHANGES IN SEXUAL AND REPRODUCTIVE FUNCTIONING

There are multiple problems related to sexual and reproductive functioning that occur in patients with renal failure. The causes of the abnormalities are multifactorial and include hormonal abnormalities, psychological problems, anemia, hypertension, medications that affect sexual function, and malnutrition. Dialysis may result in some improvement. Transplantation often results in major improvements or even in normalization of sexual functioning although some patients will continue to exhibit problems even after successful transplantation.

In males, testosterone secretion is markedly decreased in renal insufficiency. In addition, there appears to be end organ resistance to follicular-stimulating hormone, resulting in a marked decrease in spermatogenesis. This results in a low sperm count. Impotence is a significant problem among males with renal failure. Anemia, hypertension, atherosclerotic changes, low levels of testosterone, and perhaps zinc deficiency (Van Stone, 1983) have been cited as possible causes of impotence. Psychological factors such as dependency and loss of status within the family undoubtedly contribute to the incidence of impotence.

In females, ovarian hormone secretion is suppressed in renal failure. Although plasma estrogen and progesterone levels may be in the low normal range, they are abnormally low given the high levels of luteinizing hormone found in such individuals. The same end organ resistance to follicular-stimulating hormone in females results in ovulation being rare in women with renal failure. Increased prolactin levels may contribute to the high incidence of amenorrhea and infertility in these women.

Both men and women report decreased libido. In children, sexual maturation is delayed.

Nursing Care Implications. Successful transplantation is the only therapeutic modality that has been shown to result in a return to pre-ERSD sexual and reproductive functioning. Following renal transplantation, a great many of the abnormalities are resolved or improved dramatically (Emmanouel, Lindheimer, & Katz, 1984). Other therapies, particularly medications, are being evaluated but have not been proven successful.

Nurses can assist patients to explore their feelings about the changes occurring in their sexual functioning by providing a comfortable, private, and nonjudgmental environment. Offering patients the opportunity to discuss sexual concerns without forcing them to do so is vital. Often the nurse can assist patients and their significant others to express their concerns and feelings to one another and can help them find alternative methods of expressing their love and affection.

Before nurses can expect to help patients deal with problems related to sexuality and reproduction, they must be comfortable with their own sexuality and with discussing sexual issues. In addition, they must be knowledgeable. Misinformation will only add to the problems suffered by these individuals.

REFERENCES

Anagnostou, A. A., & Fried, W. (1984). The hemopoietic system. In G. Eknoyan & J. P Knochel (Eds.), *The systemic consequences of renal failure.* Orlando: Grune & Stratton.

Bernard, G. R., & Brigham, K. L. (1984). The pulmonary system. In G. Eknoyan & J. P Knochel (Eds.), *The systemic consequences of renal failure.* Orlando: Grune & Stratton.

Cummings, N. B., & Klahr, S. (Eds.). (1985). *Chronic renal disease—causes, complications, and treatment.* New York: Plenum.

Emmanouel, D. S., Lindheimer, M. D., & Katz, A. I. (1984). Endocrine function. In G. Eknoyan & J. P. Knochel (Eds.), *The systemic consequences of renal failure.* Orlando: Grune & Stratton.

Gilbert, R. J., & Goyal, R. K. (1984). The gastrointestinal system. In G. Eknoyan & J. P Knochel (Eds.), *The systemic consequences of renal failure.* Orlando: Grune & Stratton.

Kelly, R. A., & Mitch, W. E. (1984). Nutrition. In G. Eknoyan & J. P. Knochel (Eds.), *The systemic consequences of renal failure.* Orlando: Grune & Stratton.

Lancaster, L. E. (1984) End stage renal disease: Pathophysiology, assessment, and intervention. In L. E. Lancaster (Ed.), *The patient with end stage renal disease* (2nd ed.). New York: Wiley.

Massry, S. G. (1984). Disorders of divalent ion metabolism. In G. Eknoyan & J. P Knochel (Eds.), *The systemic consequences of renal failure.* Orlando: Grune & Stratton.

Tyler, H. R., & Tyler, K. L. (1984). Neurologic complications. In G. Eknoyan & J. P Knochel (Eds.), *The systemic consequences of renal failure.* Orlando: Grune & Stratton.

Van Stone, J. C. (1983). Systemic manifestations of chronic renal failure. In J. C. Van Stone (Ed.), *Dialysis and the treatment of renal insufficiency.* New York: Grune & Stratton.

Young, J. B., Krothapalli, R. K., & Ayues, J. C. (1984). The heart. In G. Eknoyan & J. P Knochel (Eds.), *The systemic consequences of renal failure.* Orlando: Grune & Stratton.

5

Nutritional Therapy

Karen L. Macheledt

OBJECTIVES

After reading this chapter on nutrition, the nurse will be able to:

1. Describe the components of a nutritional assessment
2. Describe the nutritional management of patients with acute renal failure
3. Compare and contrast the nutritional management of ESRD patients using varous treatment modalities

Nutrition plays a vital role in the treatment of patients with renal disease. As the primary care providers for these patients, nurses must understand the principles of the nutritional management of renal failure. This requires knowledge of the function of the normal kidney, the etiology and systemic manifestations of renal failure, and the practical application of nutritional therapy in this setting.

NUTRITIONAL ASSESSMENT

Since malnutrition is a common problem in patients with renal dysfunction, it is important to be aware of its manifestations and know how to assist the dietitian in its recognition and treatment. It must always be kept in mind that one assessment parameter cannot stand alone in the documentation of malnutrition: a combination of parameters, especially when evaluated periodically, is much more indicative. In addition, many nutritional parameters are influenced by the renal failure itself. Until specific nutritional parameters can be identified that are not affected by renal failure, existing indices should be interpreted with caution (Levine, 1985).

Basically, there are three body compartments that are evaluated in an assessment of a patient's nutritional status. The first is the *visceral protein compartment*. The parameters usually used as indicators are the serum albumin and transferrin levels, the total lymphocyte count, and skin antigen testing using mumps, PPD, *Candida albicans*, and streptokinase-streptodornase (Blumenkrantz, Kopple, Gutman, & Chan, 1980; Salmond, 1980). Any patient with an albumin level less than 3.5 g/dl, a transferrin level of less than 200 mg/dl, a total lymphocyte count less than 1500 cells/ml^3 and a nonreactive skin test, should be placed on an aggressive program of nutritional support. Deficiencies in these parameters suggests a recent onset of a catabolic stressor or inadequate nutritional intake (Salmond, 1980).

The second body compartment is the *skeletal protein compartment*. Arm anthropometric measurements for arm muscle circumference (AMC) and arm muscle area (AMA) and the determination of nitrogen balance or protein balance (calculated from the protein catabolic rate and the actual protein intake) are used in assessing the degree of muscle protein depletion. An AMC or AMA less than the fifth percentile, a negative nitrogen balance, or a protein catabolic rate less than 0.8 or greater than 1.4 grams of protein per kilogram of body weight per day, should alert the dietitian. Deficiencies in this compartment indicate patients with chronic catabolic illnesses and inadequate nutrient intakes (Salmond, 1980).

Finally, an evaluation of the patient's third compartment, the *energy reserves* or degree of adiposity, should be made. Although it is important to recognize the fact that malnutrition is not simply depletion of body fat stores and that many patients possessing excessive fat stores can be severely malnourished, assessing the patient's arm anthropometric measurements for triceps skinfold (TSF) and arm fat area (AFA) and weight in terms of percent usual weight and percent ideal weight, also yields information regarding the patient's morbidity. Particularly significant is the patient who has experienced an involuntary weight loss of 10 percent or more of his or her usual weight in one year, the patient weighing less that 85 percent of his or her ideal body weight, or the patient with a TSF or AFA less than the fifth percentile (Murphy & Cole, 1983; Salmond, 1980). This patient is also a candidate for aggressive nutritional support. The dietitian will have the most current anthropometric standards and height–weight tables.

In assessing any of these compartments, a diet history will elucidate whether or not the origin of the problem is dietary. If the problem is an inadequate nutrient intake, recommendations for use of a nutritional supplement can be made. The adage "if the gut works, use it" is an important one to bear in mind (Murphy & Cole, 1983). If a patient's gastrointestinal tract can tolerate food, the provision of a complete or modular supplement is preferred. When a patient cannot consume an adequate volume of nutrients, a tube feeding—used either alone or in addition to regular meals—may be in order. If the gut cannot tolerate anything, total parenteral nutrition (TPN) is appropriate. Protocols for the administration of tube feedings and TPN can be obtained from the dietitian.

Commercial dietary supplements and TPN solutions are available for patients nearing ESRD who require low-protein diets and for those on dialysis with more liberal protein allowances. In general, patients probably require more nutrients, especially calories and protein, once they have become malnourished, because the support of basic maintenance in addition to the support necessary to reverse the malnutrition must be provided.

ACUTE RENAL FAILURE

Since acute renal failure (ARF) frequently occurs in patients who are overwhelmingly catabolic, their nutritional management is complicated. The basic goal of nutritional support, however, is similar to the goal for patients in chronic renal failure: to decrease the uremia and other metabolic disorders while supporting the patient's nutritional status as aggressively as permissible. The patient's recovery may also depend on the nutritional support.

Energy requirements for stressed patients range as high as 50 calories per kilogram of body weight per day. It is usually difficult to deliver adequate calories unless the patient is nonoliguric or a decision has been made to use dialysis therapy.

Compromised patients may need as much as 2 to 4 grams of protein per kilogram of body weight per day, but the uremia usually prevents the attainment of this goal. Without dialysis, the protein delivered to the patients probably needs to be restricted to 20 to 40 grams per day (0.5g/kg body weight/day). This may be the only time essential amino acids as the sole protein source are indicated (Brown, 1983; Vennegoor, 1982). Most clinicians do not restrict the protein intake enough to prevent having to dialyze the patient.

When the patient is dialyzed, it must be remembered that amino acids and protein are also lost in the dialysate. Practical protein provisions in the acute situation are 1 g/kg body weight/day for hemodialyzed patients, and 1.2 to 1.5 g/kg body weight/day for patients dialyzed through the peritoneum (Brown, 1983). Calculating the protein catabolic rate using urea kinetics becomes invaluable in estimating a patient's protein requirements in ARF.

Patients in ARF should be provided with adequate sodium, potassium, phosphorus, magnesium, and fluid to keep their blood chemistries within normal limits. Once anabolism occurs, these requirements will increase. Calcium probably does not require supplementation, although it has not been well studied in ARF. If the recommended dietary allowances of the vitamins and remaining minerals can be administered, this is probably appropriate. Toxicity of the fat-soluble vitamins is probably insignificant in ARF (Brown, 1983).

CONSERVATIVE MANAGEMENT: CHRONIC RENAL FAILURE

Chronic renal failure (CRF) is defined for nutritional purposes as the steadily progressive, irreversible destruction of nephron mass. The three stages of CRF have been outlined as follows:

1. Renal insufficiency, or the inability to selectively filter waste from plasma, which is characterized by a glomerular filtration rate (GFR) that is 25 to 30 percent of normal
2. Frank renal failure, with steadily increasing creatinine and blood urea nitrogen (BUN) levels
3. Uremia or end-stage renal disease, in which the creatinine and BUN are high and continue rising and the overt symptoms of uremia appear (Murphy & Cole, 1983)

Although the nutritional recommendations change as renal function deteriorates and patients progress from stage I to stage III, requiring periodic re-evaluation of the diet, the goal of diet therapy remains the same: to minimize uremia and the other metabolic disorders of renal failure while attaining and maintaining good nutrition and a sense of well-being (Harem, 1984).

In general, the kidney manifests its loss of function through its inability to excrete waste products, causing them to accumulate in the blood. Since as much as 75 percent of total nephron mass can be destroyed before the accumulation of waste products becomes clinically apparent, no dietary restrictions are usually ordered.

Once frank renal failure is diagnosed, dietary intervention and nutritional support become an essential part of the patient's care. As renal function deteriorates, fluid, sodium, potassium, phosphorus, and the end products of protein metabolism accumulate in the blood. The recommended intake for each of these nutrients is subsequently limited.

Recently, there has been renewed interest in restricting a patient's protein intake to retard the rate of progression of kidney deterioration and alleviate the symptoms caused by the rising BUN and creatinine without sacrificing nutritional status. In the 1960s, Giordano and Giovanetti independently placed patients with renal insufficiency on severely restricted (20-g) protein diets that were high in calories with essential amino acids or egg protein as the only protein source. The result: the progression to ESRD (stage III) was prolonged if the diet was strictly observed (Giordano, 1963; Giovanetti & Maggiore, 1964). Currently, if a 20-g protein diet is prescribed to postpone dialysis or transplantation in symptomatic or asymptomatic patients, essential amino acids or alpha-keto analogue supplements must be used as the sole protein source with fats and carbohydrates to provide calories. The alpha-keto analogues are still classified as experimental, however. As little as 0.5 g protein/kg body weight has been alternatively suggested for patients at this stage of renal failure (Rodriguez & Hunter, 1981). Thus, the standard 70-kilogram male is allowed 35 g of protein in his diet daily. A large portion of this protein, however, must be of high biologic value (HBV) (Brenner, Meyer, & Hostetter, 1982). The *biologic value of protein* refers to its capacity to provide the proper proportion and quantity of the essential amino acids—amino acids the body cannot make and must obtain from food—required for body protein synthesis. It is calculated from controlled animal studies. In other words, most of the ingested protein from an HBV source is used by the body to synthesize proteins such as enzymes or muscle tissue. Ingested protein from food sources of low biologic value (LBV) protein ultimately contributes to the degree of waste products requiring removal by the kidneys such as urea (Harem, 1984). Eggs, milk, meat, poultry, fish, seafood, cheese, and yogurt contain HBV protein, while breads, cereals, vegetables, and fruit contain LBV protein. The protein in legumes and dried peas and beans is of intermediate quality.

When the GFR falls below 20 ml/min, low-protein diets are mandatory to minimize urea toxicity (Murphy & Cole, 1983). Table 5–1 outlines suggested dietary protein restrictions based on the GFR.

Other dietary alterations may be necessary, depending on the patient's medical condition and degree of renal function, when the GFR is 20 percent of normal or less. Sodium is allowed or restricted according to the patient's tolerance (Murphy & Cole, 1983). The average American diet contains as much as 8 g of sodium per day. Hypertension, edema, and congestive heart failure usually imply the need for a dietary sodium restriction of either 2 to 4 g daily. Hypotension, on the other hand, may indicate the need for a liberal sodium intake (Harem, 1984). Fluid intake needs to be restricted only if the patient's urine output is significantly less than normal.

As renal failure progresses, the kidney becomes increasingly efficient at excreting potassium. Fecal potassium excretion also increases. Thus, unless the urine output falls to under 1000 ml/day, the potassium content of the diet probably does not need to be restricted (Harem, 1984). Potassium blood levels should be kept between 3.5 and 5.5 mEq/L. If necessary, a dietary re-

TABLE 5–1. DIETARY PROTEIN RESTRICTIONS BASED ON GFR

GFR (ml/min)	Maximum Dietary Protein Intake (g/day)
20–25	90
15–20	70
10–15	50
Less than 5	Dialysis or transplantation

Data from Murphy, L. M., & Cole, M. J. (1983). Renal disease: Nutritional implications. Nursing Clinics of North America, 18, 57–70.

striction of 2 to 3 g of potassium a day should be sufficient, since the average American consumes between 2 and 6 g of potassium daily.

Until recently, the content of phosphorus in the urine was used to dictate the dietary phosphorus allowance, with a maximum of 400 mg of phosphorus allowed per day (Rodriguez & Hunter, 1981). With the renewed interest in low-protein diets, however, the low-phosphorus diet has enjoyed increased attention, because phosphorus may be a component in the deterioration of renal function (Levine, 1985).

The need for energy (or calories) is increased when protein intake is restricted. Patients on low-protein diets must consume at least 35 to 40 calories kg body weight/day, whereas only 25 to 30 calories/kg body weight/day are needed for weight maintenance in healthy adults. The energy needed for the increased activity level of nonsedentary patients should be added to these figures. Forty to 50 calories/kg body weight/day usually allows for weight gain (Harem, 1984; Rodriguez & Hunter, 1981). Low-protein products such as breads, cookies, and baking mixes are available to provide calories without protein. They can also be used as vehicles for carrying extra calories available in foods such as butter or jelly.

In stage II of CRF, especially if the patient is following a low-protein diet, a daily multivitamin–mineral preparation is suggested. It should not contain vitamin A. Hypervitaminosis A can result easily in individuals with significantly impaired renal function, because vitamin A is only metabolized to its excretory form (retinoic acid) in healthy kidneys, where it is subsequently excreted in the urine (Harem, 1984).

The diet is initially frustrating for a patient to follow. Patients cannot eat the same foods or amounts of foods as the rest of the family, it is difficult to eat away from home, and food preferences must be changed. As a rule of thumb, as a diet's complexity increases, adherence to the dietary regimen decreases. Nurses play a key role in a patient's acceptance of the renal diet. Most importantly, the attitude (conscious or unconscious) of the nurse about food the patient eats has a significant impact on the patient. By offering the patient support and encouragement the nurse can improve the patient's adherence to the dietary regimen. In addition, the nurse can serve as a communication link between the patient and the dietitian. See Table 5–2 for an example of a renal diet for conservative management of CRF.

ESRD (stage III or uremia) usually occurs as the creatinine clearance reaches 5 ml/min, or when less than 20 percent of the nephron mass is functioning. At this point, dietary restrictions and medications can be used to conservatively manage the uremia for a limited time, but once the BUN exceeds 100 mg/dl and the GFR is less than 3.4 mg/min, it is usually necessary to institute dialysis or transplantation.

NEPHROTIC SYNDROME

The excessive loss of plasma protein in the urine in patients with nephrotic syndrome results in reduced levels of plasma albumin if the rate of loss ex-

TABLE 5-2. AN EXAMPLE OF A RENAL DIET FOR CONSERVATIVE MANAGEMENT OF CRF

Breakfast
  4 ounces cranberry juice
  3/4 cup cold cereal and 2 teaspoons sugar
  4 ounces whole milk
  1 slice low-protein toast with 1 teaspoon margarine and 1 tablespoon jelly
  1 egg

Lunch
  Beef sandwich:
    1 ounce beef
    1 tablespoon salt-free mayonnaise
    lettuce
    2 slices low protein bread (toasted)
  6 carrot sticks
  1/2 cup canned fruit cocktail
  2 low-protein cookies
  8 ounces iced tea with 2 teaspoons sugar

Dinner
  Turkey casserole:
    2 ounces turkey
    1 cup low-protein noodles
    Salt-free seasonings
  1/2 cup green beans with 1 teaspoon margarine
  3-ounce lettuce wedge with 2 tablespoons salt-free Italian dressing
  1 piece salt-free cornbread with 2 teaspoons margarine and 1 tablespoon honey
  1 serving cherry cobbler with nondairy whipped topping
  8 ounces iced tea with 2 teaspoons sugar

Snack
  6 ounces apple juice
  2 low-protein cookies

Allow 1/4 teaspoon salt on foods or in cooking.

Nutrient Content
  2200 calories
  42 g protein, 76 percent HBV protein
  2 g (87 mEq) sodium
  1 g (39 mEq) potassium
  1000 ml (approximately 4 cups) fluid

ceeds the capability of the liver to synthesize albumin. Peripheral edema often occurs subsequently. Historically, a high-protein diet was advocated, composed of 2 g protein/kg body weight/day or 0.8 protein/kg body weight/ day plus 1.5 times the 24-hour urinary protein loss. Recently, however, with the renewed interest in low-protein diets to prolong renal function, it has been suggested that "moderate" dietary protein restrictions of 70 to 80 g protein/day be implemented to mitigate kidney damage while supporting good nutritional status in the patient. If the GFR is less than 20 ml/min, a protein restriction should be recommended. In addition, if edema becomes a problem, the sodium and fluid intake also needs to be restricted. Type IV *hyperlipoproteinemia*, the condition of elevated serum triglyceride and cholesterol levels, is also a common problem in patients with nephrotic syndrome. The dietary treatment is discussed in the following section.

HEMODIALYSIS

The loss of renal function in patients on hemodialysis provides nutritional challenges. Protein, electrolytes, water, and vitamins must all be regulated.

Protein
Typical protein requirements for patients on hemodialysis range from 1.0 to 1.5 g protein/kg body weight/day (or 1.0 g protein/kg body weight/day plus 0.2 g essential amino acids/kg body weight/day) with two thirds to three fourths of the protein being of HBV (Harem, 1984; Murphy & Cole, 1983). The use of essential amino acids is considered to be expensive with minimal benefit to the patient (Burton & Hirschman, 1983). This may seem excessive when one considers that the RDA for protein is only 0.8 g protein/kg body weight/day; however, as much as 8 to 10 g of protein plus 3 to 4 of peptides and amino acids (30 to 40 percent of which are essential) can be lost during the course of one hemodialysis run in a nonfasted patient (Food and Nutrition Board, 1980; Harem, 1984; Murphy & Cole, 1983).

There are many ways a patient's actual protein intake can be determined and evaluated in terms of adequacy. A dietitian can obtain a diet history from the patient. The patient can keep a diet record and kinetic modeling can be subsequently used to calculate the patient's protein catabolic rate. In this case, a protein catabolic rate of 0.8 to 1.4 protein/kg body weight/day indicates adequacy (Bennett, 1981). The result of the diet history or record can also be compared with the patient's BUN-to-creatinine ratio. An adequate protein intake is reflected in a BUN-to-creatinine ratio of 10 to 1. Also, nutritional assessment of the patient indirectly reveals the adequacy of the patient's diet.

Calories
An intake of at least 35 calories/kg body weight/day is recommended for patients on hemodialysis (Rodriguez & Hunter, 1981). This allows for nitrogen balance, if not anabolism. With adequate energy intake, the ingested protein is spared for tissue growth and repair. To encourage weight gain, a minimum of 40 to 50 calories/kg body weight/day is necessary.

Uremic patients frequently demonstrate an inability to metabolize exogenous glucose loads secondary to peripheral insulin resistance, making it difficult to provide adequate calories. On the other hand, some insulin-dependent diabetics may not require insulin (or as much insulin) once they reach end stage, because the kidney is one site of catabolism. The insulin in their bodies is not degraded as rapidly. The goal of glucose control is to maintain blood glucose levels below 200 or 250 mg/dl (Murphy & Cole, 1983). If the hyperinsulinism or carbohydrate intolerance precipitates lipid abnormalities, this should be treated with diet as previously discussed.

Sodium

Whether or not a patient needs a sodium restriction depends upon the degree of the patient's edema and the blood pressure status. The dietary sodium restriction can also be gauged to the amount of sodium excreted in the urine. Sodium restrictions prevent fluid overload in the extracellular compartment, overloads that can lead to hypertension and cardiac failure. Most hemodialysis patients do well on a sodium restriction of 2 to 4 g/day, although at times even 0.5 to 1.5 g/day restriction is necessary. Dietary sodium restrictions imply that salt, foods with obvious salt crystals on them, many processed and convenience foods, and some medications must be avoided. Foods to be avoided on a 4-gram sodium diet are listed in Table 5–3. One way to make

TABLE 5-3. FOODS TO AVOID ON THE 4-GRAM SODIUM (NO ADDED SALT) DIET

Seasonings

Salt	Meat tenderizers
Celery, garlic, or onion salt	Steak sauce
Monosodium glutamate (MSG)	Worchestershire sauce
Kitchen Boquet	Chili sauce
Catsup[a]	Soy sauce
Mustard[a]	

Snacks

Pretzels, potato chips[a]	Corn chips
Salted crackers[a]	Cheese curls
Salted popcorn[a]	Pickles, olives
Salted nuts[a]	Peanut butter[a]

Meats and cheeses

Ham	Canned meats or fish[a]
Luncheon meats	Smoked meat, fish
Bacon, sausage	Anchovies, sardines
Corned or dried beef	Caviar
Frankfurters, hot dogs	Pickled herring
Pastrami	Cheese spreads
Kosher meats (pickled)	Processed cheeses[b]

Miscellaneous

Buttermilk	Canned, dried, or frozen soups[a]
Sauerkraut or any foods packed in a brine	Boullion, consommé[a]
Canned, packaged, or frozen convenience entree items	Salt pork

[a]Salt-free counterparts are available in the diet sections of most grocery stores.
[b]Cheeses that can be eaten in moderation include cream cheese, cottage cheese, or naturally aged cheese.
Note: Ask your physician before using salt substitutes.

food more palatable for sodium restricted patients is to encourage them to use sodium-free seasonings. The potassium content of these seasonings should be ascertained prior to their use and counted in the daily postassium intake.

Fluid

A *fluid* is defined by nutritionists as anything that melts at room temperature. The degree of fluid restriction necessary for patients on hemodialysis depends on the kidneys' residual output, patient activity level, climate, and fecal fluid loss. The most common way to determine a patient's daily fluid allowance is to allow 500 ml of fluid in addition to the patient's 24-hour urine output. The 500 ml accounts for insensible fluid loss through the skin and lungs. As a point of reference, the suggested fluid intake for a healthy adult is approximately 2000 ml/day. In order to avoid the complications of fluid overload or dehydration, an additional 50 ml/day may be allowed for each degree (ambient temperature) above 80 F. It is important to remember that water weight can only be removed by dialysis in anephric or oliguric patients. Changes in tissue mass (muscle or adipose) are small in comparison to weight changes from fluid shifts. A patient can monitor his or her own fluid balance, because a change in body weight generally indicates fluid weight gain. Most dialysis centers consider an acceptable rate of interdialytic weight gain to be 0.5 kg body weight/day, a daily retention of 500 ml fluid. See Tables 5–4 and 5–5 for a list of foods considered to be fluids and helpful hints for fluid control.

Potassium

Dietary potassium restrictions are usually necessary for patients on hemodialysis. The degree of restriction usually required is proportional to the kidney's remaining excretory ability. The most common restrictions range from 40 to 75 mEq/day (or 1.5 to 2.0 g day). In general, if the dietary protein intake is restricted, the potassium ingested will be lower than in the average

---

TABLE 5-4. FOODS CONSIDERED TO BE FLUIDS

Any beverage
Creamers
Any soup (cream or broth-based)
Gelatin (with or without fruit or vegetables)
Syrups or water from canned fruits or vegetables
Popsicles
Sherbert, fruit ice
Ice cream, ice milk
Pudding
Custard
Yogurt
Watermelon

TABLE 5-5. HELPFUL HINTS FOR PATIENTS ON FLUID RESTRICTIONS

1. Drink only when thirsty. If you avoid high-sodium foods, you will be less thirsty.
2. Do not drink from habit or to be sociable. Try to get the most nutrition from your allowed liquids. Drink milk, juices, and other nourishing liquids before drinking coffee, tea, soft drinks, or alcoholic beverages.
3. Eat allowed fruits and vegetables ice cold between meals.
4. Try sliced lemon wedges to stimulate saliva and moisten a dry mouth. Sour hard candies and chewing gum also work well.
5. Rinse your mouth with mouthwash to refresh it.
6. Take medications with liquid at mealtimes.
7. Put lemon juice on ice cubes—you will use fewer ice cubes. Lemonade can also be frozen in an ice cube tray.
8. Measure ice allotment for the day and store it in a container in your freezer. Distribute it throughout the day.
9. Many people find ice more satisfying than the same amount of water because it stays in the mouth longer.
10. Use small cups and glasses for beverages.
11. Remember that 2 cups of retained fluid equals 1 pound of fluid weight gain.
12. Freeze allowed fruit juices in ice cube trays.
13. Try eating bread and margarine with jelly when you are thirsty before taking liquids. The sensation of thirst is often actually the sensation of a dry mouth. Food may alleviate this as well as a liquid.
14. Avoid the midday sun.
15. Take your beverages ice cold and drink in sips instead of gulps.
16. Measure your fluid allotment for the day and store it in a container in the refrigerator. Then, distribute your allotment throughout the day.
17. Keep your home well humidified. Dry air increases your thirst.
18. If you are a diabetic, high blood glucose levels will increase your thirst. Once your urine volume has decreased, it will be more concentrated and will not give a true picture of your blood glucose level.

American diet (2 to 6 g/day). Refer to Table 5–6 for a list of foods too high in potassium for hemodialysis patients to eat.

Phosphorus and Calcium

Most patients on chronic hemodialysis must keep their dietary phosphorus intake between 400 and 1200 mg/day. Fortunately, dietary protein and potassium restrictions reduce a patient's phosphorus intake as well. The goal is to maintain blood phosphorus levels between 4.0 and 5.0 mg/dl. This is slightly above the normal range. Another method of monitoring the adequacy of a patient's phosphorus restriction is to calculate the calcium-phosphorus product by multiplying the patient's serum calcium level by the serum phosphorus level. A calcium-phosphorus product of 40 is considered normal; a level greater than 70 may lead to precipitation of calcium phosphate crystals in soft tissues, blood vessels, and joints.

Control of the blood phosphorus level is not possible, in most cases, with diet alone. Aluminum hydroxide phosphate binders are usually prescribed.

TABLE 5-6. HIGH POTASSIUM FOODS

Apricots, apricot nectar	Oranges, orange juice
Avocado	Parsnips
Banana	Plums
Bran (more than 1/4 cup per day)	Potatoes
Cantaloupe	Prunes, prune juice
Dried fruits	Rhubarb
Dried peas and beans	Squash, winter
Grapefruit, grapefruit juice	Tomatoes, tomato juice
Greens (spinach, turnip, etc.)	Vegetable juice cocktail
Lima beans	Yams, sweet potatoes
Mushrooms	

Aluminum hydroxide gels bind phosphorus in the gut before it is absorbed, so they must be taken with or immediately after the ingestion of food. Some patients may develop aluminum toxicity from requiring large doses of phosphate binders. This has deleterious effects on bone metabolism and brain tissue. Calcium carbonate has been used in the past and is currently enjoying renewed attention in combination with reduced amounts of aluminum hydroxide to mitigate toxicity.

Calcium supplements may be prescribed for patients on hemodialysis. Uremic patients demonstrate decreased intestinal calcium absorption and a decreased ability to make active vitamin D, because dietary calcium is automatically reduced when protein, potassium, and phosphorus are restricted. One to 2 g of elemental calcium per day are suggested for hemodialysis patients, but supplementation should only be initiated when blood phosphorus levels are within normal limits to avoid metastatic calcification. Serum calcium levels should be monitored frequently, with 8.5 to 10.5 mg/dl considered normal.

Vitamin D deficiency is common in patients with renal failure secondary to the decreased functional renal mass. Treatment with the active form of vitamin D is recommended if the patient's phosphorus levels are within normal limits. A response to the medication can be documented radiographically in bones; biochemically by a decrease in serum alkaline phosphatase, an increase in the serum calcium level, or resolution of hyperparathyroidism; and clinically by decreased muscle weakness and bone pain.

Magnesium

The kidney is the primary organ in the body responsible for the maintenance of blood magnesium levels within normal limits. Magnesium ingestion from magnesium-containing laxatives (such as milk of magnesia), antacid therapy (magnesium hydroxide), phosphate binders, and enema solutions may cause excess magnesium accumulation in bones with deleterious side effects.

Iron

Iron supplementation is necessary due to decreased gut absorption, blood loss during dialysis, and because the intake of iron is automatically limited secondary to the protein and potassium dietary restrictions. Sixty to 100 mg of iron sulfate daily has been recommended to maintain iron stores (Rodriquez & Hunter, 1981). If oral supplementation is not well tolerated, parenteral iron is an alternative. Frequently transfused patients may not require supplemental iron as each unit of blood contains approximately 200 mg of iron (Harem, 1984). Ferritin blood levels are useful in monitoring body iron status.

Vitamins

The B complex vitamins, vitamin C, folic acid, and vitamin B_6 are routinely supplemented in patients on hemodialysis because these vitamins are water-soluble and therefore lost in the dialysate. The intake of vitamin C is usually inadequate due to the dietary potassium restriction. Fat-soluble vitamins E and K are not routinely supplemented, but the supplementation of vitamin K may be appropriate for patients receiving antibiotics. Vitamin A is never supplemented, as previously discussed. Vitamin B_{12} deficiency is uncommon in these patients. Refer to Table 5-7 for the recommended dosages of vitamin supplementation.

Zinc

Zinc is removed from the blood during dialysis. Zinc supplementation in the form of zinc sulfate (0.5 mg/kg body weight/day) may result in improved taste acuity and increased appetite if a patient complains of or exhibits these problems.

Fats

It has been estimated that as many as half of the patients on dialysis have type IV hyperlipoproteinemia (Rodriguez & Hunter, 1981). To combat this prob-

TABLE 5-7. RECOMMENDED VITAMIN SUPPLEMENTATION FOR HEMODIALYSIS PATIENTS

Vitamin	Recommended Supplementation (per day)
Vitamin C	100 mg
Thiamin	1.5 mg
Riboflavin	1.8 mg
Niacin	20 mg Niacin equivalent
Vitamin B_6	8.2 mg
Folacin	1 mg
Vitamin B_{12}	3 mcg
Vitamin D	Individualized

Data from Carron, D. (1985). A review of vitamin supplements for adults undergoing hemodialysis. CRN Quarterly, 9, 7-9.

lem, patients should attain or maintain ideal body weight, restrict their intake of concentrated sweets and alcohol, increase their polyunsaturated fat intake while decreasing saturated fat and total fat intake, and increase their activity level by exercising. Diet and exercise alone, however, may not be adequately effective, and medications may be prescribed. If the patient's cholesterol level is also elevated, foods rich in cholesterol should also be restricted.

Constipation

Constipation is a major problem for patients on hemodialysis. It can be caused by the use of phosphate binders, iron supplements, restricted fluid intakes, a lack of fiber in the diet (because most foods high in fiber are also high in potassium) and a lack of exercise. Fiber from wheat bran, 2 to 4 tablespoons per day, is fairly effective in alleviating constipation and not prohibitive in terms of its potassium content.

Food During Dialysis

Although it used to be common practice to allow patients to consume "forbidden foods" during their dialysis procedure, most centers no longer allow this. It takes approximately 7 to 9 hours for ingested nutrients to appear in the blood, which is long after the dialysis run is over (Harem, 1984). Patients may still be allowed to eat during dialysis if they wish, but they should stay within the limits of their dietary restrictions.

PERITONEAL DIALYSIS

As in hemodialysis, the nutritional objectives for patients on peritoneal dialysis include the promotion and maintenance of optimal nutritional status, the prevention of net protein catabolism, and the stimulation of the patient's well-being.

Calories

One common problem with peritoneal dialysis patients is anorexia secondary to the abdominal discomfort of dialysis. Energy intake should range between 25 and 35 calories/kg body weight/day (Kopple & Blumenkrantz, 1983). Forty to 50 calories/kg body weight/day should be provided for patients with peritonitis (Harem, 1984).

The energy available from the dextrose in the peritoneal dialysis solutions must be included in the calculations of a patient's actual caloric intake; otherwise, the patient may become obese. The maximum available caloric content of 1000 ml of the various solution concentrations is as follows: 52 calories from 1.5 percent dextrose; 85 calories from 2.5 percent dextrose; and 145 calories from 4.25 percent dextrose. On the average, patients absorb 75 percent of the dextrose in their dialysate. It may be advantageous to restrict carbohydrate intake to 35 percent of a patient's total caloric intake to account for the carbohydrate load in the dialysate (Harem, 1984).

Protein

Patients on peritoneal dialysis need to consume 1.2 to 1.5 g protein/kg body weight/day due to the protein loss (primarily albumin) of up to 10 g/day in the dialysate. At least 50 percent of the protein intake should come from HBV sources. Most patients on peritoneal dialysis are on high protein diets in comparison to patients on hemodialysis. In fact, during episodes of peritonitis, protein supplementation may be in order because protein losses increase five- to ten-fold (Harem, 1984).

Sodium and Water

Unless a patient's blood pressure or fluid balance are difficult to manage or serum sodium is increased, patients on peritoneal dialysis do not require dietary sodium restrictions (Kopple & Blumenkrantz, 1983). If hypertension is a problem, a restriction of sodium to 3 to 5 g/day (commonly referred to as a "no added salt diet") should be sufficient. Most patients on peritoneal dialysis also tolerate greater fluid intakes than patients on hemodialysis and do not need to be restricted.

Potassium and Phosphorus

Potassium restrictions are usually unnecessary for patients on peritoneal dialysis. Phosphorus intakes are restricted to 800 to 1200 mg/day, and phosphate binders are often required.

Vitamins

The water-soluble vitamins need to be supplemented because they are lost in the dialysate, especially vitamins C and B_6 and folic acid (Kopple & Blumenkrantz, 1983). Provisions of the rest of the water-soluble vitamins should at least meet the RDA. Vitamins A, E, and K do not need to be supplemented. Iron and zinc status should also be periodically monitored (Rodriguez & Hunter, 1981).

Fats

If hypertriglyceridemia is documented, the same dietary restrictions used for patients receiving hemodialysis in terms of fat and carbohydrate apply. Sweets and alcohol should be restricted. Polyunsaturated fat should be increased while decreasing saturated fat and total fat intake.

Constipation

Constipation is also a problem for patients on peritoneal dialysis who take phosphate binders and iron supplements. Dietary fiber is also recommended in the diets of these patients for its beneficial effects.

RENAL TRANSPLANTATION

Although transplantation corrects the problems of renal failure that necessitate dietary restrictions, dietary modifications are frequently still required as a result of the side effects of the immunosuppressive drugs. While this should in no way preclude transplantation, dietary modification is necessary.

Prednisone, a steroid, is usually prescribed in large doses in conjunction with cyclosporine for the first post-transplant year. Since steroids increase protein catabolism and decrease anabolism, high-protein diets providing 1.5 to 2.0 g protein/kg body weight/day are usually required when the prednisone dose is large. If the patient has a tendency to retain sodium and fluid, a 2- to 4-g sodium diet is beneficial, most likely in addition to the use of a diuretic or antihypertensive medication. In some individuals, steroids cause an increase in potassium excretion. Thus, a diet high in potassium or potassium supplementation would be warranted. The tendency of steroids to stimulate a patient's appetite may result in excessive weight gain. Steroids also induce an increase in glucose production. Some patients cannot respond with an appropriate insulin secretion, thus leading to steroid-induced diabetes mellitus (Rodriguez & Hunter, 1981).

At toxic doses, cyclosporine and azathioprine have exhibited effects such as hyperkalemia and anorexia. These effects are usually only transient; once the dosage of the drug is altered, these effects disappear.

SUMMARY

The nutritional status of patients with renal impairment is often compromised. The abilities to perform a basic nutritional assessment and to understand and assist in nutritional management are necessary components of the nephrology nurse's knowledge and expertise.

REFERENCES

Bennett, N. (1981). Urea kinetics: A dietitian's clinical tool in the nutritional management of patients with end-stage renal disease. *Dialysis and Transplantation, 10,* 332–350.

Blumenkrantz, M. J., Kopple, J. D., & Gutman, R. A., et al. (1980). Methods for assessing nutritional status of patients with renal failure. *Am J of Clin Nutr, 33,* 1567–1581.

Brenner, B. M., Meyer, T. W., & Hostetter, T. H. (1982). Dietary protein intake and the progressive nature of kidney disease: The role of hemodynamically mediated glomerular injury in the pathogenesis of progressive glomerular sclerosis in aging, renal ablation, and intrinsic renal disease. *N Eng J Med, 307,* 652–659.

Brown, R. O. (1983). Nutritional support in acute renal failure. *Journal of the American Association of Nephrology Nurses and Technicians, 10,* 25–28.

Burton, B. T., & Hirschman, G. H. (1983). Current concepts of nutritional therapy in chronic renal failure: An update. *J Am Diet Assoc, 82,* 359–363.

Carron, D. (1985). A review of vitamin supplements for adults undergoing hemo-dialysis. *CRN Quarterly, 9,* 7–9.

Food and Nutrition Board (1980). *Recommended dietary allowances* (9th ed.). Washington, D.C.: National Academy of Sciences.

Giordano, C. (1963). Use of exogenous and endogenous urea for protein synthesis in normal and uremic subjects. *J Lab Clin Med, 62,* 231–246.

Giovanetti, S., & Maggiore, O. (1964). A low-nitrogen diet with protein of high biologic value for severe chronic uremia. *Lancet, 1,* 1000–1003.

Harem, P. (1984). Renal nutrition for the renal nurse. *Am Nephrol Nurs Assoc J, 11,* 38–44.

Kopple, J. D., & Blumenkrantz, M. J. (1983). Nutritional requirements for patients un-ergoing chronic ambulatory peritoneal dialysis. *Kidney Int, 24,* S295–S302.

Levine, S. (1985). Low protein diets in chronic renal failure. *CRN Quarterly, 8,* 19–21.

Murphy, L. M., & Cole, M. J. (1983). Renal disease: Nutritional implications. *Nurs Clin North Am, 18,* 57–70.

Rodriguez, D. J., & Hunter, V. M. (1981). Nutritional intervention in the treatment of CRF. *Nurs Clin North Am, 16,* 573–585.

Salmond, S. W. (1980). How to assess the nutritional status of acutely ill patients. *Am J Nurs, 80,* 922–924.

Vennegoor, M. A. (1982). Dietary management in renal disease and transplant—2. *Nurs Times, 78,* 847–851.

6

Principles of Dialysis

Beth Tamplet Ulrich

OBJECTIVES

After reading this chapter on the principles of dialysis, the nurse will be able to:

1. Describe the principles of water movement across a membrane
2. Describe the principles of molecular movement
3. Use the principles of water and molecular movement in caring for the patient on dialysis

Several principles involving the movement of fluid or solutes apply regardless of the type of dialysis. These are diffusion, osmosis, filtration, ultrafiltration, and solute drag.

SEMIPERMEABLE MEMBRANES

All of the fluid and solute movements to be described occur across some type of *semipermeable membrane*. In hemodialysis, this membrane is the thin, pliable membrane separating the blood compartment of the dialyzer from the dialysate compartment. In peritoneal dialysis, the patient's peritoneum serves as the semipermeable membrane. Although these membranes are often depicted as looking like a flat sheet with holes, they actually look like an intricate mesh design (Fig. 6–1). Molecules maneuver through the mesh. The

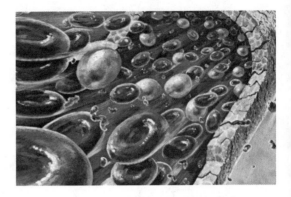

Figure 6-1. Artist's representation of a semipermeable membrane. (*From CD Medical, Inc., Miami Lakes, Florida, with permission.*)

permeability of the membrane refers to the size of the molecules that can cross the membrane. A fully permeable membrane would allow all molecules to cross. The dialyzer membrane and the peritoneum are said to be semipermeable. In the case of the peritoneum and the membranes currently used to manufacture dialyzers, molecules of up to about 5000 Daltons can cross. Smaller molecules move across easier than do larger molecules. The molecular size of molecules of particular interest in dialysis are noted in Table 6–1.

MASS TRANSFER

Diffusion

Diffusion is the transfer of solutes from an area of higher solute concentration, across a membrane, to an area of lower solute concentration. A *solvent* is a liquid that is capable of dissolving other substances to form a solution. A *solute* is

TABLE 6-1. MOLECULAR WEIGHTS

Substance	Molecular Weight (Daltons)
Water	18
Sodium	23
Chloride	35.5
Potassium	39
Urea	60
Creatinine	113
Glucose	180
Sucrose	342
B_{12}	1300
Inulin	5500
Myoglobin	17000
Hemoglobin	68000
Serum albumin	69000

Equilibrium

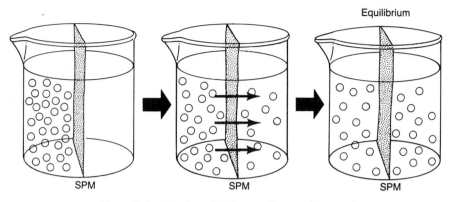

Figure 6-2. Diffusion. (SPM = semipermeable membrane.)

any substance that dissolves in a solvent to form a solution. The rate at which diffusion occurs is influenced by the concentration of the molecules on both sides of the membrane, and the permeability and size of the membrane. The relative difference in molecular concentration between solutions on both sides of the membrane is referred to as the *concentration gradient.* The larger the gradient, the faster diffusion occurs. If diffusion is allowed to continue, the concentration of molecules that can cross the membrane will be equal on both sides of the membrane. When this occurs, a state of equilibrium has been achieved (Fig. 6-2).

Osmosis, Filtration, Ultrafiltration, and Solute Drag

Osmosis. Osmosis is the movement of water molecules from an area of lower solute concentration, across a membrane, to an area of higher solute concentration. Osmosis is a function of solute concentration difference. An *osmotic gradient* occurs when the osmolality of the solution on one side of a mem-

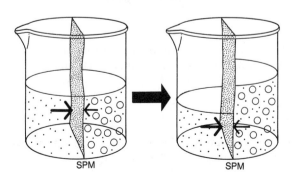

Figure 6-3. Osmosis. (SPM = semipermeable membrane.)

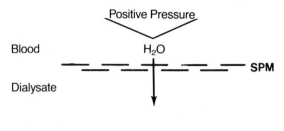

Positive Pressure

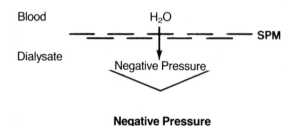

Negative Pressure

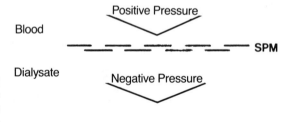

Figure 6-4. Ultrafiltration using positive, negative, and a combination of positive and negative pressure. (SPM = semipermeable membrane.)

Positive and Negative Pressure

brane is different from the osmolality of the solution on the other side of the membrane. In dialysis therapies, the osmotic gradient can be manipulated by altering the osmotic concentration on either side of the membrane (Fig. 6–3).

Filtration and Ultrafiltration. *Filtration* is the shifting of fluid from one area to another. When filtration occurs as a result of hydrostatic pressure gradients, it is known as *ultrafiltration*. In hemodialysis, *hydrostatic pressure gradients* are created by either positive pressure on the blood compartment side of the dialyzer (pushing the fluid across) or negative pressure on the dialysate side (pulling the fluid across) (Fig. 6–4).

In addition to the mechanically created pressure, hydrostatic pressure can also occur as a function of resistance to blood flow through the dialyzer. This resistance varies with dialyzer design, the blood flow rate, and the viscosity of the patient's blood. These pressures are measured in mm Hg. In peritoneal dialysis, the resistance is a function of the peritoneal membrane. The size of the gradient determines the amount of fluid removed.

Solute Drag. Solute drag results from fluid movement. When fluid moves across the membrane, it is accompanied by small amounts of small and medium-sized molecules. The amount of solute drag depends on the permeability of the membrane and the ultrafiltration rate. Although the actual amount of molecular transfer as a result of solute drag is quite small, it must be considered when molecular concentrations are critical, as in the case of dialyzing the neonate.

7

Hemodialysis and Associated Therapies

Beth Tamplet Ulrich

OBJECTIVES

After reading this chapter on hemodialysis and associated therapies, the nurse will be able to:

1. Compare and contrast vascular access alternatives for hemodialysis
2. Compare and contrast dialyzers
3. Explain water treatment options for hemodialysis
4. Perform a predialysis patient assessment
5. Understand the potential problems that may occur during hemodialysis
6. Compare and contrast associated therapies

Hemodialysis literally means the cleansing of blood. Blood is taken from the patient, passed through a dialyzer for solute and fluid removal, and returned to the patient. When used with chronic patients, the process generally takes 3 to 5 hours three times a week, and can be performed in a dialysis unit or at home. In the acute patient, the dialysis procedure may be performed daily.

HISTORICAL OVERVIEW

In 1913, Abel, Rountree, and Turner developed an experimental artificial kidney. In 1943, after advances in the purification of heparin, Dr. Willem Kolff invented the rotating drum version of the artificial kidney and used that kidney to successfully dialyze patients in Holland. Experience gained in battlefield hospitals during the Korean War further advanced hemodialysis knowledge and skills, and benefited many people with acute renal failure.

The inability to create a long-term access became the major obstacle to the successful implementation of chronic hemodialysis. That problem was solved in 1959 with the invention of the external shunt by Quinton and Scribner. Further perfection of access techniques lay ahead with the development of the subcutaneous arteriovenous fistula by Brescia and Cimino, and the ability to use bovine and synthetic graft materials. The ease of performing hemodialysis, however, gave rise to another problem. Demand for hemodialysis outweighed the public's and the insurer's ability to pay. Selection committees became the norm as the number of patients increased and the resources declined. In 1972, House Bill 95-603 legislated coverage of dialysis and transplantation under the auspices of Medicare for all individuals who qualified for Social Security. Selection committees disappeared almost overnight. In the early 1970s, capillary dialyzers and advanced membrane technology completed the resources needed to provide chronic and acute hemodialysis therapy.

VASCULAR ACCESS

In order to perform hemodialysis, a vascular access must be available that can handle the removal and return of blood at rates up to 350 cc/min. Alternatives are available for both acute and chronic access. Each has characteristics that must be considered when selecting the most desirable access (Table 7–1).

Acute Access

In the acute setting, the vascular access must be simple and quick to initiate in addition to permitting high flow rates. The alternatives for acute vascular access include femoral catheters, subclavian catheters, and external arteriovenous (AV) shunts.

Subclavian Catheters. Subclavian catheters (Fig. 7–1) are placed in the same manner as they are for uses other than dialysis. Subclavian catheters remain in place until the acute course of treatment is completed or until they need to be replaced due to poor flow, clotting, or other complications. Between dialysis procedures, the subclavian catheter must be kept heparinized and free of infection. This is usually accomplished by the postdialysis injection of enough heparin to fill the catheter. This heparin remains in place until the next dialysis procedure.

The advantages of the subclavian catheter are that it can be inserted at the bedside and that the patient's ambulation is not restricted. The disadvantages are the possibility of complications such as inadvertent puncture of the

TABLE 7-1. VASCULAR ACCESS OPTIONS

	Femoral Catheter	Subclavian Catheter	External Shunt	Internal AV Fistula	Internal Graft AV Fistula
Availability for use	Immediately after in-unit insertion	Immediately after in-unit insertion followed by chest X-ray	Instant after OR procedure	Weeks to months	Days, as soon as edema subsides
Requires Venipuncture	No	No	No	Yes	Yes, unless graft has an external access
Rate of Infection	Minimal	Minimal	High	Minimal	Moderate
Chronic Access	No	No	Yes	Yes	Yes
Access to Deep Vessels	Yes, selected	Yes, selected	Yes	Yes	Yes
Activity Restrictions	Minimal, if used for only one dialysis. Restrict only during dialysis procedure	Moderate	High	Minimal	Minimal

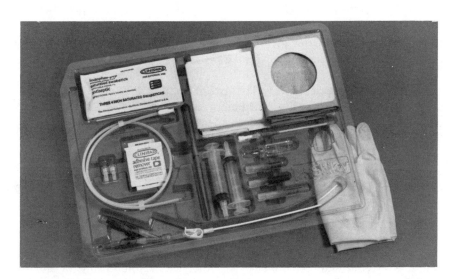

Figure 7-1. Subclavian catheter and insertion kit. (*From Shiley, Inc., Irvine, California, with permission.*)

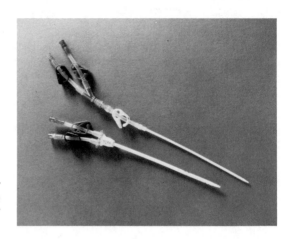

Figure 7-2. Single and dual lumen catheters. (*From Shiley, Inc., Irvine, California, with permission.*)

subclavian artery with hemorrhagic pleural effusion, perforation of the superior vena cava, pneumothorax, and subclavian vein phlebitis (Hakim & Lazarus, 1986).

Femoral Catheters. Femoral catheters (Fig. 7-2) are inserted before and usually removed after each treatment. Their placement restricts patient movement; however, many patients who have femoral catheters are already on bed rest. When the catheter is removed, pressure must be placed over the insertion site to prevent excessive bleeding. This procedure is the same as that used when arterial blood gases are drawn from the femoral artery.

Insertion of the femoral catheter is easier than insertion of the subclavian catheter. Potential complications with the use of the femoral catheter include retroperitoneal hemorrhage, femoral vein phlebitis and thrombosis, and traumatic arteriovenous fistulas (Hakim & Lazarus, 1986).

External Arteriovenous Shunt. The external shunt (Fig. 7-3), once actively used in hemodialysis has been virtually replaced by subclavian and femoral catheters for acute access except in the case of continuous arteriovenous hemofiltration (CAVH), where a resurgence in shunt use has occurred. The use of shunts as a chronic hemodialysis access has become rare.

The external shunt must be inserted surgically. The shunt consists of two pieces of silastic tubing, each with a Teflon tip on one end. The Teflon tip of one piece of the shunt tubing is placed in an artery, and the Teflon tip of the other is placed in an adjacent vein. The tubings are then brought through two puncture wounds in the skin and connected.

To initiate hemodialysis or CAVH, the shunt is clamped and disconnected. The arterial side is connected to the arterial blood line of the hemodialysis equipment and the venous side of the shunt is connected to the venous blood line. At the conclusion of the procedure, the two pieces of the shunt are reconnected.

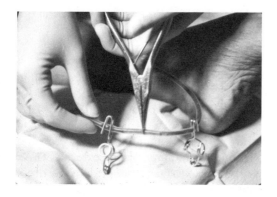

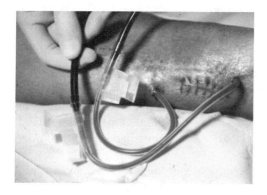

Figure 7-3. External arterio-venous shunt. **A.** Prior to dialysis procedure. **B.** After dialysis has been initiated.

Shunt Patency. The patency of the shunt must be maintained for vascular access to occur. This involves adhering to several basic principles:

1. Blood flow through the shunt must remain constant. The shunt tubing must be kept free of kinks.
2. Blood flow to the shunt must remain constant. No blood pressures or tourniquets should be placed on the shunt extremity. The shunt dressing must protect the shunt, but not restrict blood flow.
3. Infections must be prevented. The shunt site should be kept clean and dry.

The patency of the shunt must be checked periodically. If shunt clotting is diagnosed early, the shunt can often be successfully declotted. Checking shunt patency requires the use of several senses. Look at the shunt. The blood should appear red and there should be no evidence of plasma separation. Feel the shunt, though not with your thumb. A pulsation should be palpable. The shunt should also be warm to the touch. Listen to the shunt flow using a stethoscope. A gentle swish-swish (bruit) indicates a patent shunt. The nurse should also note the patient's venous resistance while hemodialysis is being performed. An increasing venous resistance often indicates decreasing patency due to venous outflow obstruction.

Shunt Complications. The most critical complication of the shunt is blood loss from a shunt separation. It should be stressed that one side of the shunt tubing is connected directly to an artery. If the shunt tubing is separated and left open, blood will gush from the shunt just as it does from a lacerated artery. Exsanguination is possible.

Shunt separation is prevented by carefully connecting the two ends of the shunt using an internal Teflon connector and tape placed externally in an overlapping technique sometimes referred to as "tabs and bridges." A dressing covers the shunt to prevent the cannulas from being snagged and dislodged. A pair of bulldog clamps should always be attached to the dressing. If the shunt separates, the bulldog clamps can be used to stop the flow by clamping the cannulas.

Shunt dislodgement is also a possibility, especially if there is erosion at the exit site. If this occurs, heavy site pressure can be used to control the resulting hemorrhage until emergency surgical correction can be accomplished.

Infections are an all too common complication with shunts. *Staphylococcus aureus* is the most frequent organism found in infected shunts. Regular cleansing with peroxide and povidone-iodine, sterile technique when handling the shunt, and maintenance of clean and dry dressings, all contribute to the prevention of infection.

Shunt clotting also occurs, more frequently in some shunts than in others. Initial attempts to declot the shunt are usually performed at the bedside or in a treatment room using a small (3 or 4 French) embolectomy catheter. Shunt declotting should only be performed by the nurse or physician who is experienced in the technique. Cerebral embolization may result if positive pressure is exerted on the arterial side of the shunt (Hakim & Lazarus, 1986). Declotting can be a painful process for the patient. Premedication with a tranquilizer is often helpful. If the declotting technique is unsuccessful, streptokinase can be infused to attempt to dissolve the clot. If the initial declotting attempts are unsuccessful, the shunt must be removed and another access developed.

Chronic Vascular Access

Chronic vascular access requires that the access not only allow delivery and return of blood at high flow rates, but also that this occur over prolonged periods of time (years). Options currently in routine use include the internal arteriovenous (AV) fistula, the internal graft AV fistula, and the internal graft AV fistula accessed by means of an external device. Fistulas, except for the latter, are accessed by the insertion of one or two large-bore needles.

Internal AV Fistula. The purpose of the internal AV fistula is to force arterial blood flow of high volume and high speed through the vein, thereby enlarging the vein. In this manner, the vein can be used for hemodialysis access.

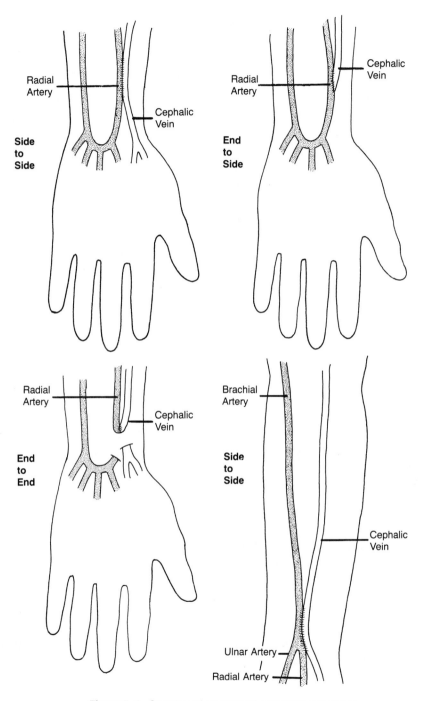

Figure 7–4. Creation of an internal arteriovenous fistula.

Surgical creation of an internal AV fistula involves the anastamosis of an artery to a vein. This anastamosis may be accomplished through an end-to-side, side-to-side, or end-to-end technique (Fig. 7–4). The most common connections are the cephalic vein to the radial artery and the basilic vein to the ulnar artery. Fistulas can also be created by connecting the cephalic vein to the brachial artery or the saphenous vein and the femoral artery.

The fistula cannot be used immediately and requires time to mature. The maturation time varies with each patient and ranges from weeks to months. In some cases, the venous enlargement never becomes sufficient for use as a hemodialysis access. The fistula can be created prior to the need for hemodialysis in the patient approaching end-stage renal failure. For patients whose fistula fails, an acute access must be used until a new fistula matures or until a graft fistula that requires no maturation can be implanted.

Internal Graft AV Fistula. The *internal graft AV fistula* may better meet the needs of patients with inadequate vessels or excessive obesity. Surgical creation of the internal graft AV fistula involves the use of a graft to connect an artery and a vein. The graft, which may be either straight or looped, is brought close to the surface of the skin for ease of venipuncture. Grafts may be biological or synthetic. Biological grafts include homologous saphenous vein grafts and bovine grafts. Synthetic grafts are usually made of polytetrafluoroethylene (PTFE) or Dacron. Grafts are most commonly placed in the upper arm, lower arm, and thigh (Fig. 7–5).

Internal Graft AV Fistula with External Access Device. The insertion of needles is traumatic physiologically and psychologically to many patients. The internal graft AV fistula with an external access device eliminates the use of needles. The synthetic graft is surgically placed in the same manner as the internal graft and AV fistula, but in a straight rather than a looped fashion. The external access device is connected to specially designed tubing to initiate dialysis (Fig. 7–6).

AV Fistula Complications. The major complications of the fistula accesses are thrombosis, peripheral ischemia, infections, and aneurysms.

Thrombosis. Although less likely than with a shunt, clotting does occur in fistulas. Blood flow to the fistula must not be restricted either by blood pressure cuffs, tourniquets, other like equipment, or constrictive clothing. Prolonged hypovolemia also contributes to fistula clotting. Although surgical repair is still the predominant treatment for clotted fistulas, the use of streptokinase is steadily increasing, with success rates of 65 to 85 percent (Van Stone, 1986).

Patency of the fistula should be assessed frequently either by palpating the fistula or using a stethoscope to hear the pulsation. As with the shunt, an

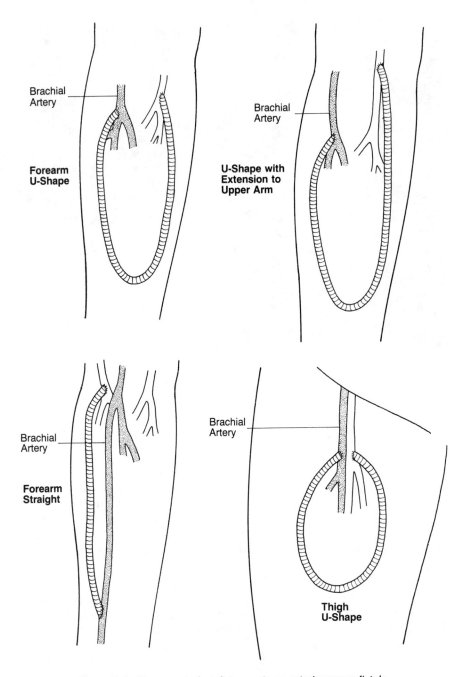

Figure 7–5. Placement of graft to create an arteriovenous fistula.

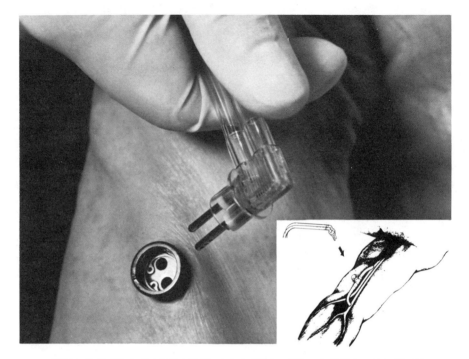

Figure 7-6. Internal graft arteriovenous fistula with external access. (*From Renal Systems, Minneapolis, Minnesota, with permission.*)

increasing venous resistance or flow problems during hemodialysis can indicate decreasing patency.

Peripheral Ischemia. Peripheral ischemia, or *steal syndrome,* results when the flow to the part of the body distal to the fistula is decreased due to the blood flow to the fistula. Usually, collateral circulation is adequate for perfusion. When it is not, the patient may exhibit a cold, possibly painful extremity. Steal syndrome can be surgically corrected by directing additional blood flow to the deprived area.

Infections. Infections occur more frequently with fistulas created using a graft than with those created by anastamosing the patient's own vessels. These graft-related infections also tend to involve the entire graft. If redness, inflammation, or exudate are observed in the fistula area, cultures should be taken. Often, the physician will initiate antibiotic therapy when symptoms of an infection are first observed.

Aneurysms. Fistula aneurysms usually result from constant use of the same venipuncture sites. Venipuncture sites must be rotated to prevent weakening of a specific graft area. The tendency to become reliant on only one or two sites for each venipuncture must be avoided.

HEMODIALYSIS EQUIPMENT

In its simplest form, hemodialysis equipment would incorporate blood access via an external shunt to a low-resistance dialyzer, continually flushed with dialysate, with the blood finally returning to the patient. Safety and efficiency, however, require more complicated equipment.

Dialyzers

The heart of a dialysis equipment set-up is the dialyzer. The dialyzer must have the capacity for blood inflow and egress, dialysate inflow and egress, and some form of semipermeable membrane to separate blood from dialysate. Dialyzer design and membrane technology are items to be considered when selecting a dialyzer.

Dialyzer Design. There are basically three types of dialyzer design: parallel plate, coil, and hollow fiber (Fig. 7-7). The parallel plate dialyzer resembles a sandwich with sheets of membrane tubing and plates layered one on top of the other. Blood enters one end of the dialyzer, flows in parallel through each of the membrane layers, and out of the other end. Dialysate enters the blood outflow end of the dialyzer, flows around the outside of the membrane tube, and out of the blood inflow end. This flow pattern is termed countercurrent flow, and creates the maximum concentration gradient.

The parallel plate dialyzer has a low resistance to blood flow, thereby creating only minimal positive pressure within the dialyzer. Compliance, or the expansion capability for the membrane, is less than that of the coil, but more than a hollow fiber design.

The coil dialyzer design consists of a long tube of membrane between two layers of flexible mesh wound in a tight spiral. Blood flows in one end of the membrane tube and out the other. Dialysate flows over and around the membranes (Fig. 7-8).

The mesh structure of the coil design creates a high resistance to blood flow, which leads to a high positive pressure within the blood compartment. This results in an obligatory ultrafiltration and a higher blood leak rate as compared to other dialyzer designs. The coil design also contributes to increased membrane compliancy, which decreases the predictability of ultrafiltration.

Originally developed by Cordis-Dow Corporation (now CD Medical) in the early 1970s, the hollow fiber dialyzer design consists of many thousands of hollow fiber membranes encased in a hard plastic tube (Figs. 7-9 and 7-10).

Blood enters the dialyzer at one end, passes through each of the hollow fibers to the other end of the dialyzer, and flows out (Fig. 7-11). Dialysate en-

124

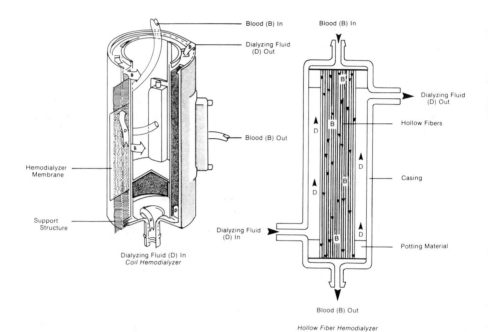

Blood (B) In
Dialyzing Fluid (D) Out
Hemodialyzer Membrane
Support Structure
Blood (B) Out
Dialyzing Fluid (D) In
Coil Hemodialyzer

Blood (B) In
Dialyzing Fluid (D) Out
Hollow Fibers
Casing
Dialyzing Fluid (D) In
Potting Material
Blood (B) Out
Hollow Fiber Hemodialyzer

Blood In
Dialyzing Fluid Out
Dialyzing Fluid In
Blood Out
Parallel Plate Hemodialyzer

Support Structure
D = Dialyzing Fluid
B = Blood

Figure 7-7. Dialyzer design. (*From Parker, J., & Wicks G. S. (eds.).* Protecting the future of quality care through an understanding of hemodialysis principles, *copyright 1984 by the American Nephrology Nurse's Association, with permission.*)

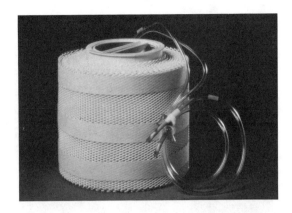

Figure 7-8. Coil dialyzer. (*From Travenol Laboratories, Inc., Deerfield, Illinois, with permission.*)

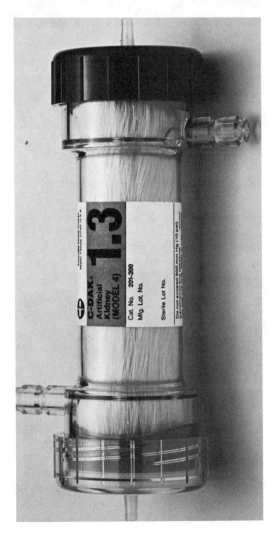

Figure 7-9. Original hollow fiber dialyzer. (*From CD Medical, Inc., Miami Lakes, Florida, with permission.*)

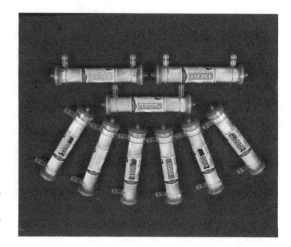

Figure 7-10. Hollow fiber dialyzer. (*From CD Medical, Inc., Miami Lakes, Florida, with permission.*)

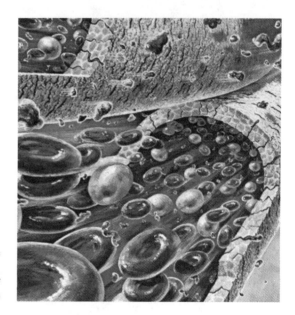

Figure 7-11. Artist's depiction of diffusion through a hollow fiber. (*From CD Medical, Inc., Miami Lakes, Florida, with permission.*)

ters the dialyzer at the blood outflow end of the dialyzer, bathes the fibers, and exits at the blood inflow end of the dialyzer. As in the parallel plate design, this flow is in the countercurrent pattern to maximize the gradient. The main advantages of the hollow fiber design are the large membrane surface area in comparison to the small blood volume, the low resistance to blood flow, the noncompliancy and therefore predictability of ultrafiltration, and the low blood leak rate. With these advantages, it is easy to see why the hollow fiber design has become the most prevalent in use.

Membrane Technology. The membranes most commonly used in dialyzers are derived from some form of cellulose. Since cellulose cannot be used in its natural state, manufacturers treat the cellulose to make the membranes for dialyzers. The various ways the membranes are treated differentiate one dialyzer from the other. In addition to cellulose, materials such as polymethyl methacrylate (PMMA), polycarbonate, polyacrylonitrile (PAN), and polysulfone have been used (Fig. 7-12). Membrane technology continues to advance.

The various types of membranes and the way they are treated during production determine the membrane characteristics. These characteristics include ultrafiltration capability, clearance capability, biocompatibility, and anticoagulation requirements. The needs of the patients can then be matched with the dialyzer membrane that best meets those needs.

Membrane–Blood Interaction. The interaction between the dialyzer membrane and the patient's blood is an area of increasing knowledge. Early during the hemodialysis procedure, there is a reduction in the patient's neutrophil count (Fig. 7-13) as well as significant arterial hypoxemia and evidence of activation of the complement system (Van Stone, 1986). The degree of this reaction varies with different membranes, with the greatest changes found using cuprophane and little changes with polyacrylonitrile. The membrane–blood effects of reprocessed, previously used dialyzers are less than those of first-use dialyzers, probably as a result of plasma proteins deposited on the membrane interrupting the interaction between the membrane and complement (Stroncek et al., 1984). The membrane–blood reaction also results in thromboxane production, which may contribute to the production of pulmonary hypertension (Cheung & Baranowski, 1984).

In addition to this overall reaction between the dialyzer membrane and the blood, an acute problem, termed *first-use syndrome,* has been identified. The syndrome occurs as soon as dialysis is initiated, and consists of chest pain, back pain, hypotension, and dyspnea. A number of patients appear to be allergic to the ethylene oxide residual that is found in new hollow fiber dialyzers after they have been rinsed with saline (Dolovich et al., 1984). Many dialysis centers reprocess dialyzers using a liquid sterilant. This is accomplished through manual techniques or automated techniques such as the one illustrated in Figure 7-14. In response to the presence of first-use syndrome, some units have instituted the practice of reprocessing all dialyzers before use.

Dialysate

As discussed in the previous chapter, both diffusion and osmosis rely on gradients between the blood on one side of the semipermeable membrane and the dialysate on the other side. The gradient is generally controlled by altering the composition of the dialysate.

Dialysate, like blood, is composed mainly of water. By recalling the elec-

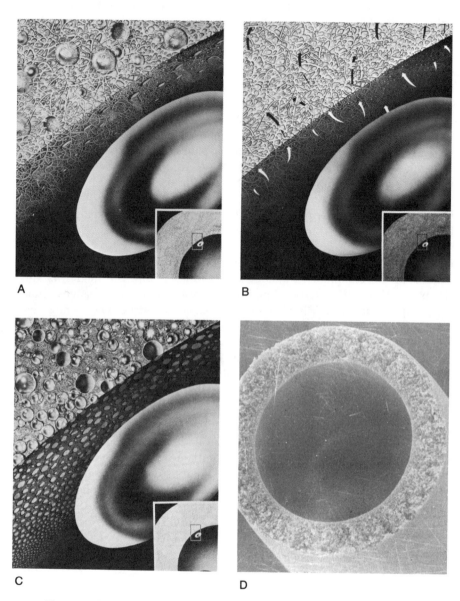

A

B

C

D

Figure 7-12. Dialyzer membrane technology. **A.** Saphonated cellulose ester (SCE). **B.** Regenerated cellulose. **C.** Cellulose acetate. **D.** Polysulfone. (*A, B, & C from CD Medical, Inc., Miami Lakes, Florida; D from Seratronics/Fresenius USA, Inc., Concord, California, with permission.*)

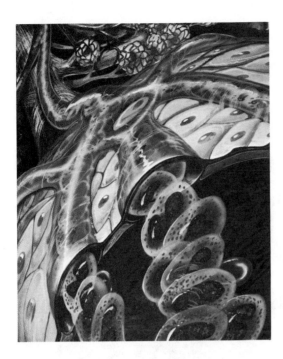

Figure 7-13. Artist's representation of neutrophils collected in pulmonary capillaries resulting in a transitory decrease in lung capacity (bioincompatibility). (*From CD Medical, Inc., Miami Lakes, Florida, with permission.*)

trolyte imbalances that occur in renal failure, one can easily surmise the other components of the dialysate and their approximate concentrations. Electrolytes generally found in dialysate include sodium, chloride, potassium, calcium, and magnesium. Glucose is sometimes present to increase dialysate osmolality and thereby increase ultrafiltration. The concentration of these elecrolytes in dialysate is found in Table 7-2.

A buffer is required to maintain the electrolytes in solution. Either acetate or bicarbonate is used for this purpose. Both also serve to improve the metabolic acidosis seen in patients with renal failure. Some patients tolerate dialysis better with a bicarbonate dialysate, whereas others tolerate acetate-buffered dialysate better.

Bicarbonate dialysate is generally associated with improved hemodynamic stability. It has been shown to be especially beneficial in patients with acute renal failure, patients with severe infection, and children (Van Stone, 1986). Bicarbonate dialysis is also useful in patients who have demonstrated acetate intolerance. Problems with routine usage of bicarbonate dialysate appear to occur when no attempt is made to individualize the dosage of bicarbonate.

The sodium composition of the dialysate is also a topic of debate. Higher dialysate sodium concentrations have been shown to be directly correlated with better preservation of extracellular fluid and plasma volumes (Brunois et al., 1984). Improved vascular stability has also been associated with higher

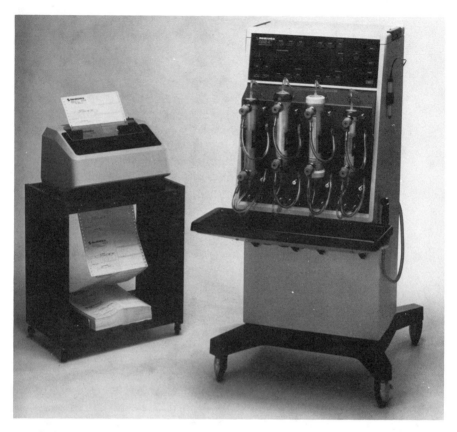

Figure 7–14. Dialyzer reprocessing system. (*From Seratronics/Fresenius USA, Inc., Concord, California, with permission.*)

TABLE 7–2. COMPOSITION OF DIALYSATE

Component	Dialysate Level
Sodium	133 to 142 mEq/L
Potassium	0.0 to 4.0 mEq/L
Chloride	103 to 105 mEq/L
Calcium	2.5 to 3.5 mEq/L
Magnesium	1.0 to 1.5 mEq/L
Glucose	0.0 to 200 mg/100 ml
Acetate	33 to 38 mEq/L
Bicarbonate	As ordered

concentrations of dialysate sodium. The problem with higher sodiums, however, is that the positive aspects are often accompanied by an increased interdialytic weight gain.

The dialysate is usually delivered to the facility in the form of concentrate. This concentrate is then reconstituted either manually or by the hemodialysis proportioning system.

Water Treatment

The water used to reconstitute the dialysate must be free of electrolytes, and without bacteria or particulate matter. This "pure" water is obtained by subjecting regular water to one or more forms of water treatment.

Deionization. Deionization, a common water treatment method, refers to the use of an ion exchange resin to remove electrolytes from the feed water. The cation resins exchange cations for hydrogen ions, and the anion resins exchange anions for hydroxyl ions (Fig. 7–15).

Reverse osmosis. Reverse osmosis uses a semipermeable membrane. The water is passed over the membrane under high pressure. This procedure removes particles and organic matter over 200 Daltons in size, and electrolytes, from the water (Fig. 7–16.)

Filtration. Filtration removes suspended matter and large bacteria. It does not remove dissolved particles or ions. Sediment filters usually incorporate a 5-micron filter so that anything over 5 microns is filtered out. Carbon filters are used to remove chloramines, pyrogens, endotoxins, and other organic matter.

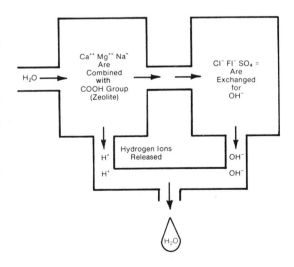

Figure 7–15. Deionization. (*From Parker, J. & Wicks, G. S. (Eds.). Protecting the future of quality care through an understanding of hemodialysis principles. Copyright 1984 by the American Nephrology Nurse's Association, with permission.*)

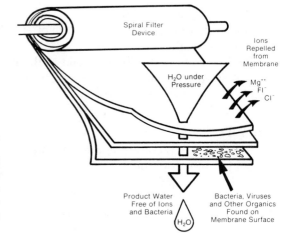

Figure 7-16. Reverse osmosis. *(From Parker, J. & Wicks, G. S. (Eds.).* Protecting the future of quality care through an understanding of hemodialysis principles. *Copyright 1984 by the American Nephrology Nurse's Association, with permission.)*

Water Softeners. Water softeners use an ion exchange mechanism to exchange hard ions, such as calcium and magnesium, for soft ions such as sodium.

Distillation. Distillation, although not often used because of the cost and time involved, removes ions and organic materials by heating the water and rapidly cooling the vapor.

The purity of the water used for dialysate is critical. No one method of water treatment appears to be adequate alone. To determine the treatment required in a particular location, the water is first analyzed. Based on the water analysis, several water treatment methods are installed in a series. Methods of water treatment are compared in Table 7-3.

Quality Assurance. The water treatment system must be continually monitored to assure that the quality of the water remains adequate. This involves routine visual monitoring and systematic culturing of the treated water at locations throughout the unit. Both the Association for Advancement of Medical Instrumentation (AAMI) and the Centers for Disease Control (CDC) have developed standards for water treatment. (AAMI standards are given in Table 7-4.) If the system becomes contaminated, it must be sterilized, generally using formaldehyde.

Hemodialysis Machines

The hemodialysis machine has traditionally been called a delivery system because originally its main function was to deliver dialysate to the dialyzer

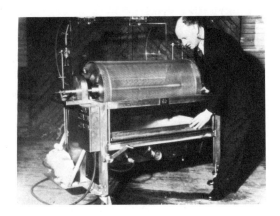

Figure 7-17. One of the first hemodyalysis machines, the rotating drum. (*From Travenol Laboratories, Inc., Deerfield, Illinois, with permission.*)

(Fig. 7-17). Machine functions have now expanded to include intricate monitoring systems and onboard computers. With regard to the delivery of dialysate, there are two main designs of hemodialysis machines, the batch or recirculating design and the proportioning or single-pass design. Several other designs are a combination of these two.

The first "mass-produced" hemodialysis machine was the 100-liter tank. Dialysate concentration, in liquid or powdered form, was mixed with water manually in the tank. To determine if the dialysate mixture was correct, the nurse measured the conductivity of the dialysate using a hand-held conductivity meter. *Conductivity,* the ability of a solution to conduct electricity, is determined by the solute concentration of the solution. Measuring conductivity, therefore, told the nurse that the total number of ions in the dialysate was correct, but it did not tell her whether the correct mixture of ions was present. The coil dialyzer was placed in a holder in the tank, and dialysate flowed around and through it. Partway through the treatment, the tank was emptied and refilled with fresh dialysate.

The 100-liter tank evolved into the Travenol RSP (recirculating single pass) when the need to increase efficiency became apparent (Fig. 7-18). Dialysate was still manually mixed in a holding tank, and then heated and pumped to a smaller (8-liter) cannister that contained the dialyzer. The dialysate recirculated in the canister and was pumped out to the drain at a rate of 500 to 600 cc/min. By incorporating the cannister, the blood in the dialyzer was subjected to higher concentration gradients than provided with the 100-liter tank. The problem of manually mixing the dialysate and refilling the tank mid-treatment remained. The RSP had simple blood leak, temperature, dialysate flow, and pressure monitors.

A major advance in hemodialysis machines occurred with the advent of the proportioning, true single-pass machine (Fig. 7-19). The machine auto-

TABLE 7–3. COMPARISON OF WATER TREATMENT METHODS

	Sediment Filter	Carbon Filter	Softening
Design	Rigid core with porous fabric wound around	Activated charcoal housed in pressure cannister through which water flows	
Method	Acts as a strainer; keeps particles larger than pore size from passing through fabric	Adsorptive filter; activated charcoal adsorbs specific impurities like a magnet attracts iron filings	Ion exchange; hard ions are exchanged for soft ions
Removes	Undissolved particulate matter larger than pore size of filter	Free chlorine, chloramine, pyrogens, endotoxins, and other organics	Calcium, magnesium, iron, manganese, aluminum
Does Not Remove	Particulate matter smaller than pore size of filter	Anything except those listed above	Substances organically bound to aluminum; anything not listed above
Equipment Maintenance	Minimum; can become clogged and overloaded, requiring replacement and service	Minimum, can become overloaded, requiring replacement and service	Minimum; routine regeneration of resin bed to replenish sodium supply
Potential Problems To Dialysis Equipment If Malfuncion Occurs	Particles >5µ plug tubing and orifices in equipment	Unlikely	Iron can foul equipment
Potential Problems To Patient If Mal-Function Occurs	Unlikely	Pyrogenic reaction, if housing bacteria; hemolytic anemia, if chloramine present	Hard water syndrome (headache, nausea, and vomiting) High levels of aluminum may lead to dialysis dementia

Deionization	Reverse Osmosis	Distillation
Resin beds in cannisters; cation bed treated with strong acid; anion bed treated with stong base; cation, anion, and mixed bed cannisters	150 to 200 molecular weight; semipermeable membrane of cellulose or nylon; pressure pump, product water collection device; reject water collection device; cellulose membrane spirally wound, nylon membrane hollow fiber	Heat source, evaporation vapor separation, collecting apparatus, condensing chamber and distillate collection device
Ion exchange; cation bed exchanges all cations for hydrogen ions; anion bed exchanges all anions for hydroxyl ions $H + OH = H_2O$	Water under high pressure passed over membrane to produce ultrafiltrate	Heating water and rapid cooling of vapor; vapor rises in evaporation chamber; impurities do not vaporize; rapid cooling of pure vapor creates condensation (liquid distillate)
All cations (i.e., sodium, potassium, magnesium, calcium); all anions (i.e., sulfate, nitrates, chloride, fluoride)	All ions; organics with molecular weight > 150 to 200	Ions and organics
Organics (pyrogens); Chlorine, chloramine; inert substances	Chloramine; all of feed water chlorine	
Moderate; routine regeneration of resin beds using acid and caustic solutions; requires pretreatment of water to prevent organic fouling; can be costly; may house bacteria; anion bed usually the first to be exhausted	Considerable; membrane deteriorates with excess chlorine, iron, and manganese; cellulose membrane deacetylates with pH > 8; nylon membrane deaceytlates with pH > 11; bacteria do not digest but clog fibers	Considerable
Unlikely	Organics can foul equipment	Organics can foul equipment
Pyrogenic reactions if contaminated	Pyrogenic reactions; hemolytic anemia if carbon filter attached to R.O. only and not to bypass line	Pyrogenic reactions

(Continued)

TABLE 7-3. (CONTINUED)

	Sediment Filter	Carbon Filter	Softening
Additional Comments	Often used in tandem with adsorptive filter to pretreat water going to expensive water treatment equipment	Essential for city water treated with chloramine; often used in tandem with sediment filter to pretreat water going to expensive water treatment equipment	Essential for pretreatment of water going to reverse osmosis equipment

TABLE 7-4. WATER TREATMENT GUIDELINES

Contaminant	Suggested Maximum Allowable Level (mg/L)
Calcium	2.0 (0.1 mEq/L)
Magnesium	4.0 (0.3 mEq/L)
Sodium	70.0 (3.0 mEq/L)
Potassium	8.0 (0.2 mEq/L)
Fluoride	0.2
Chloride	0.5
Chloramines	0.1
Nitrates	2.0
Sulfate	100.0
Copper	0.1
Barium	0.1
Zinc	0.1
Aluminum	0.01
Arsenic	0.005
Lead	0.005
Silver	0.005
Cadmium	0.001
Chromium	0.014
Selenium	0.09
Mercury	0.0002

Data from the Association for Advancement of Medical Instrumentation (AAMI). (1982). The American national standard for hemodialysis. Arlington, Va.: AAMI.

Deionization	Reverse Osmosis	Distillation
Product water 2 to 3 ppm; often used to complement R.O.	Product water 50 ppm; often used to complement deionization	Product water 5 ppm; most expensive and time consuming

matically mixes dialysate concentrate with treated water, heats the dialysate, delivers it to the dialyzer, and then discards the dialysate down the drain. The standard for dialysate mixture is 34 parts water to one part dialysate concentrate. This single-pass design establishes the optimal concentration gradient when the dialysate is connected in a countercurrent flow path. In the rare cases, such as dialyzing a neonate or very small infant, where it may actually be beneficial to minimize the gradient, the dialysate path can be connected concurrently. Because this is a closed system, negative pressure can be created to increase ultrafiltration with hollow fiber and plate dialyzers.

In addition to being more efficient, the proportioning machines are also safer for the patient. These machines incorporate visual and audible monitors for blood leaks, conductivity, dialysate temperature, and positive and negative pressure.

Ancillary Equipment

Other equipment for hemodialysis includes the blood pump, heparin pump, air and foam detector, and, on occasion, single-needle machine. A blood

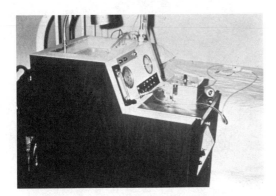

Figure 7–18. Recirculating single-pass hemodialysis machine. (*From Travenol Laboratories, Inc., Deerfield, Illinois, with permission.*)

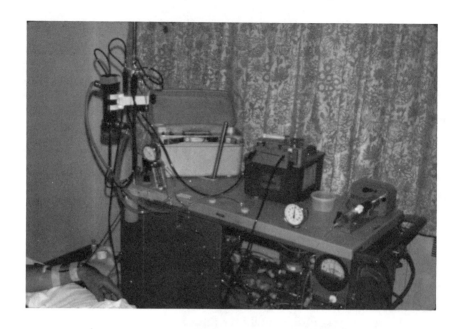

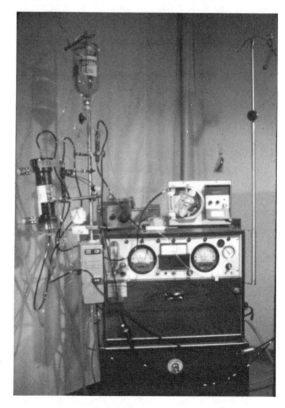

Figure 7-19. Early designs of single-pass hemodialysis with ancillary equipment.

pump is used to circulate the blood from the patient to the dialyzer and back. Blood flows in the range of 200 to 350 cc/min are required to obtain an adequate dialysis in a short time (less than 8 hours). The blood pump is a simple roller pump.

The heparin pump is used in most facilities to provide the heparinization required so that the dialyzer does not clot. This is a small pump that holds a syringe of heparin or heparin and saline solution, and delivers that solution through the bloodline to the patient.

The air detector was developed to detect air in the extracorporeal system and to prevent air emboli, which had been known to occur as a result of an intravenous bottle running dry, a leak in the bloodline, or at the end of dialysis when an air rinse was being used while returning blood to the patient. Even though intravenous solutions are now supplied in bags and air rinses are no longer used, the air detector continues to be an important safety device in dialysis, and has virtually eliminated the occurrence of air emboli during hemodialysis.

The single-needle machine allows the use of one access needle rather than two. There are several designs for single-needle machines. In each case, the nurse must be aware that using one access site may decrease the efficiency of the hemodialysis treatment. Often this decrease can be overcome by using a more efficient dialyzer.

Recent developments in hemodialysis machines have incorporated the ancillary equipment into the hemodialysis machine (Fig. 7–20). In addition to the ancillary equipment noted above, the hemodialysis machines now have the ability to calculate required and actual ultrafiltration, perform individual sodium modeling, and perform automated dialyzer rinsing. Each new model of machine brings a higher level of sophistication.

CARING FOR THE PATIENT ON HEMODIALYSIS

Hemodialysis may be used as an acute or chronic treatment modality. In the acute setting, hemodialysis can serve to decrease the imbalances created by acute renal failure or to remove certain toxins from the bloodstream. In the chronic setting, hemodialysis intermittently removes excess electrolytes and water. The hemodialysis procedure remains virtually the same regardless of the setting, but the intensity and critical nature of the procedure increase in acute hemodialysis and in chronic hemodialysis of unstable patients.

Assessment
Prior to initiating the hemodialysis procedure, the nurse must perform a complete physical assessment of the patient and record the pertinent details.

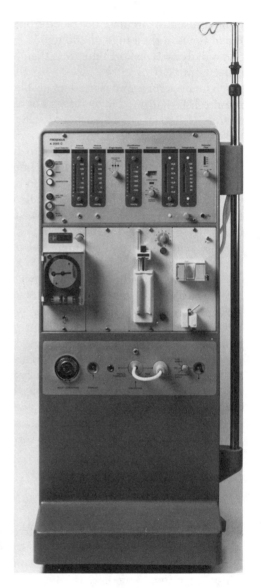

Figure 7-20. Modern dialysis system. (*From Seratronics/Fresenius USA, Inc., Concord, California, with permission.*)

Weight. The patient must be weighed before dialysis. This should occur using the same scales each time and, if the patient is dressed, in the same amount of clothes. Ideally, underbed or underchair scales should be used. The predialysis weight is then compared to the last postdialysis weight to determine the *interdialytic weight gain.* A weight gain of 1 kg/day between dialysis treatments is generally accepted as the desired weight gain. This weight gain represents excess body fluid, and should not be confused with actual tissue weight gain. The nurse should be attentive to any pattern of alterations in weight over time.

The term *dry weight* or *ideal weight* refers to the estimated weight of the patient with no excess fluid, and is manifested by clear breath sounds, absence of edema, and normotension. The dry weight can be thought of as the target postdialysis weight when initiating dialysis. The goal is to dialytically remove the excess fluid during the dialysis procedure so that the patient walks out of the unit carrying no excess fluid. This is often easier in theory than it is in practice, because individual patients respond quite differently to fluid removal techniques.

Vital Signs. Vital signs will vary with the patient's fluid gain and other coexisting conditions. Independent of comorbidities, the blood pressure, pulse, and respirations serve as indicators of fluid status. The patient who presents with an increased blood pressure, pulse, and respirations, and is short of breath, is likely to be fluid overloaded. The patient's temperature can be used to alert the nurse to the existence of a possible infectious process.

Fluid Volume Indicators. Other fluid volume indicators include the status of the neck veins, the presence or absence of edema, skin turgor, and breath sounds. Neck vein engorgement is a clear indicator of fluid overload, as is the presence of pitting edema. Periorbital edema may be observed if excess fluid is present and the patient has been supine for a prolonged period of time. Otherwise, the nurse must rely on the classic sites for edema checks. Overall skin turgor, although more subtle, is also indicative of fluid status. Breath sounds are one of the best assessment tools for fluid volume assessment. With experience, the nephrology nurse can become adept at distinguishing even minimal fluid changes in the lungs.

Cardiovascular Assessment. One of the disadvantages of hemodialysis is the strain it places on the cardiovascular system. It is not uncommon, therefore, for hemodialysis patients to exhibit changes in the cardiovascular status either intra- or interdialytically. In addition to the need for assessing cardiovascular indicators for fluid status, the nurse must also assess the patient for general cardiovascular changes and abnormalities.

Neurological Assessment. It is generally not necessary to do a complete neurological check. An assessment should be performed if the patient is unstable or if the nurse has any doubt as to the neurological status.

Gastrointestinal System. In the early stages of chronic hemodialysis, the patient may experience nausea and vomiting as a result of an increased urea load. At other times, simple nausea, vomiting, or diarrhea can result in electrolyte problems. Acute renal failure patients have a relatively high incidence of ulcers. These patients also frequently have nasogastric tubes. Constipation is a GI problem frequently experienced by chronic hemodialysis patients taking large doses of aluminum hydroxides.

Integumentary System. Pruritis may be observed in the face of someone who has undergone inadequate dialysis. Skin color should also be assessed. A yellow skin tone (not previously observed) would alert the nurse to the possibility of hepatitis. Skin turgor is an indicator of fluid status.

Vascular Access. The vascular access should be checked for patency and any indication of infection. See the "Vascular Access" section earlier in this chapter for the information on assessing specific accesses.

Psychosocial System. In the final analysis, imbalances in the psychosocial system may be equally as devastating to the patient as imbalances in the physical systems. The patient requiring chronic hemodialysis is under a tremendous strain on his or her psychosocial system. Areas of potential psychosocial problems and nursing interventions are detailed in Chapter 11.

Planning

When the assessment has been completed and the pertinent results documented, the nurse can plan the hemodialysis treatment. Physician's orders should have already been written for the specific dialyzer, length of dialysis, dialysate composition, laboratory specimens to be obtained, and medications to be administered intradialytically. The physician should be notified prior to beginning the hemodialysis procedure if the patient assessment has revealed any data that would contraindicate the written orders.

The ideal hemodialysis treatment would have an evenly distributed removal of fluid and electrolytes with no incidences of hypotension, nausea and vomiting, cramps, and so on. The goal of the nurse in planning the treatment is to come as close to the ideal as possible (Table 7–5).

TABLE 7–5. HEMODIALYSIS OUTCOME STANDARDS

1.	Dialysis procedure will meet the fluid and metabolic needs of the patient.
2.	Dialysis procedure will be safe for the patient.
3.	Patient and significant others will be knowledgeable in the ESRD disease process and its treatment including, but not limited to, all treatment options, necessary dietary modifications, access care, available services, and emergency procedures.
4.	Patient will not experience dialysis-related complications such as hypotensive episodes, cramps, arrhythmias, nausea and vomiting, headaches, bleeding, disequilibrium syndrome, seizures, or cardiac arrest.
5.	Patient will not experience mechanically induced complications such as air embolism, hyperthermia, hemolysis, line separations, or clotted dialyzer or bloodlines.
6.	Vascular access will be free of infections.
7.	Patient will be rehabilitated to the degree possible based on physical limitations.

Implementation

Pre-hemodialysis Initiation. Prior to initiating hemodialysis, the nurse must assure the correctness of the hemodialysis setup. The dialyzer and bloodline setup assessment must include checking the presence of the correct dialyzer. This is particularly important when the unit reprocesses dialyzers or bloodlines. The dialyzer and bloodlines must be checked to assure the absence of any sterilant. If the patient is able, the patient should jointly check the dialyzer and bloodlines. The correct dialysate is also of primary importance. All hemodialysis machine monitors should have their alarm limits set according to unit policy, and all monitors should be registering safe. All checks must be documented on the patient's record.

Anticoagulation. Anticoagulation is generally required to prevent clotting of blood in the dialyzer and bloodlines. Heparin is the anticoagulant of choice, and is obtained from pork or beef lung. Heparin has a half-life of 30 to 90 minutes in the patient with renal failure and 90 minutes for the patient with adequate renal function. Metabolism occurs in the liver by heparinase, so consideration must be given when the patient's hepatic system is compromised.

There are several methods of heparinizing the patient. Because of the potential bleeding that can occur with anticoagulation, it is preferable to use as little heparin as possible. Many units use activated clotting times (ACTs) to determine the heparin requirements of a patient. These ACTs can be done either manually or using portable equipment. Most chronic units have a routine heparinization procedure established, which consists of a loading dose given at the initiation of dialysis and smaller doses given throughout the hemodialysis treatment. The smaller doses may be administered by means of intermittent injection or continuous infusion into the bloodline. If intermittent injections are used, the last dose is usually given at least 1 hour before the termination of the procedure. If continuous infusion is used, the infusion is discontinued at least 1 hour prior to termination. These times may be increased if the patient experiences excessive access site bleeding postdialysis. Bleeding problems may be encountered if the hemodialysis treatment is terminated early and the heparin has not yet been discontinued or as a result of heparin rebound. Care must be taken to assure adequate clotting at access sites, and the patient must be aware of the increased tendency towards bleeding until the clinical effect of the heparin has diminished. Patients should routinely be instructed to avoid sharp objects and, in general, to avoid activities that could cause bleeding on hemodialysis days. If necessary, protamine can be used to counteract the effects of the heparin, but extreme care must be taken as allergic reactions to protamine administration have been observed and an overdose of protamine can actually increase anticoagulation.

Infection Control. The patient on hemodialysis is especially susceptible to infection transmission, given a compromised total body function resulting from the effects of ESRD and the potential direct accesses to the vascular system created during the hemodialysis procedure. Extreme care must be taken to optimally protect the patients and the staff. Handwashing before, after, and between patients is a necessity and, while it is the simplest technique, it is often the most neglected. Screening of patients and staff is also important. It is best to assume that the patient may be infected until it has been shown that the patient is infection free.

Hemodialysis Treatment. With the assessment, planning, and pre-hemodialysis checks completed, the nurse is ready to initiate hemodialysis. The vascular access is prepared and connected to the arterial bloodline. Blood flow is initiated slowly. When the blood reaches the end of the venous bloodline, the blood pump is turned off and the venous bloodline is connected to the vascular access. Blood flow is reinitiated and gradually increased until it reaches the desired level, usually between 200 and 350 cc/min. The hemodialysis initiation time is the time at which blood flow is reinitiated or when the target blood flow is reached, depending on unit policy.

Intradialytic Monitoring. If the patient is unstable, the blood pressure is monitored every 15 to 30 minutes and prn, depending on the status of the patient. Stable patients do not require as frequent monitoring. The policy in many chronic units is to monitor the blood pressure every 30 minutes and prn if the patient becomes unstable. The monitors on the dialysis machine and the continuous heparin infusion, if used, are checked at least every 30 to 60 minutes and more often if necessary. These blood pressures and monitor checks are documented on the hemodialysis flow sheet.

Potential Hemodialysis Complications. There are a number of complications that may occur to the patient as a result of the hemodialysis procedure. Hakim and Lazarus (1986) note that these complications result from the complex interaction between the patient and the dialysis procedure as well as from the hemodialysis process itself; and that the incidence of complications increases with age and the presence of comorbidities.

Hypotension is a frequent complication. The pathophysiology of hemodialysis hypotension is due to a decreased venous return to the heart by ultrafiltration-induced hypovolemia. This results in a decrease in filling pressures, cardiac output, and left ventricular work index (Kinet et al., 1982). Decreases in plasma osmolality can contribute to hemodialysis hypotension by creating an osmotic gradient that favors the movement of water from the vascular and interstitial spaces to the intracellular spaces (Rosa, Shideman, McHugh, Duncan, & Kjellstranal, 1981). These and other factors associated with hemodialysis hypotension are illustrated in Figure 7–21.

With careful observation and blood pressure monitoring, hypotension can usually be discovered and treated early. The patient would then have either no complications from the hypotension or only minor nausea or a tired

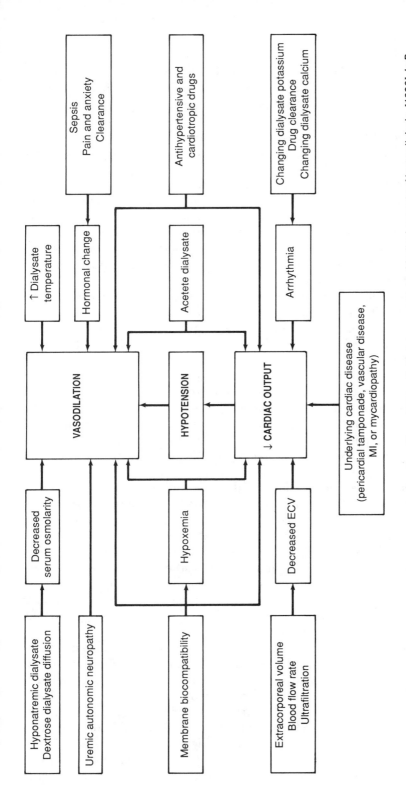

Figure 7-21. Factors associated with hemodialysis hypotension. (*From Hakim, R. M. & Lazarus, J. M., Medical aspects of hemodialysis. [1986]. In B. M. Brenner & F. J. Rector, Jr. The Kidney. Philadelphia: Saunders, with permission.*)

145

feeling following dialysis. More severe hypotension can result in vomiting, headache, and cramps, and can progress to seizures and ultimately cardiac arrest if not treated promptly. Research has further suggested that dialysate temperature has a significant effect on the occurrence of hemodialysis hypotension. When the dialysate temperature is decreased to 34.4C, the frequency of hypotention significantly decreases (Lindholm, Thysell, Yamamoto, Forsberg, & Gullberg, 1985; Sherman, Rubin, Cody, & Eisinger, 1985). The problem is that many patients cannot tolerate such low temperatures.

The immediate treatment for hypotension is to place the patient in Trendelenburg's position, decrease the ultrafiltration pressures, and administer replacement fluids. Depending on the philosophy of the individual unit, the fluids may be a saline solution or a vascular volume expander. Long-term treatment involves reassessing the patient's dry weight, dialysate composition, and dietary regimen.

Arrhythmias are another hemodialysis complication. The causes of hemodialysis arrhythmias include a rapid shift in the serum potassium level, an increase in the serum calcium, and the clearance of antiarrhythmic drugs (MacDonald, Uldall, & Buda, 1981; Morrison, Michelson, Brown, & Morganroth, 1980).

Severe complications, such as hemolysis, air embolism, and hyperthermia, are rare; but all require immediate corrective measures when they do occur. *Hemolysis* is the destruction of red blood cells. It can occur when the patient's blood is exposed to hypotonic solutions such as incorrectly mixed dialysate or hypotonic chemicals such as formaldehyde and chlorox.

The patient experiencing hemolysis will present with chest pain, arrhythmias, hypotension, shortness of breath, and burning at access entry and exit sites. The hemolyzed blood in the extracorporeal circuit is often described as looking like liquid cherry jello. The treatment for hemolysis is to immediately clamp the extracorporeal bloodlines and disconnect the patient without returning the blood in the bloodlines and dialyzer; monitor the patient's vital signs including pulse and respirations; administer oxygen if the patient is short of breath; obtain hematocrit and electrolyte specimens; and notify the physician. Hemolysis can be prevented by carefully checking conductivity before and during the dialysis procedure, making sure that alarm limits are set in the correct positions, and always remaining aware that mechanical monitoring equipment can fail.

An *air embolism* can occur when an air bolus is introduced into the patient's vascular system. The patient with an air bolus will generally have chest pain, shortness of breath, pallor, hypotension, confusion, and disorientation, and may also have visual problems. The treatment for an air embolism is to stop the infusion of air, place the patient on the left side in the Trendelenburg position, monitor vital signs, administer oxygen, and notify the physician. Like hemolysis, air embolisms can usually be prevented by careful attention to details such as arming the air detector; making sure that clamps are always close at hand; taping all connections securely; never administering solutions from bottles unless the administration is carefully observed throughout; and, as with the prevention of hemolysis, remembering that mechanical devices are not foolproof.

Hyperthermia can occur with a malfunction of the temperature control devices on the hemodialysis machine. The patient will complain of feeling hot and hemolysis may occur. Treatment includes monitoring the patient's temperature, checking the temperature of the dialysate, discontinuing dialysis, observing for and if necessary treating hemolysis, and notifying the physician.

Medication Dialyzability. An important consideration, especially when using the relatively rapid-acting treatment modality of hemodialysis is the dialyzability of the medications the patient is taking. Dialyzability is determined by the molecular weight of the medication, the abilities of the drug to be soluble in water and protein bound, and the plasma clearance of the drug.

While the nephrologists generally consider medication dialyzability when ordering the medication, the dose, and the time of administration, the nephrology nurse must be alert as not all healthcare professionals share the nephrologists' knowledge of the mixing of medications and dialysis. When dialyzable intravenous medications must be administered during the dialysis procedure, it is usually advisable to administer the medication on the "venous" side of dialyzer. Often, the nephrologist will request that medication administration not occur until the end of the procedure.

It is equally as important to know the medications that are not dialyzed as it is to know those that are. Knowing these properties of the medications administered prior to or during dialysis allows the nurse to better plan the treatment and to anticipate potential patient problems.

Potential Hemodialysis Equipment Problems. Although the hemodialysis equipment of today is very sophisticated, it is not perfect. Dialyzers still leak or clot, bloodlines still leak, and machines still malfunction. Though the incidence of these problems has certainly decreased since the early years of nephrology nursing, the nurse must be constantly aware of the potential for equipment failure. Most problems can be prevented by an adequate preventative maintenance program and careful monitoring.

Terminating the Hemodialysis Treatment. The hemodialysis procedure is terminated when the preestablished length of treatment is completed or in the event of an emergency. In a true emergency, such as a cardiac arrest or a fire in the dialysis unit, termination is accomplished by stopping the blood pump, clamping both access lines and both bloodlines, and disconnecting the patient. Obviously this is not the preferred method of termination, but it is effective. Emergency termination procedures should be reviewed with each patient routinely and that review documented.

Termination of a routine hemodialysis treatment should begin at the time the treatment is to be over; if a 4-hour treatment started at 7:30 AM, the blood pump should be turned off to initiate termination at 11:30 AM. Routine termination of the hemodialysis procedure involves stopping the blood pump, clamping the arterial bloodline and access line, disconnecting the arterial bloodline from the arterial access line, slowly restarting the blood pump, returning the blood to the patient using a saline infusion into the arterial bloodline, and finally clamping and then disconnecting the venous bloodline and access line.

If the access lines are removable, they are taken out and pressure placed on the site until the bleeding has stopped. If the access lines are not to be removed after each procedure, they must be either reconnected in the case of an AV shunt, or flushed and clamped in the case of subclavian and femoral catheters.

Post-hemodialysis Assessment. After the hemodialysis treatment has been terminated, the patient's vital signs are taken as well as a post-hemodialysis weight. The nurse compares the actual weight to the dry weight to determine the degree to which the patients must limit fluids until the next treatment. Fluid input is totaled. The overall treatment plan, process, and outcome are then evaluated. Any changes that need to be made in future treatments are noted in the patient's record. The patient's ability to ambulate should be assessed, especially if hypotensive episodes have occurred during the treatment.

PROGNOSIS

Patients always want to know, and rightly so, the survival rates on hemodialysis. Although the prognosis for each patient cannot be accurately predicted, there are some factors that have been found to influence survival. Actuarial survival data analysis reveals that survival is heavily influenced by the age of the patient and the presence of comorbidities prior to the initiation of dialysis (Blagg, Wahl, & Lamers, 1983; Shapiro & Umen, 1983; Volmer, Wahl, & Blagg, 1983). However, despite a marked rise in mean patient age and in the percentage of patients experiencing serious multiorgan diseases between 1965 and 1980, Kjellstrand (1983) found that the first-year mortality dropped from 50 to 15 percent during that period of time. Shapiro and Umen (1983) have reported that when ESRD is not complicated by comorbidities, the 5-year survival of patients beginning dialysis when they are under 46 years of age is as high as 97 percent, and is 84 percent for patients under 61 years. Between 1965 and 1975, the year when the patient began dialysis was a factor in actuarial survival data, but with the advent of advanced technology this is no longer the case.

In terms of total length of survival, Franklin (1987) has reported the survival of several patients for over 20 years. As knowledge and technology progress further, increased survival times can be expected.

ASSOCIATED THERAPIES

Since the advent of hemodialysis, several associated therapies have been developed. These include hemoperfusion, hemofiltration, and continuous arteriovenous hemofiltration.

Hemoperfusion

Hemoperfusion is a treatment alternative for use in patients who have severe poisoning that is associated with a high mortality. This includes instances in which a large amount of the poison are converted by the body into more toxic substances, the poisoning agent is known to produce severe toxicity, or the poison is a narcotic agent that produces profound coma (Winchester, 1983).

Hemoperfusion uses a cartridge made of activated charcoal, activated carbon, or resin. These substances have high porosity, a large surface area, and high adsorption capability. *Adsorption* is the physical attachment of a solute or gas molecule directly to the surface of the substance by secondary bonding. The adsorptive capacity of the cartridge decreases over time as toxin is adsorbed. Hemoperfusion does not remove fluid, urea, or electrolytes from the blood. It does adsorb water-soluble poisons and drugs. Fat-soluble poisons and drugs are adsorbed slowly. Some large-molecule drugs such as antibiotics are not adsorbed. It is important to determine the adsorption potential of all medications the patient is receiving and to compensate for adsorption or lack of adsorption.

The hemoperfusion procedure is much like hemodialysis, requiring a vascular access, blood pump, bloodlines, the hemoperfusion cartridge, a heparin pump, and pressure monitors. Heparinization is important. Since the patient will usually have normal clotting factors, the cartridge will clot if the patient is not well heparinized. A blood flow of about 200 cc is generally required. The length of the hemoperfusion procedure varies depending on the poison level of the patient. The procedure may need to be repeated if the poison has rebound capability. Side effects associated with hemoperfusion include hypotension, hypothermia, hypocalcemia, hypoglycemia, and thrombocytopenia.

Hemofiltration

Hemofiltration uses a device similar to a dialyzer except that it has a much higher ultrafiltration rate and is not designed for diffusive transport. The hemofilter uses special membranes that are more permeable to water and plasma solutes. Hemofiltration works on the principle of convection, where small solutes pass freely through the filter at a rate proportional to their concentration in the blood, but very large solutes are retained. The so-called middle molecules with a weight between 500 and 5000 Daltons are removed at a higher rate in hemofiltration than in hemodialysis. Frei and Koch (1982) proposed that this improved middle molecule removal rate may account for the improved vascular stability with hemofiltration. An alternative explanation by

Schuenemann and associates (1982) regarding the improved vascular stability is that hemofiltration allows better control of water volume and electrolyte balance. Because hemofiltration removes very large amounts of fluid, a major portion of that fluid must be replaced during the procedure.

Continuous Arteriovenous Hemofiltration
Continuous arteriovenous hemofiltration (CAVH) is an extracorporeal process in which fluid, electrolytes, and small and middle molecules are removed from the patient by ultrafiltration over an extended period of time. At the same time, a replacement solution is administered to reconstitute the blood volume. CAVH is especially useful in patients with fluid overload, regardless of the cause of the overload; it can also be used to remove urea nitrogen and control or maintain electrolyte balance.

The filters used for CAVH look quite similar to those used in hollow fiber or parallel plate dialyzers. The blood inlet and outlet ports are connected to bloodlines. The ultrafiltrate outlet port is connected by a line to a collection bag. An arteriovenous shunt is often used for vascular access. Femoral catheters and internal AV grafts can also be used. The patient's arterial pressure moves the blood through the extracorporeal circuit. Ultrafiltration is flow dependent at rates between 90 and 250 cc/min (Bosch, 1986). The ultrafiltration, in general, is determined by the hydrostatic pressure inside the filter and the oncotic pressure exerted by plasma proteins (Lauer et al., 1983).

REFERENCES

Association for Advancement of Medical Instrumentation. (1982). *The American National Standard for Hemodialysis.* Arlington, Va.: AAMI.

Blagg, C. R., Wahl, P. W., & Lamers, J. Y. (1983). Treatment of chronic renal failure at the Northwest Kidney Center, Seattle, from 1960 to 1982. *J Am Soc Artif Intern Organs, 6,* 176.

Bosch, J. P. (1986). In L. W. Henderson, E. A. Quellhorst, C. A. Baldamus, & M. J. Lysaght (Eds.), *Hemofiltration.* Berlin: Springer-Verlag.

Brunois, J. P., Toupance, O., Vistelle, R., et al. (1984). Role of sodium in the control of compartmental distribution of water during hemodialysis: Measurement of water transfer. *Nephrologie, 5,* 27–31.

Cheung, A. K., & Baranowski, R. L. (1984). The role of thromboxane in pulmonary hypertension (PHTN) induced by cuprophan-activated plasma (CAP). *Abstracts of the 17th Annual Meeting of the American Society of Nephrology.* Thorofare, N.J.: Charles B. Slack.

Dolovich, J., Marshal, C. P., Smith, E. K., et al. (1984). Allergy to ethylene oxide in chronic hemodialysis patients. *Artif Organs, 8,* 334–337.

Franklin, T. (1987). Kidney patient lives "miracle." *The Torchbearer,* Summer, 3.

Frei, U., & Koch, K. M. (1982). Fever and shock during hemofiltration. *Contrib Nephro, 36,* 107–114.

Hakim, R. M., & Lazarus, J. M. (1986). Medical aspects of hemodialysis. In B. M. Brenner & F. J. Rector, Jr. (Eds.), *The kidney* (3rd ed., pp. 1791–1845). Philadelphia: Saunders.

Kinet, J. P., Soyeur, D., Ballard, N., et al. (1982). Hemodynamics study of hypotension during hemodialysis. *Kidney Int, 21,* 868.

Kjellstrand, C. M. (1983). Introduction to a workshop on morbidity and mortality in hemodialysis, hemofiltration, and continuous ambulatory peritoneal dialysis. *J Am Soc Artif Int Organs, 6,* 167.

Lauer, A., Saccaggi, A., Ronco, C., et al. (1983). Continuous arteriovenous hemofiltration in the critically ill patient. *Ann Intern Med, 99,* 455.

Lindholm, T., Thysell, H., Yamamoto, Y., et al. (1985). Temperature and vascular stability in hemodialysis. *Nephron, 39,* 130–133.

MacDonald, I. L., Uldall, P. R., & Buda, A. J. (1981). The effect of hemodialysis on cardiac rhythm and performance. *Clin Nephrol, 15,* 321.

Morrison, G., Michelson, E. L., Brown, S., & Morganroth, J. (1980). Mechanism and prevention of cardiac arrhythmias in chronic hemodialysis patients. *Kidney Int, 17,* 811.

Parker, J., & Wicks, G. S. (Eds.). (1984). *Protecting the future of quality care through an understanding of hemodialysis principles.* Pitman, N. J.: American Nephrology Nurses' Association.

Rosa, A., Shideman, J., McHugh, R., et al. (1981). The importance of osmolality fall and ultrafiltration rate on hemdialysis side effects. *Nephron, 27,* 134.

Schuenemann, B., Quellhorst, E., Kaiser, H., et al. (1982). Regeneration of filtrate and dialysis fluid by electro-oxidation and absorption. *Trans Am Soc Artif Intern Organs, 28,* 49–53.

Shapiro, F. L., & Umen, A. (1983). Risk factors in hemodialysis patient survival. *J Am Soc Artif Int Organs, 6,* 176.

Sherman, R. A., Rubin, M. P., Cody, R. P., & Eisinger, R. P. (1985). Amelioration of hemodialysis-associated hypotension by the use of cool dialysate. *Am J Kidney Dis, 5,* 124–127.

Stroncek, D. F., Keshaviah, P., Craddock, P. R., et al. (1984). Effect of dialyzer reuse on complement activation and neutropenia in hemodialysis. *J Clin Lab Med, 104,* 304–311.

Van Stone, J. C. (1986). Hemodialysis. In H. C. Gonick (Ed.), *Current nephrology (vol. 9).* Chicago: Year Book Medical Publishers.

Volmer, W. M., Wahl, P. W., & Blagg, C. R. (1983). Survival with dialysis and transplantation in patients with end stage renal disease. *N Engl J Med, 308,* 1553.

Winchester, J. F. (1983). Active methods for detoxification: Oral sorbents, forced diuresis, hemoperfusion, and hemodialysis. In L. M. Haddad & J. F. Winchester (Eds.), *Poisoning and drug overdose.* Philadelphia: Saunders.

8

Peritoneal Dialysis Therapy

Janel Parker and Beth Tamplet Ulrich

OBJECTIVES

After reading this chapter on peritoneal dialysis therapy, the nurse will be able to:

1. Understand the general principles of peritoneal dialysis
2. Compare the principles of peritoneal dialysis with the principles of hemodialysis
3. Compare the methods of performing peritoneal dialysis
4. Describe the various peritoneal catheters and the methods used to insert them
5. Describe the potential complications of peritoneal dialysis

Peritoneal dialysis is a form of intracorporeal hemodialysis that uses the peritoneum for the semipermeable membrane. Gantner first used the concept in humans in 1923. The relatively low efficiency of the procedure, coupled with the lack of a chronic access, limited peritoneal dialysis to the acute setting when hemodialysis was contraindicated or not available. Tenckhoff's development of a permanent peritoneal catheter solved the chronic access problem; and, in the late 1970s, Popovich developed the concept of continuous ambulatory peritoneal dialysis (CAPD). In CAPD, a method had been discovered to use the relative low efficiency of peritoneal dialysis to the patient's advantage. Automated peritoneal dialysis further advanced the procedure in the early 1980s. Today peritoneal dialysis is relied upon as a safe and effective treatment modality for the treatment of chronic or acute renal failure.

GENERAL PRINCIPLES

Anatomy and Physiology of the Peritoneum

It is necessary to have an in-depth knowledge of the anatomy and physiology of the peritoneum in order to fully understand the process of peritoneal dialysis.

Peritoneal Membrane. The peritoneal membrane outlines the peritoneal cavity (Fig. 8–1). A thin layer of mesothelial cells composes the side of the membrane adjacent to the organs located in the peritoneal cavity. A basement membrane lies between the mesothelium and the endothelial lining of the capillary bed. Blood vessels and connecting tissue are sandwiched in between the two cell layers. In the adult, the peritoneal membrane measures about 2.2 m². All or part of the membrane may be useable for peritoneal dialysis. Membrane injury due to disease processes, surgical scarring, infections, and so forth, can render the peritoneum ineffective as a semipermeable membrane. For this reason, one usually refers to the *effective surface area* rather than the surface area of the peritoneum. Compared to the synthetic membrane used in hemodialysis, the peritoneal membrane has larger but fewer pores. As a result, peritoneal dialysis plasma clearances of large molecular weight substances such as inulin usually exceed the plasma clearances of similar substances by hemodialysis. Clearances of smaller solutes are usually lower in peritoneal dialysis.

Vascular Structure. The amount of effective peritoneal capillary blood flow has not yet been conclusively determined. The total abdominal splanchnic blood flow in adults usually exceeds 1200 ml/min at rest (Wade et al., 1956). This amount is exclusive of the blood flow to the parietal peritoneum. The total capillary endothelial area available for exchange in the peritoneum may represent only a small portion of all capillary beds supplied by the splanchnic blood flow. Almost 80 percent of the capillaries may be nonperfused because of capillary sphincters, except during vasoconstriction (Nolph et al., 1977). This would make blood flow to peritoneal capillaries that can participate in solute exchange during peritoneal dialysis very low (Nolph et al., 1978). Indirect evidence indicates that the effective peritoneal capillary blood flow may only be about 60 to 70 ml/min (Aune, 1970; Nolph et al., 1978).

Clearance and Ultrafiltration

Exchange between peritoneal capillaries and the peritoneal cavity involves diffusion of solutes and the convective transfer of water and solutes through the capillary endothelium and peritoneal mesothelium. Given adequate blood

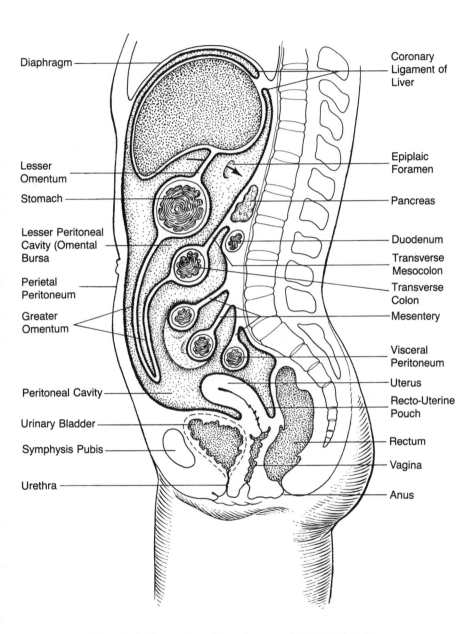

Figure 8-1. The peritoneal membrane and peritoneal cavity.

flow rates, membrane resistance appears to be the major limitation on small and large solute clearances.

Membrane Resistance

Solutes must cross six sites of resistance in their movement across the peritoneal membrane (Nolph, 1980). These resistances are shown in Figure 8-2.

Solute Transport

Solute transport for peritoneal dialysis is similar to solute transport in hemodialysis or in the human kidney. Diffusion accounts for virtually 99 percent of the solute transport, with the remainder resulting from solute drag. The rate of transport is affected by the permeability of the peritoneal membrane, the molecular weight of the solutes, the temperature of the dialysate, and the concentration gradient that is established between the dialysate and the blood. As stated previously, the peritoneal membrane, in comparison to the synthetic hemodialysis membrane, has pores that are fewer in number but larger in size. Peritoneal dialysis is therefore less effective for small molecular weight substances, about the same for solutes between 500 and 5000 Daltons, and more effective for molecules larger that 5000 Daltons. Increased dialysate temperature has been shown to increase clearances. Gross and McDonald (1967) demonstrated a 30 to 35 percent increase in clearances by increasing the temperature of the dialysate from 20 to 37C. Another method of increasing peritoneal clearance involves the intraperitoneal administration of vasoconstrictors, which open new channels in the peritoneal capillary beds, thereby increasing the effective surface area.

Ultrafiltration

Ultrafiltration in peritoneal dialysis is accomplished with hyperosmolar dialysis solutions that have high glucose concentrations ranging from 1.5 to 4.25 g/dl and osmolalities from 340 to 490 mosm/kg of water (Nolph, 1986). The ultrafiltration rate is highest immediately after the infusion of new dialysate into the peritoneal cavity and decreases as the solutions equilibrate in osmolality.

DIALYSATE

Dialysate is the critical controllable element in peritoneal dialysis therapy. The concentration of the dialysate, the dialysate flow, and the size and number of dialysate exchanges are all important factors.

Dialysate Composition

The approximate composition of peritoneal dialysis fluid is shown in Table 8-1. Glucose is used as an osmotic agent in peritoneal dialysis. Dialysate is avail-

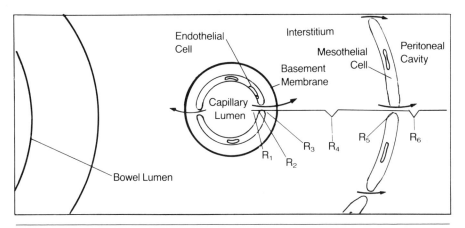

Resistance	Description	Estimated distance represented μ	Major mechanisms of solute movement[a]	Factors causing changes in resistance
R_1	Intracapillary fluid films	1 to 3	C + D	Capillary flow rate, turbulence, blood viscosity
R_2	Endothelial intercellular channels ("pores")	<0.5	C?	Vasodilation may open more permeable capillaries (increase number of pores and mean pore area)
R_3	Capillary basement membranes	0.2 to 0.5	C?	Diseases such as diabetes mellitus may cause thickening
R_4	Peritoneal interstitium	0.1 to 100	D	Inaccessible stagnant fluid may be the resistance least subject to change
R_5	Mesothelial intercellular	<0.9	D	Unknown in clinical setting may be influenced by drugs that interfere with cell metabolism and/or dialysate osmolality
R_6	Fluid films in peritoneal	Variable	D, stagnant C, mixing	Subject to influence of rapid cycling and better mixing juxtamesothelial layers may be inaccessible

[a]D is diffusive; C is convective.

Figure 8-2. Factors that may alter peritoneal resistances to solute movement. (*From Nolph, K. D. et al. [1980]. New directions in peritoneal dialysis concepts and applications. Kidney International, 18, p. 2111, with permission.*)

TABLE 8-1. APPROXIMATE COMPOSITION OF PERITONEAL DIALYSIS FLUID

Glucose	0.5 – 4.5 g/dl
Sodium	130.0 – 141.0 mEq/L
Chloride	96.0 – 107.0 mEq/L
Magnesium	0.5 – 1.5 mEq/L
Calcium	3.0 – 3.5 mEq/L
Acetate or lactate	35.0 – 45.0 mEq/L
pH	5.0 – 5.8
Osmolality	340.0 – 490.0 μosm ≠ kg

able in several different glucose solutions, ranging from 0.5 to 4.25 percent dextrose. An infusion of 2000 cc of 1.5 percent glucose will usually yield a return volume of about 2100 to 2200 cc. A 4.25 percent glucose solution of the same amount of influx will result in a return of 2500 to 3000 cc. Many facilities now recommend periodic use of the 4.25 percent solution; however, care must be taken with such hypertonic solutions because the possibility exists of dehydration, hyperglycemia, and hypernatremia. Sodium concentrations below 130 mEq/L can be used to prevent hypernatremia when excessive amounts of hypertonic dialysate are necessary to remove excessive fluid. Another less serious problem that may result from the use of high concentration glucose solutions is patient weight gain, because the glucose in the dialysate can provide one third or more of the necessary calories each day.

Most peritoneal dialysate solutions do not contain potassium. There is a net sieving effect such that potassium is removed with the ultrafiltrate.

Either acetate or lactate is used as a buffer in peritoneal dialysis solutions. The advantages of acetate are its use in lactic acidosis and its high final pH. The disadvantages are the potential reduction of ultrafiltration and increased glucose uptake. Lactate has the advantage of reducing carmelization of dextrose during heat sterilization (Winchester, 1986).

Dialysate Flow

Optimal peritoneal clearance and ultrafiltration would be achieved with a continuous flow of dialysate in and out of the peritoneum. The method of peritoneal dialysis that most closely approximates this situation is that which uses a cycling device. CAPD is slower, but allows the patient freedom from a machine.

Dialysate flow is controlled through the number and amount of exchanges and the dwell time. The optimal ultrafiltration and clearance rates occur when the concentration gradient is the largest. Any combination of numbers of exchanges, amount of exchanges, dwell time, and composition of exchanges, that maximizes the concentration gradient will make the peritoneal dialysis procedure more efficient.

Dialysate Exchanges

Regardless of the method of performing peritoneal dialysis (to be discussed next), the exchange of dialysate remains conceptually the same. A certain amount of warmed peritoneal dialysate is inserted into the peritoneal cavity through a catheter. The dialysate remains in the peritoneal cavity for a predetermined period of time, and is then allowed to drain out of the cavity, usually into the same bag that was used to hold the fresh dialysate. The bag is disconnected, a new bag of dialysate is connected, and the procedure is repeated.

The critical element in peritoneal dialysate exchanges is the maintenance of sterile technique. Several tubing connection designs and devices assist in the maintenance of a sterile system (Fig. 8-3).

METHODS OF PERITONEAL DIALYSIS

The methods for performing peritoneal dialysis include continuous ambulatory peritoneal dialysis (CAPD), intermittent peritoneal dialysis (IPD), and continuous cycling peritoneal dialysis (CCPD).

CAPD

In 1976, Popovich proposed CAPD as a modification of the peritoneal dialysis technique being performed in hospitals at the time. CAPD consists of exchanging approximately 2 L of dialysate 4 to 5 times a day, 7 days a week. The amount of dialysate and the number of exchanges will vary with the size, clearance, and ultrafiltration needs of the individual patient. The continuous nature of the dialysis closely simulates the results of normal renal function. This is advantageous in a number of clinical situations, because the patient does not experience the extreme shifts associated with hemodialysis. Dietary restrictions are also fewer with this treatment modality.

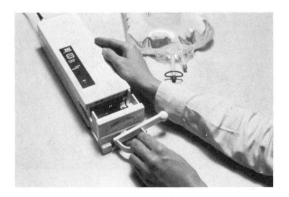

Figure 8-3. Ultraviolet light device. (*From Travenol Laboratories, Inc., Deerfield Illinois, with permission.*)

Perhaps the major advantage of CAPD, at least from the patient's perspective, is the freedom the procedure allows. There is no machine to feel connected to or dependent on. A partner is not necessary. The exchanges can be done almost anywhere. Perhaps the only limiting factor in CAPD is the need to transport heavy bags of peritoneal dialysate wherever the exchanges will take place.

IPD and CCPD
IPD and CCPD are methods of performing peritoneal dialysis over an established period of time with frequent exchanges. For efficiency purposes, IPD and CCPD are done using a machine (described later). With IPD, the patient may come to the dialysis unit several days a week. The procedure ends after a drainage. In CCPD, the patient is connected to the machine for a period of time, usually while sleeping, and disconnected after a dialysate instillation. The dialysate remains in the patient's abdomen until the next time he or she is connected to the machine. CCPD is usually done 6 or 7 days a week. CCPD has been used very effectively in small children.

Cycler. The cycler is either partially or totally automated (Fig. 8-4). The foreruners of current cyclers were developed by Bosch, and Lasker, and associates in the mid-1960s. These machines, many of which are still in use, consist of 8 to 10 containers of dialysate hung from a multiprong metal pole and connected to a tubing system that supplies the dialysate to the delivery system. A series of clamps, controlled by electronic timers, regulates the dialysate flow. Dialysate flows from the bag into a heater bag or other reser-

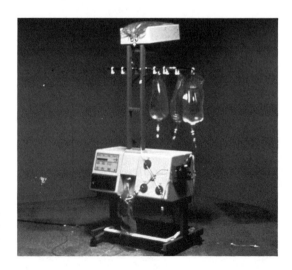

Figure 8-4. Automated peritoneal dialysis machine. (*From Travenol Laboratories, Inc., Deerfield, Illinois, with permission.*)

voir, flows into the patient's peritoneal cavity, remains for the preset dwell time, and is drained by gravity into a weigh bag and then a drainage bag. The weigh bag is attached to an electronic scale that measures the effluent dialysate. If the weight (and therefore volume) is too low, an alarm will sound. Other alarms on the system include a temperature alarm and an alarm to indicate a failure of the weigh bag to empty. Newer models of these machines have included improved control and monitoring capabilities.

On-line Proportioning Machines. The on-line proportioning system seeks to correct the biggest problem with cyclers, that of dialysate storage and disposal. McDonald (1965) first described such a system. The on-line proportioning system is designed to work much like the hemodialysis system. Reverse osmosis is used to prepare purified water, which is then mixed with concentrate and delivered to the patient.

Potential Machine Problems. As with hemodialysis equipment, equipment problems can occur. Dialysate contamination is usually due to human error in tubing connections rather than to equipment malfunction. Inadequate temperature control affects clearances and causes patient discomfort. Malfunctioning in conductivity controls can result in delivery of the wrong dialysate and can be life-threatening. Failure in the timing mechanisms can cause the patient to receive an incorrect amount of dialysate.

PERITONEAL CATHETERS

Peritoneal catheters may be inserted on an acute or chronic basis. Basically, the peritoneal catheter is a catheter made of silastic tubing with some form of anchor device (Fig. 8–5). The anchor may be in the form of cuffs, soft disks, or a balloon. Perforations are spaced throughout the tubing to allow fluid flow in and out the catheter.

Catheter Insertion

The insertion of the peritoneal catheter can be performed at the bedside under local anesthesia using a trocar or stylet to puncture the abdominal wall, or in the operating room using either local or general anesthesia. In either case, strict sterile technique must be maintained. General preinsertion preparation of the patient includes the administration of an enema or cathartic to clear the colon, and voiding to empty the bladder.

Bedside Insertion. The insertion of the catheter at the bedside is usually performed when acute access is required. The abdominal area is surgically pre-

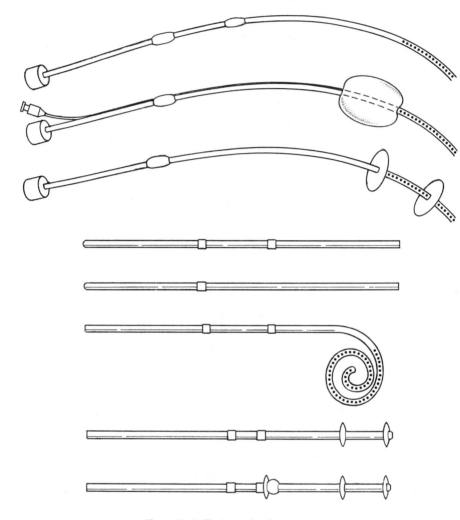

Figure 8-5. Peritoneal catheters.

pared, and a sterile field established. In addition to the trocar or stylet and the catheter, the surgeon will need local anesthetic, a scalpel, 4 × 4s, heparinized dialysate, tubing, and the antibiotic flush to be administered postinsertion.

After the administration of local anesthesia, a midline incision of about 2 mm in length is made 2 to 5 cm below the umbilicus. Any incisional bleeding is stopped before the catheter is placed. The patient is asked to tighten the abdominal muscles. The stylet or trocar is inserted into the incision site until it penetrates the peritoneum (Fig. 8-6). Most surgeons prefer to expand the peritoneal cavity by inserting dialysate at the earliest opportunity. This makes threading the catheter easier and safer. The catheter is threaded into the peritoneal cavity. There should be no resistance to fluid flow if the catheter has been properly placed. The trocar is then removed and a subcutaneous tunnel is created between the incision site and a stab wound that is created as a catheter exit site. The catheter is brought outside the skin via the stab wound and sutured in place. The peritoneal cavity is flushed with an antibiotic solution.

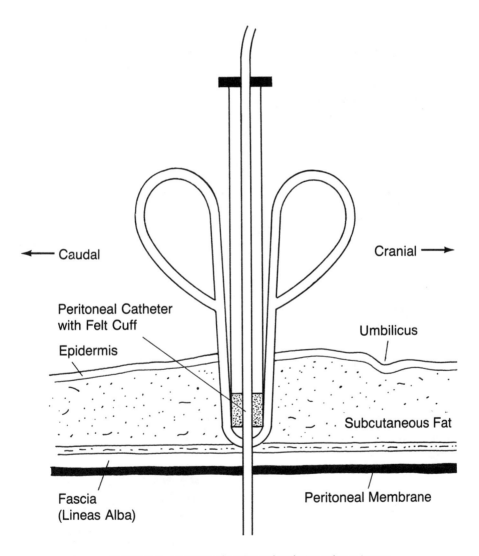

Figure 8-6. Insertion of peritoneal catheter using a trocar.

Operating Room Insertion. The insertion procedure is quite similar in the operating room. The notable difference is the placement of the catheter visually rather than through the use of a trocar. This type of insertion is preferred for chronic catheters; patients with an ileus, extensive previous abdominal surgery, coma, cachexia, or scaphoid abdomen; and is necessary with some of the catheters that have disks for stabilization (Nolph, 1986).

Postinsertion Care. Although chronic peritoneal catheters have been used immediately after insertion (Tenckhoff, 1976), it is generally preferable to allow a waiting period of 3 to 7 days. During that time, small amounts of heparinized dialysate are inserted intermittently. The nurse may administer this dialysate in the hospital or the patient may do it at home.

Potential Catheter Complications

There are a number of potential catheter complications. These include perforations, catheter movement, catheter malfunctions, infections, and skin erosion (Table 8–2).

TABLE 8-2. TECHNICAL COMPLICATIONS OF PERITONEAL DIALYSIS

Complication	Probable Causes
Fluid will not flow into the patient	Kink in tubing Air lock in tubing Fibrin clot Constipation Dialysate bag below abdomen Encapsulation of catheter
Fluid will not flow out of the patient	Kink in tubing Air lock in tubing Fibrin clot in catheter No fluid in peritoneal cavity Constipation Dialysate bag above abdomen Catheter malpositioned Encapsulation of the catheter
Outflow less than inflow	Reabsorption of the fluid into the vascular space Clotting catheter Catheter malpositioned
Accidental disconnection of tubing from catheter	Poor connection technique Equipment failure
Catheter leakage	Inadequate seal between catheter and peritoneum Immature catheter (too early after insertion for large volume dialysate)

Intra-abdominal Perforations. There is always a risk of intra-abdominal perforation when insertion of a peritoneal catheter is attempted. The most common perforations are those of the bowel and bladder. As noted previously, preinsertion emptying of the bowel and bladder will decrease the chance of perforation. Should perforation occur, the patient may suffer an acute blood loss (if a vessel is punctured), peritonitis (if the bowel is punctured), or surgical risks due to repair of the perforation.

Catheter Obstruction. Catheter obstruction may be temporary or permanent, one-way or two-way. Often in one-way temporary obstructions, inflow is adequate but outflow is not. One-way obstructions can be caused by something as simple as constipation or as complicated as the formation of omental flaps over the drainage holes or the presence of fibrin or blood clots in the catheter. The most common cause of a true catheter obstruction is the migration of the catheter from the pelvis to the upper quadrants of the abdomen (Veitch, 1986).

If constipation is the problem, stimulating bowel peristalsis may alleviate the flow problems. Otherwise, catheter irrigation can be attempted with heparinized saline. If neither of these techniques is effective, a new catheter may be required.

Total permanent catheter obstruction may result from encapsulation of the catheter by fibrous adhesions or the omentum. These adhesions can occur from surgical procedures, peritonitis, or the presence of the catheter. Permanent obstruction requires replacement of the catheter.

Catheter Leakage. The leakage of dialysate from the catheter at the exit site is a common complication, especially with acute catheters. Leakage may result from an inadequate seal between the catheter and the peritoneum or not allowing the catheter insertion to mature adequately before progressing to large volume dialysate exchanges. In addition to occurring at the exit site, fluid leakage may also occur subcutaneously into the abdominal wall, eventually spreading to the thigh, scrotum, or labia. Temporarily discontinuing the use of the catheter may allow creation of an adequate tissue seal.

Exit Site or Tunnel Infection. Exit site and tunnel infections must be diagnosed and treated quickly to prevent peritonitis. The chance of having one of these types of infections is increased with dialysate leakage, repositioning of the catheter either intentionally or accidentally, and poor site care.

The signs and symptoms of exit site infections include redness, tenderness, and drainage at the site. The patient is generally treated with antibiotics and a review of the protocols on exit site care, and is carefully observed for any indications of peritonitis.

Tunnel infections often exhibit redness, tenderness along the tract, and swelling. As with the exit site infection, the patient is usually treated with antibiotics and observed for signs of peritonitis.

Catheter Removal

Catheter complications may necessitiate removing the catheter. To remove the catheter, a buttonhole incision is made around the catheter exit site for catheters with cuffs in that area and an incision over the site of the deeper cuff. The physician dissects down to the deeper cuff, severs the catheter into two pieces, removes the two pieces, and closes the incisions (Nolph, 1986).

POTENTIAL COMPLICATIONS OF PERITONEAL DIALYSIS

The potential complications of peritoneal dialysis include peritonitis, fluid imbalance, and protein loss (Table 8-3).

Peritonitis

Peritonitis is the major complication of peritoneal dialysis, and also the most preventable. Peritonitis usually results from a break in sterile technique or a failure of the equipment. It can also result from a catheter site infection that

TABLE 8-3. PATIENT COMPLICATIONS OF PERITONEAL DIALYSIS

Complication	Probable Cause	Signs and Symptoms
Peritonitis	Break in sterile technique	Cloudy outflow Abdominal pain Nausea and vomiting Fever
Fluid overload	Inaccurate assessment of patient's dry weight Imbalance of intake and output	Hypertension Edema Shortness of breath Increase in weight Congestive heart failure or pulmonary edema
Dehydration	Inaccurate assessment of patient's dry weight Removal of too much fluid from patient	Hypotension Cramping Orthostatic hypotension Dizziness Decrease in weight
Muscle cramps	Too much fluid removed Fluid removed rapidly	Cramping in legs, feet, and hands
Exit site infection	Break in sterile technique	Redness at site Tenderness at site Drainage at site
Tunnel infection	Break in sterile technique	Redness along track Tenderness along track

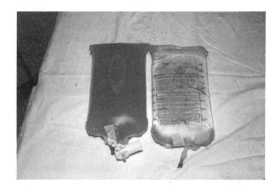

Figure 8-7. Peritonitis dialysate (*left*).

progresses through the tunnel into the peritoneal cavity. Prompt detection and treatment of these infections can, however, prevent peritonitis.

The signs and symptoms of peritonitis include abdominal pain, cloudy dialysate outflow (Fig. 8-7), fever, nausea and vomiting, chills, and catheter flow problems due to fibrin. Cultures, gram stains, and dialysate white blood cell counts are used to confirm the diagnosis of peritonitis. A dialysate white blood cell count over 50 cells per thousand is generally accepted as diagnostic of peritonitis.

Although the use of antibiotics to treat peritonitis is standard, the method of administration is not. One method involves intermittent flushing of the peritoneal cavity with antibiotics in the dialysate. A second method involves the same type of flushing, but with a short dwell time. The most common method is to administer antibiotics intraperitoneally for several days with no alteration in dialysate cycles. This may or may not be combined with systemic antibiotic administration. Regardless of the treatment method, the patient must be observed carefully. Complications of peritonitis include massive protein loss, increased glucose absorption, fibrin formation, decreased leukocytes with lavage, and constipation. If the peritonitis does not respond to the therapy, removal of the catheter must be considered.

Fluid Imbalance

Fluid imbalance may be manifested as fluid overload or fluid depletion. Fluid overload may be caused by the catheter problems described earlier or by fluid abuse by the patient. Regardless of the cause, hypertension can occur if the fluid overload is allowed to persist. Fluid depletion, on the other hand, most often results from the improper or overaggressive use of hypertonic dialysate solutions. Hypotension may occur if the fluid depletion is not treated in a timely fashion. Treatment includes increasing fluid and salt intake and decreasing the tonicity of the dialysate solutions.

Protein Catabolism

Protein is lost in the dialysate fluid. Up to 0.5 to 1.0 g may be lost with every exchange. With situations of increased catabolism, such as peritonitis, protein losses can increase further. The treatment for excessive protein catabolism is to increase the protein intake.

NURSING CARE OF THE PATIENT ON PERITONEAL DIALYSIS

The nursing care of the patient on peritoneal dialysis is usually performed on an outpatient basis except in the acute patient or the chronic patient who is hospitalized temporarily. Much of the nurse's time with the peritoneal dialysis patient is spent in teaching the patient how to perform the procedure at home, and in serving as a resource when problems arise.

Home Training

Home-training the patient in peritoneal dialysis is generally less time-consuming than training the patient in home hemodialysis. Two weeks or 10 training days are usually sufficient. Because the peritoneal procedure occurs more slowly, there is less chance of acute problems that must be corrected immediately. Training takes place in the outpatient setting, in an unhurried and relaxed environment. The patient is taught how to perform a basic physical assessment, with special emphasis on fluid and electrolyte balance, sterile technique, the exchange procedure, machine operation if on IPD or CCPD, and troubleshooting. When the patient is competent in each of these areas, he or she may perform the procedures at home. Posttraining clinic visits serve to reinforce learning, to determine the effectiveness of the dialysis prescription, and to alter the prescription if necessary.

Inpatient Care

In the hospital setting, the peritoneal dialysis nurse is responsible for assessing the patient's status with regard to dialysis, and for performing the dialysis procedure or assisting the staff in performing the procedure. The efficiency of the peritoneal dialysis staff is increased greatly if all of the peritoneal dialysis patients, or at least all of the nonintensive care patients, can be housed on one nursing unit. The peritoneal dialysis nurses can then serve as clinical specialists for peritoneal dialysis. A set of typical physician's orders, as seen in Figure 8–8, illustrates the dialysis care required for the hospitalized peritoneal dialysis patient.

Drugs and Peritoneal Dialysis

The nurse caring for the patient on peritoneal dialysis must be aware of the potential need to adjust drug dosages, both as a result of the presence of ESRD and the use of peritoneal dialysis as a treatment modality. ESRD alters

PHYSICIAN'S ORDERS

To Primary Nurse or General Nursing Staff:
1. Begin ____ Acute ____ Chronic Peritoneal Dialysis per ____ machine at ____ A.M./P.M.
2. Pre Dialysis Lab: HbsAg ____
3. Pre dialysis check & record: Weight, BP ____ lying & standing or sitting, TPR volume status: include any signs of dyspnea edema or venous distention.
4. During dialysis: TPR, BP q ____ hr or ____ daily at ____
   Weight q ____ hr ____
   Measure output q ____ hr ____
5. Notify PD nurse of start time and dialysis related questions or problems. Contact PD nurse on call through page operator
6. Notify physician if:
   a. Fluid retention greater than ____ in ____ hr
   b. Fluid drainage greater than ____ in ____ hr
   c. Systolic BP greater than ____ in ____ hr
   d. Pulse greater than ____ or less than ____
   e. Temperature greater than ____
   f. Appearance of cloudy or bloody dialysate
7. Post dialysis check & record: Weight, BP—lying & standing or sitting, TPR, volume status: include any signs of dyspnea edema or venous distention
8. Post dialysis Lab:

To Peritoneal Dialysis Nurse:
1. Dialysate solution ____ % Addidtives: ____
2. Length of treatment ____ hrs or ____ exchanges
   a. Inflow time ____
   b. Dwell time ____ Infuse ____ cc/exchange
   c. Drain time ____
3. Desired Wt. ____ Remove ____ cc Dry Wt ____
4. Obtain baseline cellcount and differential. If dialysate cloudy or if accidental disconnection of the line occurs obtain cell count and differential, C & S gram stain of effluent
5. Change dialysate K+ to ____ if K+ of patient ____
6. Change dialysate solution to ____ % when patient weight ____
7. Irrigate peritoneal catheter with Normal Saline and ____ p.r.n. obstruction
8. Obtain signed PD consent and file on chart
9. Post dialysis orders:

_____ M.D.

Figure 8-8. Typical physician's orders for hospitalized peritoneal dialysis patients.

the metabolism of many drugs. In addition, some drugs are removed by the peritoneal dialysis process and some are not. The method of peritoneal dialysis must also be considered. The constant nature of CAPD allows increased consistency in drug administration, whereas the fluctuations in blood levels of IPD patients may require more dosage adjustments.

It is also possible to administer drugs by means of a peritoneal dialysis solution. Antibiotics are routinely administered in this manner when peritonitis is present or suspected. The use of the peritoneal solution as a transport for insulin to diabetic patients has been shown to be quite effective.

PROGNOSIS

Peritoneal dialysis is newer than hemodialysis as a chronic treatment modality, so historical evidence on which to base prognoses is limited. The Office of Technology Assessment has reported that in the United States, 1 and 2-year survival rates are comparable for CAPD and hemodialysis; but only 50 to 80 percent of the patients who start on CAPD are still using CAPD at the end of 1 year (Stasen & Barnes, 1985). Kurtz and Johnson (1984) compared CAPD and home hemodialysis patients at the Mayo Clinic in terms of adequacy of dialysis, morbidity, and survival. Survival was similar in both groups at 32 months of therapy. The number of hospitalized days was, however, twice as large in the peritoneal dialysis group. Peritonitis accounted for the difference. Moore and associates (1984) studied the results of CAPD in Europe and found that 1-year patient survival was 87 percent. Additionally, this study found improved survival rates in dialysis centers with more peritoneal dialysis experience.

REFERENCES

Aune, S. (1970). Transperitoneal exchange. II. Peritoneal blood flow estimated by hydrogen gas clearance. *Scad J Gastroenterol, 5,* 99.

Gross, M., McDonald, Jr., H. P. (1967). Effect of dialysate temperature and flow rate on peritoneal clearance. *JAMA, 202,* 363–365.

Kurtz, S. B., & Johnson, W. J. (1984). A four-year comparison of continuous ambulatory peritoneal dialysis and home hemodialysis: A preliminary report. *Mayo Clin Proc, 59,* 659–662.

McDonald, H. P. (1965). An automatic peritoneal dialysis machine: Preliminary report. *Trans Am Soc Artif Intern Organs, 11,* 83–83.

Moore, R., Brunner, F. P., Jacobs, C., et al. (1984). Comparison of the results of CAPD treatment in "experienced" versus "inexperienced" centers in Europe. *Peritoneal Dialysis Bull, 4,* 159–168.

Nolph, K. D. (1983). Peritoneal dialysis. In W. Drucker, F. Parsons, & J. Maher (Eds.), *Replacement of renal function by dialysis.* The Hague: Martinus Nijhoff.

Nolph, K. D. (1986). Peritoneal dialysis. In B. M. Brenner & F. J. Rector, Jr. (eds.), *The kidney* (3rd ed., pp. 1847–1906). Philadelphia:P Saunders.

Nolph, K. D., Ghods, A.J., Brown, P., et al. (1977). Factors affecting peritoneal dialysis efficiency. *Dial Transplant, 6,* 52–90.

Nolph, K. D., Popovich, R. P., Ghods, A. J., & Twardowski, Z. J. (1978). Determinants of low clearances of small solutes during peritoneal dialysis. *Kidney Int, 13,* 117–123.

Nolph, K. D., Miller, F. N., Rubin, J., & Popovich, R. (1980). New directions in peritoneal dialysis concepts and applications. *Kidney Int, 18,* 93.

Renkin, E. M. (1969). Exchange of substances through capillary walls. Circulatory and respiratory mass transport. In Wolstenholme (Ed.), *Ciba Found Symp.* Boston: Little, Brown.

Stasen, W. B., & Barnes, B. A. (1985). *The effectiveness and costs of CAPD.* Health Technology Case Study 35 (OTA-HCS-35). Washington, D.C.: Office of Technology Assessment, U.S. Government Printing Office.

Tenckhoff, H. (1976). Home peritoneal dialysis. In S. G. Massry & A. L. Sellars (Eds.), *Clinical aspects of uremia.* Springfield, Ill.: Chas. C. Thomas.

Veitch, P. (1986). Surgical aspects of CAPD. In R. Gokal (Ed.), *Continuous ambulatory peritoneal dialysis.* Edinburgh: Churchill Livingstone.

Wade, O. L., Combes, B., Childs, A. W., et al. (1956). The effect of exercise on the splantic blood flow and splantic blood volume in normal man. *Clinical Science, 15,* 457–463.

Winchester, J. F. (1986). CAPD systems and solutions. In R. Gokal (Ed.), *Continuous ambulatory peritoneal dialysis.* Edinburgh: Churchill Livingstone.

9

Transplantation

Betty Irwin Crandall

OBJECTIVES

After reading this chapter on renal transplantation, the nurse will be able to:

1. Describe the usual process for assessing and preparing a recipient for renal transplantation, including:

   - Candidacy requirements
   - Contraindications
   - Information needed
   - Tests to be performed

   the personnel usually involved in the process

2. Explain the tissue typing and histocompatibility testing performed prior to transplantation, including the ABO and HLA typing, MLC/MLR test, and cross-matching

3. State at least four criteria used to evaluate the suitability of kidney donors (living-related or cadaver)

4. Describe the usual surgical placement of a transplanted kidney and at least two reasons for its placement in that area

5. State the mechanism of action and major adverse effects of steroids, azathioprine, cyclosporine, antithymocyte preparations, and monoclonal antibodies

6. Describe at least four major complications that may occur following renal transplantation

7. Name the four types of rejection and briefly describe each in terms of its timing, immunologic basis, and clinical characteristics

Renal transplantation has clearly emerged as a universally accepted treatment modality for end-stage renal disease (ESRD). In the decades that have passed since the first transplant was performed in the United States in 1954, significant advances have occurred in surgical techniques, immunology, immunosuppression, and organ preservation. Such developments have allowed renal transplantation to become a treatment modality that compares favorably to hemodialysis and peritoneal dialysis. Patient mortality rates, excessive in the early days of transplantation, have improved dramatically. Graft survival has also significantly improved. Advances continue to be made and one can expect even greater successes in renal transplantation in the near future.

In this expanding era of organ transplantation, it is tempting to consider renal transplantation as the cure for ESRD. Care must be taken not to misrepresent transplantation to patients and their families. There is no real "cure" for ESRD, only several alternative modes of treatment. One of them is renal transplantation. It must be viewed, along with hemodialysis and peritoneal dialysis, as an option. These treatment modalities may be used alone or in combination to provide comprehensive quality care to those suffering from ESRD. Movement from one modality to another must be facilitated and encouraged based upon ongoing individual patient assessment.

No longer is transplantation limited to a few large teaching institutions. Most nurses in nephrology will have some involvement in renal transplantation: referring and preparing patients for transplant, providing posttransplant care, or providing dialysis care if a transplant is unsuccessful. The growth of renal transplantation as a treatment option and the rapid expansion of scientific knowledge in the field demand that nephrology nurses be educated and well prepared to provide care to this patient population.

RECIPIENT SELECTION AND PREPARATION

Candidacy

Renal transplantation is a treatment option for most patients with ESRD. There are few conditions that are absolute contraindications. Patients with other end-organ disease, such as severe pulmonary or cardiac disease, may be too ill to safely undergo surgery, and so may not be candidates. Such persons include those with a recent myocardial infarction and those with severe chronic obstructive pulmonary disease. Active or incurable malignancy is also a contraindication to transplantation.

Age is a consideration; however, it is the physiological rather than chronological age that is important. In the past, most transplant centers held

55 to 60 years as the upper age limit for eligibility. With recent developments in immunosuppressive therapy, many centers report a willingness to transplant older individuals. Transplantation remains the preferred method of treating children with ESRD. There is no lower age limit, although recipient size may severely limit donor organ availability and tax the technical skill of the surgeon.

Transplantation must not be undertaken in an individual with an active infectious process of any kind. Hepatitis is often a concern. A prior history of hepatitis or hepatitis B antigenemia need not preclude transplantation, although active hepatitis is a contraindication and may delay transplantation for an indefinite period. Other common sites of infection in dialysis patients include the pulmonary system, vascular access sites, and the peritoneum in those treated by peritoneal dialysis.

Candidacy for renal transplantation is decided on the basis of multiple physiological, psychological, and sociological factors. Transplantation should be discussed with all ESRD patients. For those in the early phases of renal failure, especially those with a living-related donor, transplantation without the need for frequent dialysis (known as primary transplantation) may be an option. For other patients, dialysis may need to be initiated prior to consideration of transplantation. The patient's desire for a transplant is an important factor. There are no guarantees and many potential problems. No patient should be "talked into" pursuing transplantation against his or her wishes.

The final issue to be addressed is adherence to the prescribed therapeutic regimen. To the extent possible, assessment must be made of an individual's capacity and willingness to comply to the medical regimen after transplant. Although a history of nonadherence to the many restrictions of a dialysis regimen need not exclude an individual from transplantation, it must be considered and discussed prior to transplantation. Because transplantation is a less restrictive regimen than that during dialysis, adherence is often less of a problem. Those expressing great concern about changes in physical appearance and body image should be identified as a greater risk for nonadherence with a posttransplant regimen due to the changes caused by immunosuppressive medications.

Assessment and Preparation of the Recipient

Patients are referred for transplant evaluation by the nephrologist, primary physician, or dialysis unit, and are seen by the members of the transplant team during a visit to the transplant institution. Extensive medical, psychosocial, and immunologic evaluations are conducted and the patient and family are educated about renal transplantation.

In most transplant centers, the evaluation process occurs in the outpatient setting over a 1- to 2-day period. Records from the patient's referring nephrologist and dialysis unit are reviewed. Patient and family interviews are conducted. Blood is usually drawn for tissue typing and screening of the potential recipient and any possible living-related donors. Other lab testing is performed as indicated. Members of the transplant team usually involved are the transplant surgeon, nephrologist, transplant nurse, and social worker. A psychologist or psychiatrist may also see the patient.

The purpose of the evaluation visit is to individually assess each patient as a candidate for transplantation, taking into consideration his or her individual risk factors. Particular attention must be paid to the following factors (Table 9-1).

Renal Disease. If possible, the patient's primary renal disease should be determined. No disease that causes ESRD categorically excludes a patient from consideration for transplantation. Certain diseases do, however, warrant special consideration. Patients with polycystic kidney disease may require a

TABLE 9-1. ASSESSMENT AND PREPARATION OF THE RECIPIENT

Systems and Areas of Consideration	Factors to Be Evaluated
Etiology of renal disease	Need for bilateral nephrectomy (polycystic disease, chronic pyelonephritis, refractory hypertension) Likelihood of reoccurrence of original disease (lupus nephritis, Goodpasture's syndrome, hemolytic uremia)
Function of urinary tract	Bladder size and emptying Evidence of reflux Enlargement of the prostate Patency of uretha
Cardiovascular system	Patency of iliac vasculature Degree of atherosclerotic disease Cardiac function Degree of coronary artery disease
Gastrointestinal system	Evidence of peptic ulcer disease, pancreatitis, gall bladder disease, diverticulosis Liver function
Pulmonary system	Evidence of COPD History of tuberculosis History of smoking
Endocrine and metabolic systems	Diabetes mellitus Evidence of hyperparathyroidism
Oral cavity and dental evaluation	Evidence of dental caries or other infections in mouth
Psychosocial evaluation	History of psychiatric illness Desire and motivation to undergo transplantation

bilateral nephrectomy pretransplant to avoid posttransplant complications such as infection and bleeding from the cysts once the patient is immunosuppressed. Patients who have had chronic pyelonephritis will have the potentially infected kidneys removed prior to instituting immunosuppressive therapy. Likewise, patients with hypertension refractory to medical management may require a bilateral nephrectomy prior to transplant, in order to control renin production and thus blood pressure. This is desirable to assure that the transplanted kidney is not damaged by uncontrolled hypertension. Patients with Goodpasture's syndrome, hemolytic uremia, and lupus nephritis, generally must wait until the disease process is quiescent or "burned out" so that the original disease does not damage the newly transplanted kidney.

Urinary System. The patient's bladder must be functional and the lower urinary tract must be patent and allow for complete emptying of the bladder. Cystoscopy, voiding cystourethrograms, and cystometrograms may all be useful in this evaluation. These tests should be considered in any patient with a history of reflux and chronic infection and in those with a neurogenic bladder. Diabetic neuropathy may affect bladder control and emptying and these patients should also undergo a urologic workup. Children with congenital anomalies of the urinary tract must be completely evaluated pretransplant. Elderly men may have prostatic enlargement, which partially obstructs outflow. Recognition and surgical correction of these problems prior to transplantation will help prevent postoperative complications.

Cardiovascular System. Patients with renal failure have accelerated atherosclerosis, with an increased incidence of myocardial infarction, cerebrovascular accidents, and hypertension. As such, they are at increased risk to undergo general anesthesia and major surgery. Pretransplant evaluation should include studies to determine cardiac function, the patency of the iliac vasculature, and the degree of atherosclerotic disease present. Those with severe coronary artery disease may require bypass surgery prior to transplant. In some instances, cardiovascular disease may be so advanced as to be a contraindication to transplantation.

Gastrointestinal System. Peptic ulcer disease and intestinal diverticuli may cause life-threatening complications following transplantation. Steroids increase the risk of gastrointestinal bleeding and perforation. These conditions must be recognized pretransplant. They may require aggressive medical management or even surgical correction. Studies such as an upper GI series, barium enema, or endoscopy may be required.

Liver function should be carefully evaluated with the usual laboratory studies (bilirubin, LDH, SGOT, SGPT, alkaline phosphatase). Chronic hepatitis and cirrhosis may be contraindications to transplant. Chronic hepatitis B antigenemia need not exclude a patient. Because both azathioprine and cyclosporine may be hepatotoxic, careful assessment of baseline hepatic function is essential pretransplant. Pancreatitis and gall bladder disease may also require pretreatment.

Pulmonary System. Infections of the pulmonary system are common after transplantation. Preoperative evaluation should identify patients such as smokers, those with chronic obstructive pulmonary disease (COPD), and those with a past history of tuberculosis who are at an increased risk for postoperative pulmonary problems. Smoking should be discouraged. Patients with tuberculosis may require indefinite treatment. The risk of morbidity and mortality may be so high for patients with severe COPD or other pulmonary compromise as to exclude transplantation.

Endocrine and Metabolic Systems. The complications associated with systemic endocrine or metabolic diseases may increase the risks of transplantation. Most centers now transplant diabetics with ESRD in great numbers because the success of treating them with transplantation is greater than the success of long-term dialysis in such patients. These patients are at greater risk for developing complications. Wound healing is delayed in diabetic recipients. Infections are seen more frequently in diabetics and tend to be more difficult to treat. The atherosclerotic process is accelerated in diabetic renal transplant recipients. Despite a successful transplant, peripheral vascular disease, coronary disease, and cerebrovascular disease may result in limb loss, myocardial infarctions, and cerebrovascular accidents. Steroids increase insulin requirements in these patients and make glucose control an even greater challenge.

Many ESRD patients have evidence of hyperparathyroidism due to poor control of calcium and phosphorus over a number of years. The pretransplant evaluation process should include an assessment of the degree of parathyroid involvement. Some patients will require surgical removal of the glands prior to transplant. Unrecognized and untreated, hyperparathyroidism can result in an excessive level of serum calcium posttransplant when renal fuction normalizes. Calcium can then be rapidly deposited in the kidney and cause irreparable damage.

Oral Cavity and Dental Evaluation. Dental caries and other untreated infections in the mouth may result in major complications posttransplant when the patient is on immunosuppressive therapy. The administration of cyclosporine may result in gingival hyperplasia, bleeding and soreness in the gums. Patients should be examined by a dentist or oral surgeon pretransplant and have all preventive and corrective dental work performed.

Psychosocial Evaluation. No standard criteria or tests exist to determine psychosocial suitability for transplant. As stated previously,two major areas to be explored are the patient's desire and motivation to undergo transplant and his or her ability to adhere to the prescribed regimen. Formal psychological or psychiatric evaluation may be helpful in the assessment of these two areas.

Patients with a history of psychiatric illness are at risk for further complications because of the stress associated with the surgery and treatment and because of the effects of steroid therapy. Steroids may produce emotional lability and aggravate an underlying psychiatric condition. In these cases, pretransplant psychiatric evaluation is essential and continued treatment posttransplant is indicated.

TRANSPLANTATION IMMUNOLOGY

The success of transplantation depends upon being able to surgically place a foreign tissue in a recipient and then alter the individual's immune response so that rejection does not occur. As transplantation has evolved, efforts have been directed to two separate but related aspects of transplantation immunology: matching of donor tissue to the recipient and altering the recipient's ability to recognize and respond to the foreign tissue. The second of these, the rejection response and preventing and treating rejection with various immunosuppressive regimens, will be discussed later in the chapter. The present section concentrates on identifying the transplant antigens, matching of donor and recipient, ABO compatibility, and pretransplant immunologic modifications.

ABO Compatibility

For successful transplantation to occur, the donor and recipient must be compatible for the major blood group. *ABO typing*, performed on red blood cells, must be done. Minor red blood cell antigens (such as Rh) do not seem to play a role in transplantation. ABO compatibility for transplantation follows the rules used to assure compatibility for blood transfusion. Thus, those with blood type O are universal organ donors while those with blood type AB are universal recipients.

The HLA Region and Tissue Typing

Understanding transplant immunology requires a basic knowledge of human genetics. Each human ovum and spermatozoan has 23 chromosomes. When they are joined at fertilization, 46 chromosomes (23 pairs) are present. Individuals thereby inherit one half of their genetic material from each parent. *Genes* are structures located on the chromosome that carry the inherited code for protein and enzyme synthesis. *Antigens* are protein molecules on the surfaces of cells. Their structure is determined by genes located on the chromosomes. Antigens are the structures that stimulate an immune response. Antigen expression is an inherited trait.

Antigens expressed on almost all body cell surfaces, but most readily identified on white blood cells (leukocytes), have been determined to be those most important in transplantation. They have been named the *human leukocyte antigens (HLAs)* and are known as the major histocompatibility

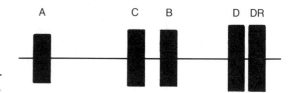

Figure 9-1. Portion of sixth chromosome showing four HLA loci.

complex. *Histocompatibility* refers to the compatibility between donor and recipient. A single genetic region located on the sixth chromosome controls the expression of these antigens. Experts are now able to identify antigens coded at four regions (or *loci*) of the sixth chromosome. These loci, shown diagramatically in Figure 9-1, are known as the A, B, C, and D (or DR) regions. Because each individual has a pair of number 6 chromosomes, we are then able to identify eight specific HLA antigens, four coded on each chromosome. Many other antigens are coded at other loci on that portion of the chromosome but have not yet been identified.

The HLA region is inherited as a haplotype, one of a pair of chromosomes from each parent. Each haplotype contains an A, B, C, and D (or DR) gene coding for the respective antigen. Figure 9-2 shows diagrammatically the inheritance of HLA antigens in a family. Each offspring of the same biological parents can be seen to have a 25 percent chance of being the same HLA type as another of the offspring (HLA identical); a 25 percent chance of being totally HLA dissimilar; and a 50 percent possibility of sharing half of the HLA identity of a sibling (1-haplotype match). Because of this inheritance pattern, when two close family members are found to share antigens found on the same haplotype, it is known that even the antigens we cannot yet identify but that are located on that haplotype will be identical. Unrelated individuals may share one or more HLA antigens. However, because they did not inherit the genetic codes as a haplotype, one cannot expect that they share any other unidentified antigens. This helps to explain why HLA matching between unrelated donors and recipients has not been as successful as between related donor-recipient pairs.

HLA typing is done by lymphocytotoxicity testing performed on a venous blood sample. Lymphocytes are exposed to antisera with known antibodies. If the lymphocytes carry a cell surface antigen that is recognized by

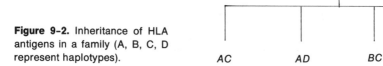

Figure 9-2. Inheritance of HLA antigens in a family (A, B, C, D represent haplotypes).

the antibodies, the lymphocytes are lysed. One can then identify the specific HLA antigen to which the antibody is reacting. The antisera used for HLA typing are internationally standardized, and sharing mechanisms are established for obtaining serum containing rare antibodies. In renal transplantation, recipients and donors are typed to identify their HLA antigens. Once an individual has been HLA-typed (sometimes referred to as tissue typing), this study need not be repeated. One's HLA antigens are genetically determined and do not change.

Other Histocompatibility Tests

Two tests, in addition to ABO and HLA typing, provide the basis of histocompatibility testing in renal transplantation: white blood cell cross-matching and the mixed lymphocyte culture. The *white blood cell cross-match* is performed to detect preformed antibodies in the recipient directed against the antigens expressed on the donor cells. This test, which resembles the red blood cell cross-matching done prior to administering a blood transfusion, is performed by mixing donor lymphocytes with recipient serum. If antibodies to the donor HLA antigens are present in the recipient serum, the cross-match will be positive and transplantation must not occur. The transplanted kidney would be rejected immediately. The presence of these antibodies in the serum varies over time. Therefore, specimens must be drawn on a regular basis to screen development of new antibodies. In addition, in the case of cadaveric transplantation, a current sample must always be available to test for antibodies against potential donors.

The final test, the *mixed lymphocyte culture or reaction* (MLC/MLR), is performed only in the case of living-related donor transplantation. It is used to determine the degree of D-locus compatibility between the donor and recipient. Lymphocytes from both donor and recipient are incubated for a 5-day period. Cell surface differences are determined by measuring the proliferative response of these lymphocytes in vitro. The MLC is used to confirm HLA identity and to determine the degree of compatibility at the D-locus between living-related donor-recipient pairs. Because of the time required for incubation, an MLC is not feasible for cadaveric donor transplants.

Methods of Pretransplant Immunologic Modification

Most efforts aimed at preventing rejection of a transplanted kidney consist of drug therapy administered after transplantation. However, a few pretransplant interventions are directed to modifying the immune response prior to transplanting the organ. These include pretransplant blood transfusion, splenectomy, total lymphoid irradiation, and thoracic duct drainage.

Pretransplant Blood Transfusions. Many studies, beginning with Dr. Terasaki in 1973, have demonstrated the beneficial effects of pretransplant blood transfusions on graft survival in patients receiving renal transplants (Opelz, Sengar, Mickey, & Terasaki, 1973; Opelz, 1985). The exact mechanism by which these beneficial effects are achieved is not understood. In fact, transfusing patients prior to transplant, and thus exposing them to foreign antigens, would seem to be contrary to basic immunologic principles. It would seem that such patients would become sensitized and in fact have a decreased graft survival rate. However, in patients treated with conventional immunosuppressive agents (not cyclosporine), most centers in the world have demonstrated that graft survival rates are significantly improved in those patients who have received multiple blood transfusions prior to transplant (Spees et al., 1980). These beneficial effects are greatest for those who receive cadaveric kidneys. The evidence of the beneficial effects of pretransplant blood transfusions is not as compelling in cyclosporine-treated patients (Klintmalm et al., 1985). Perhaps cyclosporine will be shown to improve graft survival so significantly that no additional advantage would be achieved by encouraging multiple pretransplant blood transfusions. The data to substantiate this claim are still being generated.

More recently, many centers have adopted a protocol of *donor-specific transfusion* (DST) between HLA-mismatched living-related donors and recipients. The original reports of improved graft survival to that of the HLA-identical donor-recipient population were generated at the University of California, San Francisco where the protocol was first implemented in 1978 (Salvatierra et al., 1980). According to the standard protocol, a unit of blood from the donor is divided into aliquots (usually three) and transfused to the recipient over a 6-week period of time. Immune responsiveness of the recipient is measured by cross-match testing. If the recipient does not develop antibodies to the donor during the transfusion process, the transplant is performed within a month of the last transfusion. Graft survival rates in the 85 to 90 percent range can be expected (Salvatierra et al., 1983).

There are two potential benefits of pretransplant blood transfusion: improved success of transplantation and correction of the patient's anemia. The major risk is that the patient may develop cytotoxic antibodies, making transplantation more difficult. The other risk is the transmission of infections such as hepatitis, cytomegalovirus (CMV), and AIDS.

Splenectomy. Splenectomy prior to transplantation or at the time of transplant is advocated by a few centers. It reduces lymphoid mass, thus decreasing lymphocyte production (Briggs, 1984). It is a major surgical procedure with the potential for many complications. Most centers do not routinely perform splenectomy.

Total Lymphoid Irradiation. Total lymphoid irradiation is also a procedure performed to reduce lymphocyte production in an attempt to prevent graft rejection. It involves low-dose radiation of the thoracic-abdominal lymphatic system (Hopper, Sweeney, & Pierce, 1984). Few centers currently advocate its use because of problems with over-immunosuppression and the development of life-threatening infection.

Thoracic Duct Drainage. Like splenectomy and total lymphoid irradiation, thoracic duct drainage is performed to deplete the lymphatic system of lymphocytes. It involves draining the lymphatic system through an indwelling catheter in the right or left thoracic lymph duct. The fluid drained undergoes pheresis to remove the lymphocytes and then is returned to the patient (Taylor, 1981). It is a cumbersome procedure that may place the patient at greatly increased risk from infection. In addition, the timing of the transplant must be such that the patient is in a lymphocyte-depleted state when he or she receives the kidney. For these reasons and with the advent of improved immunosuppressants, few centers now employ thoracic duct drainage.

SOURCES OF DONOR KIDNEYS

Both living-related and cadaver donors may be the source of kidneys for transplantation. Currently, about two thirds of the kidneys transplanted in the United States are from cadaver donors (U.S. ESRD Program, 1984). Kidneys do not need to be matched between donor and recipient for age, sex, or race. Matching for size between donor and recipient is rarely necessary. Kidneys from pediatric donors hypertrophy within a few months to be functionally suitable for adult recipients. Except in the case of very small children, pediatric recipients can accommodate an adult-sized kidney. Sometimes, in order to do so, the kidney must be placed in the abdominal cavity rather than as usual in the retroperitoneal space.

The Living-related Donor

When a patient with ESRD is evaluated for transplantation, the potential for living-related donors is usually explored with the patient and family. Most centers currently operate under the belief that a well-matched living-related donor offers the best chance of successful transplantation to patients with ESRD. In addition, the significant shortage of cadaveric donor organs nationwide makes it difficult to adopt a policy of using no living-related donors. A few centers have achieved such success with cadaveric donor transplantation and have an ample supply of donor organs locally that they prefer not to use living-related donors. Although some animal studies have shown proteinuria and hypertension developing as a result of unilateral nephrectomy (Brenner, 1983), studies of living-related kidney donors have failed to show significant health problems developing even many years after donation (Velosa et al., 1985). Therefore, most experts agree that the use of living-related donors is safe and ethical.

Except in unusual circumstances (for example, in cases of identical twins), minors are not allowed to be living-related donors. If a child is to be considered, permission must be obtained through the courts or by appointing a guardian. Current practice also discourages the use of living donors other than close blood relatives, because the success rates with living nonrelated donors have not differed significantly from those with cadaver donors. Studies currently underway, most involving donor specific transfusion, may alter that practice in the future. Recent legislation outlaws the sale of organs for transplant.

Selection and Evaluation of the Living-related Donor. A reasonable first step in the evaluation of potential living-related donors is to perform an initial health screening to exclude persons with obvious health problems (such as diabetes and hypertension) that would prevent donation. Very early in the evaluation process, ABO and HLA typing are performed to determine histocompatibility. Of those willing and medically suitable to be donors, the person who is the best HLA match will most often be chosen.

Once the most likely living-related donor has been identified, that person will undergo an extensive medical evaluation designed to assure the presence of normal kidney function and that there are no other health problems that could place the donor at increased risk to undergo nephrectomy. The medical evaluation will include a complete history and physical examination, chest x-ray, electrocardiogram, and blood studies for hematology, chemistries, and coagulation. Urine studies including urinalysis, urine culture, urinary protein excretion, and creatinine clearance are performed and must be within normal limits. Other studies, such as a glucose tolerance test, pulmonary function tests, or stress ECGs, may be performed if the potential donor's history or initial medical evaluation warrant them. If there is a history of familial renal disease, special studies such as genetic testing or even a renal biopsy may be indicated.

Renal anatomy and functioning must be evaluated with great care. Sonograms, renal scans, and intravenous pyelograms may be used. The decision about the particular tests to be performed is made by those involved in donor evaluation at a given center. A renal arteriogram to outline the renal vasculature is performed as a final step in the evaluation process. This is important so the surgeon performing the donor nephrectomy knows prior to surgery of the existence of any accessory vessels.

Throughout the evaluation process, it is important to assess the individual's motivation to donate. There must be no evidence that an unwilling person is being coerced into becoming a donor. Psychological evaluation may be helpful in this regard. If a potential donor indicates an unwillingness to proceed, the reasons for his or her decision must be kept confidential so as not to disrupt family relationships. The donor will require information, education, and emotional support throughout all phases of the evaluation process as well as pre- and postoperatively.

Living-related Donor Nephrectomy. The donor nephrectomy is a major surgical procedure that takes 3 to 4 hours. A traditional flank incision is used. Care must be taken to prevent ischemic damage to the kidney as well as to assure an adequate length of renal artery, renal vein, and ureter to facilitate anastomosis in the recipient.

Postoperative care of the living-related donor is the same as for anyone undergoing a unilateral nephrectomy. Early ambulation, good respiratory toilet, adequate pain relief, and adequate hydration are important aspects of the nursing role. Nurses must also remember to provide support to the donor, as he or she often becomes the forgotten patient when the family's attention focuses on the recipient.

Results of Living-related Donor Transplantation. If a patient receives an HLA-identical renal transplant, one can expect a 1-year graft survival of 95 to 99 percent. Long-term graft survival should remain well above 90 percent. In HLA-mismatched living-related renal transplants, the graft survival averages 85 to 90 percent at one year if donor specific transfusion is performed pre-transplant. Without DST, graft survival rates for the 1-haplotype living-related donor transplant are 70 to 80 percent at 1 year (Morris, 1984).

The Cadaveric Donor

Cadaveric donors account for most of the kidneys used for transplantation. These donors are usually healthy children or young adults who are victims of sudden trauma or other cerebral injury that results in brain death. To preserve organ viability, these individuals must be maintained on life-support systems.

Specific criteria for cadaveric renal donors vary among centers. However, the following general criteria apply:

1. Age 1 year to 65 years
2. No history of malignancy (except for primary brain tumor)
3. No history of renal disease or hypertension
4. No systemic infections
5. Adequate renal function (generally measured by urine output, creatinine, and blood urea nitrogen)
6. Diagnosis of brain death

Brain Death. The diagnosis of brain death is made by the patient's primary physician or by a neurologist or neurosurgeon acting as a consultant. Members of the transplant and procurement teams must not be involved in the declaration of brain death. The medical community generally recognizes brain death as a legitimate set of criteria for determining death. However, not all states have passed legislation making it a legal form of death. In those states that have not, organ recovery efforts have been hindered by fear of litigation unless cardiopulmonary arrest occurs.

Brain death is a clinical determination. The patient must not be hypothermic and must be free of all central nervous system depressants for the diagnosis to be made. Careful evaluation of the patient must demonstrate:

1. Complete apnea despite levels of CO_2 sufficient to trigger respiration
2. Absence of all spontaneous movement
3. Unresponsiveness
4. Absence of all cephalic reflexes (spinal cord reflexes may continue to be present)

An electroencephalogram (EEG) may be used to confirm the clinical findings. An EEG shows electrocerebral silence in the brain dead individual. Increasingly, studies to demonstrate the absence of cerebral blood flow are being employed to confirm the diagnosis. This is particularly important if it cannot be established with certainty that the patient is free of all possible drug intoxicants. Death occurs once a qualified physician, often a neurologist or neurosurgeon, determines that the individual meets all of the appropriate criteria for brain death. The bodily functions of the individual are then maintained until consent for organ donation can be obtained and until any organs that can be transplanted can be surgically removed.

Donor Maintenance. While the appropriate clinical and laboratory tests are being performed to make the diagnosis of brain death, attention must be directed to maintaining organ viability. Maintaining adequate urine output and sustaining the patient's blood pressure are key to preserving viable organs for transplant. In most instances, adequate hydration and the use of low doses of vasopressors will accomplish these goals. Because diabetes insipidus frequently occurs in brain-dead individuals, vasopressin may need to be administered.

During this time, additional tests may be performed to assure that no systemic infections are present. These tests should include screening for syphilis, hepatitis, and AIDS as well as cultures of the blood, urine, and respiratory secretions.

Consent for Donation. Although some adults may have indicated their desire to be organ donors by signing a uniform organ donor card, organ procurement agencies and transplant programs request agreement from the family. In most instances, there will be no evidence of the wishes of the deceased in the form of a donor card. In such cases, permission from the next of kin is required by law. Consent from the legal next of kin may be obtained by members of the transplant or procurement teams or by the patient's primary physician. Many physicians prefer that the organ procurement team obtain consent so that there is no hint of a conflict of interest.

The majority of family members are willing to consent to donation when they are approached about organ donation compassionately and at an appropriate time and when they understand that there is no chance for the deceased to recover. As a result of heightened public awareness of the need for organ donors, an increasing number of families actually introduce the topic of organ donation themselves.

Activities surrounding the declaration of brain death and obtaining consent for donation are stressful for the families as well as for members of the health care team. Organ donors are generally healthy young individuals who have suffered a sudden tragic death. This is devastating for all concerned. Support for the family and friends of the deceased must be provided by nursing and medical personnel, social workers, crisis intervention workers, and members of the clergy. It is also vital to remember the support needs of the nurses and physicians caring for the potential donor.

Organ Recovery and Preservation. The bilateral nephrectomy is performed under sterile conditions in the operating room. Oxygenation and circulation are maintained until all transplantable organs have been removed. The goal is to minimize warm ischemic time. Thus, the kidneys are usually flushed in situ with a cold intracellular solution high in potassium prior to their removal. Heparinization prevents blood clotting in the small vessels of the kidney. Regitine or Dibenzyline are administered to reduce vasospasm. Diuretics may be given to the donor to increase urine flow.

Specific techniques for bilateral nephrectomy vary depending on the surgeon's preference and on whether other organs for transplant are being recovered. The multiorgan donor presents a special challenge in coordination to assure that all organs remain viable. Despite the particular surgical technique, the kidneys must be carefully dissected. It is important that multiple renal arteries and veins be identified and preserved. The ureter must be dissected free to the bladder. Particular attention must be directed to preserving the vasculature of the ureter.

Once the kidneys are removed, one of two methods of renal preservation is employed. The simplest and least expensive is the cold storage technique. Here, the kidneys are flushed and instilled with a cold synthetic intracellular solution. In this hypothermic state, cellular metabolism is slowed and ischemic damage to the cells of the kidney minimized. The kidneys are packaged in sterile containers, submerged in solution, and packed in ice. Kidneys preserved using cold storage are viable for 24 to 36 hours, and some centers have reported successful transplantation of kidneys preserved in this way for 72 hours.

The other method of renal preservation is pulsatile perfusion, in which a machine pumps a cooled nutrient solution (plasmanate, albumin, or cryoprecipitated plasma) through the renal vasculature. This method decreases cellular metabolism as well as providing nutrients and oxygen to the cells and removing the waste products of metabolism. In addition, it allows for monitoring of the temperature, pressure, and rate of flow of the perfusate. These parameters provide information about organ viability. Kidney viability may be maintained for 48 to 72 hours using pulsatile perfusion.

Both methods of preserving cadaveric donor kidneys allow sufficient time for HLA typing of the donor and selection of a suitable recipient from the national computerized listing. Potential recipients for cadaver kidneys can be listed on the national computerized list maintained by the United Network for Organ Sharing (UNOS). Each transplant center and procurement team has access to a computer terminal through which they can access the system. In this way, donated kidneys can be matched with the most suitable recipient anywhere in the country. Once the recipient has been located, the kidney can be transported to the appropriate location for transplantation.

Results of Cadaveric Donor Transplantation. With recent developments in immunosuppression, specifically cyclosporine, the results of cadaver donor transplantation have improved dramatically. Most centers now report 1-year graft survival rates of 65 to 85 percent. This compares quite favorably with graft survival rates of 50 to 60 percent in most centers using conventional immunosuppressive therapy (Schoenberg, 1984).

RECIPIENT TRANSPLANT SURGERY

The transplanted kidney is usually placed in the anterior iliac fossa on either the right or left side. This position is preferred over the usual anatomic position for several reasons. The vascular and ureteral anastomoses are easier because the kidney is closer to the blood vessels and bladder. The recipient need not undergo nephrectomy to allow placement of the transplant. The recipient's postoperative recovery is less complicated because the abdominal cavity is not entered. Assessment of the kidney by palpation, auscultation, and renal biopsy is made much easier, aiding in the diagnosis of rejection or other complications. Finally, reoperation to repair or remove the kidney, if necessary, is facilitated.

The renal artery is anastomosed end-to-end to the hypogastric artery or end-to-side to the external iliac artery. The renal vein is sewn to the iliac vein (end-to-side). Usually, the donor ureter is implanted into the recipient's bladder using a technique known as a ureteroneocystostomy. Some surgeons prefer to connect the donor ureter to a stump of the recipient's own ureter (ureteroureterostomy). Occasionally, the donor ureter may be damaged or too short to allow ureteroneocystostomy. In such cases, a ureteroureterostomy must be performed. The donor ureter is tunneled through the submucosal layer of the bladder. This tunnel acts as a one-way valve to prevent reflux of urine when the bladder contracts to empty. By preventing reflux, the danger of infection in the transplanted kidney is reduced.

When a small child receives a kidney from an adult donor, the kidney may be so large that it must be placed in the abdominal cavity. In such cases, the renal artery and renal vein are anastomosed end-to-side to the aorta and vena cava. Such patients usually have a slightly longer recuperation period after surgery because the abdominal cavity has been entered.

Transplant surgery usually takes 3 to 5 hours. Postoperatively, recipients go to a unit where they can receive intensive nursing care and monitoring.

IMMEDIATE POSTOPERATIVE CARE

The care of a patient immediately after transplantation is essentially that of any patient who has undergone major surgery and has had general anesthesia. Nursing care involves careful monitoring of the patient to assure that cardiovascular function is stable and that respiratory efforts are sufficient to adequately oxygenate the tissues. Transplant recipients will return from surgery with a urinary catheter in place to drain the bladder and to accurately measure urine output. A wound catheter is often placed to allow for drainage of any blood, lymph, or other fluid from the area where the kidney was placed. This helps to prevent the accumulation of fluid that could obstruct the flow of urine or that could later become infected. Frequently, a central venous pressure line will have been inserted to more adequately assess fluid replacement needs. Arterial lines and other lines for invasive monitoring may be present if the patient's condition warrants.

In addition to the care necessary for any patient after major surgery, the transplant recipient has some special needs. Care focuses on three specific objectives: assessing renal function, assuring fluid and electrolyte balance, and preventing infection.

Assessment of Renal Function

Immediate Function or Acute Tubular Necrosis (ATN). The newly transplanted kidney may function immediately or it may take days or weeks before it clears wastes adequately to allow dialysis to be discontinued. Immediate function is ideal and simplifies the management of the patient. However, many patients who receive renal transplants do not experience immediate function. Acute tubular necrosis (ATN) due to ischemia is the most common reason for nonfunction after transplantation. This is especially likely if a cadaver donor kidney was transplanted 24 hours or longer after surgical procurement. ATN involves damage to the tubules of the nephron and is a reversible condition, but the damage repair cannot be hastened by treatment. The tubular cells almost always regenerate and renal function returns. This process may take 6 weeks or longer to complete. During this time the patient usually must remain on dialysis to control fluid and electrolytes and to clear uremic wastes.

Acute tubular necrosis may take two forms: oliguric or nonoliguric. In oliguric ATN, urine volumes are less than 400 cc daily (for an adult). Potassium and fluid balance are more difficult to control. Dialysis two or three times weekly is required. For those with nonoliguric ATN, potassium levels and fluid balance are usually less of a problem. Dialysis may or may not be required.

Evaluation of Renal Function. The assessment of renal function for a transplant recipient is performed on a continual basis. It begins in the immediate postoperative period. Many parameters are considered in evaluating the function of the transplanted kidney. These include:

1. Urine output
2. Blood urea nitrogen (BUN)
3. Serum creatinine
4. Creatinine clearance
5. Fluid balance (as determined by daily weights, blood pressure, and the presence or absence of edema)
6. Ultrasound studies (sonograms). A sonogram is frequently done in the first few days after transplantation especially if oliguria or anuria is present. Ultrasound studies can be used to exclude obstruction as a cause of reduced urine volumes. Obstruction can occur as a result of a ureteral kink, a clot lodged in the urinary tract, or from external compression. Sonography can also be used to exclude a large perinephric collection such as a urinoma, lymphocele, or hematoma
7. Renal scans (renograms). A baseline renal scan is usually performed in the first 24 to 48 hours postoperatively. Renal scans allow evaluation of perfusion to the transplanted kidney as well as assessing the function of the graft. Problems with the vascular anastomoses can often be seen on renal scan. If problems are suspected, angiography can be used to more clearly delineate the vasculature. Rejection can also be demonstrated by using nuclear medicine studies
8. Renal biopsy. A percutaneous renal biopsy may be performed to aid in the determination of the reasons for less than optimal renal function. The results of a biopsy may assist in making a differential diagnosis when rejection, acute tubular necrosis, cyclosporine toxicity, or recurrence of the patient's original disease may be possibilities

Nursing care in the immediate postoperative period must include careful assessment of renal function. Accurate records of intake and output, daily weights, and vital signs are essential. Nurses should monitor the patient's laboratory studies such as BUN and creatinine. When special studies are planned, patients must be prepared physically as well as having the exam carefully explained to them. The recipients of renal transplants require much education and explanation. If the kidney is not functioning immediately after surgery due to ATN, patients need to understand that such primary nonfunction will not alter their chances for an ultimately successful kidney transplant.

Assurance of Fluid and Electrolyte Balance

In the immediate postoperative period, careful attention must be paid by nurses and physicians to fluid and electrolyte balance. Common problems include fluid overload or dehydration, hyperkalemia, and hyperglycemia.

Fluid balance may be assessed by keeping accurate hourly records of intake and output, monitoring the patient's central venous pressure (CVP), and recording weights daily at the same time and using the same scale. If the kidney functions immediately, urine volumes may be excessive and it is easy for the patient to become dehydrated. Replacement fluids must be administered. The CVP gives a good indication of intravascular volume and may be used to judge fluid needs. When the kidney does not function immediately, fluid overload may quickly appear, because patients usually receive large volumes of fluid in the operating room and during the first few postoperative hours. Dialysis may be required to remove fluid and prevent complications such as congestive heart failure and pulmonary edema.

Hyperkalemia may rapidly become a life-threatening problem if not closely monitored. A poorly functioning kidney compounded by tissue destruction during surgery and stored red blood cells transfused in surgery or immediately thereafter may result in dangerously high levels of serum potassium. Potassium levels must be closely monitored and hyperkalemia aggressively treated.

In many patients, hyperglycemia may become a problem if large volumes of dextrose-containing intravenous fluids are administered. If this is noted, intravenous fluids without dextrose may be used as replacement fluid.

Other electrolyte abnormalities may occur depending on the patient's urine output and the types of intravenous fluids used as replacement. Nurses must frequently monitor electrolytes and advise physicians of abnormalities present.

Prevention of Infection

Immediately after a transplant, patients are particularly vulnerable to the development of infectious complications. High doses of immunosuppressive medications are being administered. Many invasive lines and catheters offer an easy access for organisms to enter the body. Great care must be taken to use aseptic technique and to assure a clean environment so that the risk of infection is minimized.

REJECTION

Rejection is a normal physiological reaction of the immune system to a foreign organ. Unchecked, it will result in destruction of the graft. All the studies previously mentioned to match donor and recipient, and the interventions performed to modify the immune system before transplantation, have one

purpose—to prevent rejection. Although helpful, they alone are not sufficient. Immunosuppression posttransplantation using potent medications is
essential. Even with these agents, prevention of rejection remains a major
problem in transplantation. Rejection remains the primary reason for graft
loss.

The response of the human immune system to a foreign antigen is extremely complex and not as yet completely understood. The lymphocytes
predominate although other cells do play a role in an immune response. Two
types of lymphocytes are involved: T-lymphocytes, so called because they are
thymus dependent; and B-lymphocytes, called such because they arise from
the bursa of Fabricus in the chicken (and from an unknown source in
humans). B-lymphocytes form antibodies and are the basis of humoral immunity. T-lymphocytes are responsible for cell-mediated immunity. Both T-
and B-lymphocytes are formed from bone marrow stem cells. All types of
allograft rejection are caused by an interaction of these two types of cells.
Figure 9–3 shows diagrammatically our current understanding of an immune
response. Note the interaction between T- and B-lymphocytes and between
the various subsets of T-lymphocytes (helper, cytotoxic, and suppressor cells).

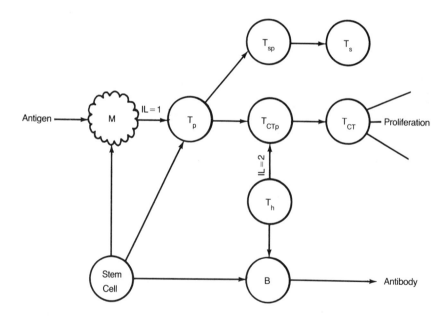

Figure 9–3. Diagram of the immune response showing T-cell and B-cell activity.
(M = macrophage; T_p = T-cell precursor; T_{sp} = suppressor T-cell precursor; T_s
= suppressor T-cell; T_{CTp} = cytotoxic T-cellprecursor; T_{CT} = cytotoxic T-cell; T_h
= helper T-cell; B = B-cell.)

The stimulus for the immune response (rejection) is provided by the antigens found on the cells of the transplanted kidney.

Types of Rejection

Rejection may take many forms depending on the timing of the reaction and the immunologic processes involved. Rejection is commonly categorized into four types based primarily upon the timing of the response and the clinical picture expected.

Hyperacute rejection occurs within minutes or hours of the reestablishment of blood flow to the transplanted organ. It results from preformed antibodies to the donor antigens already circulating in the recipient's serum. Hyperacute rejection is extremely rare now that cross-matching techniques have improved so greatly and antibodies are usually detected prior to a transplant being performed. Hyperacute rejection is a humoral immune response and is not responsive to treatment. Tissue destruction occurs immediately because of the antigen-antibody response and the activation of the complement and coagulation systems. This results in thrombosis and necrosis of the kidney. Classic hyperacute rejection causes the transplanted organ to become necrotic in the operating room. Removal of the kidney is necessary.

Accelerated rejection usually occurs 3 to 5 days following transplantation. It too is thought to involve a humoral immune response. Instead of preformed circulating antibodies, however, accelerated rejection is believed to be a secondary response that results in antibody formation after contact with an antigen to which the recipient has already been sensitized. It presents as a severe sudden episode of graft dysfunction occurring within a few days of transplantation. Accelerated rejection can sometimes be reversed, but large doses of potent immunosuppressives are required.

The most common type of rejection is *acute rejection.* It is primarily a cellular immune response involving T-lymphocytes. Immunosuppressive therapy is aimed primarily at preventing and treating this form of rejection. Acute rejection may occur at any time, but it is most likely after 7 to 10 days following transplantation and during the first year. After contact with an antigen, T-lymphocytes, by direct contact and through the release of chemicals called lymphokines, cause the activation of so-called cytotoxic or killer T-lymphocytes. These cells actually destroy the cells of the kidney that express the antigen to which they have been sensitized. Most renal transplant recipients will experience at least one episode of acute rejection. Immunosuppressive therapy is quite effective at reversing such episodes.

The fourth type of rejection, *chronic rejection,* is believed to involve both humoral and cell-mediated immunity. It is a slow, gradual process that results in the destruction of the graft primarily due to ischemia. Chronic rejection usually occurs years after transplantation and is not responsive to treatment. Because it occurs slowly, it often produces no clinical symptoms. The only evidence that is occurring may be a gradual deterioration in graft function.

Clinical Picture of Acute Rejection

As stated previously, most transplant recipients will undergo at least one episode of acute rejection. Nurses must be alert to the signs and symptoms of acute rejection and must be certain that patients and their families are taught the signals for which to watch once the patient has been discharged. Early diagnosis and treatment are key to successful treatment.

Nonspecific clinical signs of rejection are those typical of any immune response. They include fever (usually greater than 100F but rarely greater than 102F), general malaise, and tenderness over the graft. More specific signs show deterioration of the function of the transplanted kidney. Common findings include decreased urine output, weight gain, the development of edema, rises in BUN and serum creatinine, decreases in creatinine clearance, and hypertension. Clinical findings can often be confirmed by radiological tests. Sonography often documents enlargement of the kidney while excluding obstruction as a cause of the deterioration in renal function. Renal scans show reductions in the perfusion of the graft.

IMMUNOSUPPRESSIVE MEDICATIONS

Acceptance of the transplanted kidney is primarily determined by the immunologic responsiveness of the recipient to the antigens expressed on the donor kidney. Attempts are made prior to transplantation to match donor and recipient tissues and to alter the immune responsiveness of the recipient. However, for most transplant patients, manipulation of the immunosuppressive medications prescribed postoperatively is the factor most important in assuring graft survival. Several medications may be used to alter immunologic responsiveness. All of these medications must be considered two-edged swords, capable of preventing or treating graft rejection but also capable of rendering the patient incapable of mounting a response to an infection.

Steroids

Adrenocorticosteroids have been used as immunosuppressants for almost as long as transplantation has been performed. Intravenous steroids are often administered during the immediate perioperative period. Oral steroids (prednisone or prednisolone) are usually begun within two days of surgery. Individual transplant units have widely varying protocols for determining the doses of steroids used posttransplant. Steroid doses are gradually tapered over time. Rejection may be treated with boluses of intravenous steroids or with an increase in oral steroids and a tapering over several days or weeks back to maintenance doses.

Adrenocorticosteroids have a very general immunosuppressive effect. They are anti-inflammatory agents and help to stabilize cell membranes and prevent the infiltration of T-lymphocytes. They also have a cytotoxic effect on T-lymphocytes.

Clinicians attempt to minimize the total amount of steroid administered to a given patient because of the very nonspecific action and multiple adverse effects of these drugs. Worrisome and sometimes life-threatening adverse effects of steroids include an increased susceptibility to infection, Cushing's syndrome, salt and water retention, cataracts, hypertension, diabetes mellitus, weight gain, and aseptic necrosis of joints. Other effects include ulceration and GI bleeding, delayed wound healing, acne, and psychotic changes.

Azathioprine (Imuran)

Azathioprine has also been used since the early days of transplantation. It is an antimetabolite, a derivative of 6-mercaptopurine, that interferes with nucleic acid synthesis. As such, it interferes most with the replication of cells that are rapidly dividing. In a transplant recipient, the most rapidly multiplying cells are those of the immune system that are attempting to respond to the introduction of foreign antigens. Thus, azathioprine acts by preventing the rapid growth of lymphocytes and other immunologically active cells. It slows the body's response to the transplanted organ.

The most worrisome adverse effects of azathioprine are clearly related to its mechanism of action. Bone marrow toxicity with resulting leukopenia, thrombocytopenia, and occasionally anemia is the most common and potentially life-threatening adverse effect noted. Myelotoxicity can render a transplant recipient defenseless against infection. Other frequently seen effects include alopecia and liver toxicity.

Cyclophosphamide (Cytoxan)

Cyclophosphamide is also an antimetabolite and a 6-mercaptopurine derivative sometimes used as an immunosuppressive agent in transplant recipients. It is most often used in substitution for azathioprine when an individual has developed hepatotoxicity. Cytoxan is less toxic to the liver than azathioprine. Unfortunately, it appears to be a less effective immunosuppressant.

Cyclosporine (Sandimmune)

The latest development in the immunosuppressive therapy to achieve widespread use is cyclosporine. This naturally occurring substance is the metabolite of *fungi imperfecti*. It is the most specific of any of the commonly used immunosuppressive medications. Since its discovery in the early 1970s, it has undergone extensive laboratory and clinical evaluations. Late in 1983 it received approval from the FDA for general use. It is now used in nearly all transplant centers, although protocols for its use vary widely.

Cyclosporine acts to prevent rejection of a transplanted organ by interfering with the production, release, and action of interleukin 2, a chemical necessary for the growth and activation of T-lymphocytes. It seems to particularly inhibit T-helper cells while sparing the suppressor arm of the immune response. Because of its specific action, cyclosporine does not interfere as greatly as many other immunosuppressants with an individual's ability to fight infection, particularly bacterial infection.

The major factor limiting the use of cyclosporine in renal transplantation has been nephrotoxicity. Early in the posttransplant period, the nephrotoxicity appears to be dose related and to respond well to dose reduction. However, many clinicians fear the effects of long-term use. Much of the difficulty in successfully using cyclosporine in clinical renal transplantation relates to the problem of differentiating nephrotoxicity from rejection. There are no absolute rules for making the diagnosis. Generally, within the first month after the transplant, rejection is more likely than toxicity. Later after transplantation, toxicity is more likely. With rejection, the rise in BUN and creatinine tends to be more rapid than with toxicity. Toxicity is usually, but not always, associated with elevated cyclosporine blood levels. However, some patients show evidence of toxicity with levels that in most patients would be considered subtherapeutic. A biopsy may or may not be helpful. Often, all that can be done is to reduce the dose of cyclosporine and see if the BUN and creatinine fall. If not, treatment for rejection is begun.

Other side effects of cyclosporine that have complicated its use include hypertension, hepatotoxicity, paresthesias, tremors, seizures, hirsuitism, and gingival hyperplasia. The high cost of the drug has prevented some patients from receiving it or from continuing the drug past a few months.

Antithymocyte Preparations

There are many antithymocyte preparations, both serums and globulins, available for use in transplant patients. Most are not approved by the FDA and must be administered under protocol. Only Atgam, a horse antithymocyte globulin produced by the Upjohn company, has received FDA approval. All of these preparations act in a similar manner to prevent or treat rejection. They are preparations of antibodies to human T-lymphocytes produced in sensitized animals such as horses, rabbits, sheep, or goats. When administered to a transplant recipient, antithymocyte preparations cause T-cell depletion, resulting in a decreased ability of the individual to mount an immune response.

Because one is administering an animal protein, an anaphylactic reaction, though rare, is possible. Equipment to handle such an emergency must be readily available. Skin testing prior to the first dose is recommended. Other adverse reactions to antithymocyte preparations include fever, chills, and increased susceptibility to infection, phlebitis at the site of administration, and a serum sickness response (fever, malaise, joint pain).

Antithymocyte preparations are used in many transplant centers. Some clinicians administer them for a specific period of time after transplant to prevent early rejection. Others use them to treat diagnosed rejection episodes. Because these preparations must be administered intravenously or intramuscularly, they cannot be used for long-term immunosuppression.

Monoclonal Antibodies

The technology of monoclonal antibodies is being developed and applied to the field of transplantation. Several monoclonal antibodies are being tested. One, OKT3, produced by Ortho Pharmaceuticals, has shown the most promise to date.

Monoclonal antibodies are administered intravenously to treat a diagnosed rejection episode. They are given for a defined period of time (usually 7 to 14 days). Presently, they cannot be used to treat a second rejection episode because the patient develops antibodies to the preparation. This limits their usefulness.

These preparations contain antibodies specific for an antigen found on the cell surface of a subset of immune reactive cells. Most preparations developed to date contain antibodies that recognize an antigen found on the surface of T-lymphocytes. When given to a transplant recipient, these preparations treat rejection by destroying or inactivating T-lymphocytes. They are highly effective. In clinical trials, OKT3 was effective in reversing rejection in over 90 percent of patients tested (Goldstein, Schindler, Sheahan, Barnes, & Tsai, 1985). As our understanding of the immune response grows, one can imagine developing monoclonals directed against only that subset of T-lymphocytes responsible for rejection, leaving the remainder of the immune system intact.

The adverse reactions seen initially with the administration of OKT3 (fever, chills, respiratory distress) have been mitigated with various pretreatment regimens and more careful attention to the hydration status of the patient. Commonly, fever, chills, diarrhea, and headache are seen with the first few doses. Subsequent doses usually are given without adverse effects.

COMPLICATIONS FOLLOWING RENAL TRANSPLANTATION

The complications that occur following renal transplantation may be divided into four major categories: technical or surgical, infection, irreversible rejection, and malignancy.

Technical Complications

Vascular Complications. Thrombosis of the graft by emboli that completely block the arterial supply to the kidney most often results in loss of graft. When infarction occurs, the kidney must usually be removed on an emergency basis. It is a very uncommon complication and usually occurs early in the posttransplant period.

Renal vein thrombosis is also rare and usually results in graft failure. It is difficult to detect, because it may mimic a rejection episode with edema, fluid retention, and deterioration of renal function. Renal vein thrombosis most often results in the need for removal of the kidney.

Vascular leakage may occur in the early posttransplant period and is a life-threatening complication. It is caused by technical problems at surgery or by poor healing of the tissues at the vascular anastomoses. Patients must be closely monitored for evidence of bleeding postoperatively. Evidence of significant bleeding should make one suspicious of vascular leakage. Attempts at repair of the vessels are often unsuccessful and nephrectomy results.

Renal artery stenosis is a more common vascular complication. It usually occurs at the anastomosis itself or distal to the anastomosis in the transplanted artery. Renal artery stenosis is believed to be related to the surgical technique itself or to the process of rejection occurring in the donor artery, resulting in vascular endothelial proliferation. This complication usually presents with worsening hypertension, the development of a bruit over the iliac arteries, and sometimes deterioration in renal function. When this picture presents, angiography is warranted to rule out a renal artery stenosis. If detected, a stenosis in the transplant artery can sometimes be successfully dilated using balloon angioplasty. Otherwise, surgical repair is indicated using vascular grafting material or the patient's own saphenous vein.

Graft Rupture. Rupture of the transplanted kidney is usually caused by swelling of the kidney during a rejection episode. Surgery is nearly always required. Repair of the kidney may be attempted, but removal is usually required. Some clinicians perform a capsulotomy at the time of transplantation to allow more room for swelling during rejection. They believe that this reduces the incidence of rupture by preventing the buildup of pressure when swelling does occur.

Urologic Complications. Urine leaks may occur because of ureteral leakage, ureteral disruption, or a leak from the bladder. These complications occur primarily because of poor tissue healing or poor vascularity with tissue necrosis. Careful attention must be paid during procurement to maintaining the vascular supply of the ureter. Postoperatively, it is vitally important to assure adequate drainage of urine so that the bladder does not become distended and exert pressure on the suture line in the bladder wall or on the ureteral-vesicle anastomosis.

Ureteral obstruction may be caused by blood clots, stone formation, stricture, or kinking of the ureter. This condition must be carefully watched for so that obstruction and hydronephrosis do not result in damage to the kidney or in a life-threatening infection. Sonography is especially useful in monitoring for obstruction.

Wound Complications. Perinephric hematomas, urinomas, lymphoceles, and abscesses can exert external pressure on the kidney or ureter and result in deterioration of renal function. More commonly, they can serve as a medium for infection. Wound infections are a relatively common cause of morbidity in transplant recipients because of their immunosuppressed state. Wound infections can result in septicemia and death.

Prevention of wound infections is vitally important. Prevention begins during organ procurement and preservation. Donors are carefully screened and cultures performed to eliminate this source of contamination. Organ retrieval and preservation are performed under absolute sterile conditions. In the operating room preoperative skin washing with antibacterial agents, preoperative shaving, strict aseptic technique in surgery, and prophylactic wound irrigation have contributed to a decreasing incidence of wound infections. Many centers also employ perioperative antibiotics to reduce the incidence of infection. Postoperatively, aseptic technique must be used when caring for incisions and drains until the skin layer has healed and can serve as a barrier to bacterial invasion.

Close monitoring for evidence of perinephric collections is important after surgery. Wound drains are often placed for 24 to 36 hours to remove any blood or lymph and prevent the formation of a collection that could later become infected. With fevers or other evidence of wound infection, sonography is a valuable tool to detect perinephric collections noninvasively. If a collection is found that could be infected or could cause obstruction, it should be drained and cultured. If infected, the wound will usually need to be opened and packed. Antibiotics will be administered according to the sensitivities of the organisms cultured.

Infection

Infectious complications continue to be the primary cause of mortality in the first year after transplantation (Winearls, Lane, & Kurtz, 1984). The most common sites of infection include the urinary tract, wound, pulmonary system, vascular access, peritoneal cavity (in those with an indwelling peritoneal dialysis catheter), and the mouth and mucous membranes. When infection invades any of those local sites, systemic infection and death may result.

In the early posttransplant period, bacterial infections with common hospital pathogens are most likely to occur. Wound infections, urinary tract infections, pneumonia, and infection of the vascular access site or access for peritoneal dialysis may be seen. Aseptic technique, early ambulation, and careful patient surveillance will prevent infections or detect them early and prevent life-threatening systemic complications.

Long-term transplant recipients are most susceptible to opportunistic infections, particularly fungal and viral. With the use of cyclosporine and the reduction in the amount of steroids administered, transplant patients are more able to maintain immunity to bacterial infections. Their compromised immune system remains susceptible to infection with *Pneumocystis carinii*, *Nocardia*, *Cytomegalovirus* (CMV), *Herpes zoster*, and *Herpes simplex* organisms. Other pathogens include fungi such as *Candida*, *Aspergillus*, *Mucor*, and *Cryptococcus*.

Prevention and early detection of infection are vital. Surveillance cultures, particularly of the urine, are commonly collected. Any febrile episode must be thoroughly evaluated to exclude infectious causes. Immunosuppressive therapy must be kept at a minimum, sufficient to prevent rejection but not so much as to prevent the patient from warding off infection. If a serious infection presents, immunosuppressive therapy must be reduced. It must always be remembered that the patient's life is much more important than preserving the transplanted kidney. Return to dialysis and retransplantation are preferable to death from over-immunosuppression.

Infectious complications remain a significant risk in transplantation. Hopefully, as immunosuppressive agents are developed that are more specific in their action, we will be able to preserve more of the patient's ability to ward off infection while reducing the risk of rejection.

Irreversible Rejection

Nearly all transplant recipients will experience at least one episode of acute rejection. The diagnosis and treatment of acute rejection has been previously discussed. Some patients will have multiple episodes of rejection and will reach a point when further treatment of rejection exposes them to too great a risk of complications, especially infection. In other patients, attempts at reversing a particularly aggressive episode of rejection will be unsuccessful. Finally, some patients will have gradual deterioration of renal function due to chronic rejection. Chronic rejection is not generally responsive to treatment. These three groups of patients will all lose the transplanted kidney due to irreversible rejection.

Nursing care during a rejection episode must include a careful assessment of renal function. As kidney function deteriorates, fluid retention, weight gain, hypertension, uremia, and electrolyte disturbances result. Dietary restrictions of protein, salt, potassium, and fluid may need to be reinstituted. Dialysis treatments may be resumed temporarily or permanently. Medications such as phosphate binders and antihypertensives may be prescribed. Patients will require much explanation and support during this time. It is an uncertain time as, at least initially, it may be unclear whether this is a reversible rejection episode or rejection that will result in graft loss. During a rejection episode, patients also suffer the side effects of increased doses of immunosuppressive agents, especially steroids. These adverse effects can be quite debilitating and disturbing to patients. It is also at this time that the patients are most susceptible to infectious complications.

If the rejection cannot be reversed, the patient will return to dialysis. The transplanted kidney may be left in place and immunosuppressive medication gradually tapered and discontinued. Quite frequently, especially in the case of an acute rejection episode, as immunosuppression is reduced the patient develops fever and pain over the kidney, which necessitate its removal.

Transplant nephrectomy is a relatively easy surgical procedure to perform and only takes 1 to 2 hours. However, because of the immunosuppressed state of the patient and because it involves reopening a surgical incision, the risk of wound infection and hematoma formation is higher than with the original transplant surgery. Following transplant nephrectomy, immunosuppressive medications are rapidly tapered and discontinued. Care must be taken not to reduce steroids too quickly, an an Addisonian crisis can result.

When patients are discharged from the hospital following a failed transplant, arrangements for chronic dialysis must be made. Usually, the patient is referred back to the unit where he or she was receiving dialysis prior to transplantation. Occasionally, a patient may have been tranplanted prior to beginning dialysis. Such patients must be referred to a chronic dialysis facility. It is important that transplant nurses convey adequate information about the patient's physical and psychological condition to the dialysis staff. After a failed transplant, patients may return to dialysis in a more debilitated state than when they were referred for transplantation. Particular attention should be paid to their ability to return to home dialysis or self-care. Communication between the transplant and dialysis staffs is essential.

Malignancy

An increased incidence of neoplastic disease is seen in transplant recipients (Sheil, 1984). These malignancies are most commonly skin cancers or malignancies of the lymphoreticular system. No one immunosuppressive agent has been shown to be responsible. Rather, the total amount of immunosuppression seems to be important.

Patients need to be advised of this increased risk. Careful attention to warts or moles on the skin is advised. Measures such as monthly breast self-examination and regular gynecological examinations with Pap smears are encouraged so that malignancies are detected early. Overexposure to the sun is discouraged because this increases the risk for developing skin cancer. Those caring for transplant recipients must remain aware of the risk of malignancy and include it in the list of things that are continually assessed.

PATIENT EDUCATION

An important part of the nursing care of renal transplant recipients is patient education. Successful outcomes depend on the patient understanding the actions of the medications prescribed, their effects, and their side effects. Rejection will occur without appropriate immunosuppression. After discharge from the hospital, patients must be able to accurately administer their own medications, recognize the signs of rejection, and identify symptoms that may indicate adverse effects of their medications.

Patient and family education begins before transplantation during the evaluation process. Following transplant, intensive teaching is started as soon as the patient has recovered from surgery and anesthesia. Many centers have a protocol of self-medication administration whereby patients give their own medications while in the hospital. This allows for a safe method for patients to learn their medications under supervision. They are then better prepared to administer those medications following discharge from the hospital.

In addition to medication administration, patients must be instructed in their dietary restrictions, limitations on activity, follow-up care, and clinical signs and symptoms for which they should seek medical care. The resumption of sexual activity, contraception, and pregnancy should be discussed openly with all patients.

The goal of patient education is to prepare the patient for independence after discharge. Individualized methods of teaching must be employed based upon an assessment of the patient's abilities and readiness to learn. Family members may be included in the teaching program to reinforce learning and help to assure compliance.

FOLLOW-UP CARE

Transplant recipients usually remain in the hospital one to three weeks. After discharge it is essential that the overall condition and laboratory results are closely monitored. This has become increasingly important with the shortened lengths of in-hospital stay. Patients usually are followed very frequently for several weeks after discharge. The frequency of visits to the clinic is then gradually reduced. Some centers return patients to the care of their primary nephrologist and follow the patient jointly with this physician. These patients return to the transplant center for evaluation periodically. Other transplant programs retain primary responsibility for following all transplant patients.

Prior to discharge it is vital that patients understand fully the importance of continued medical follow-up and the schedule of visits planned for them. They must also clearly know how to reach a physician in an emergency.

SEXUAL ACTIVITY AND PREGNANCY AFTER TRANSPLANTATION

Fertility and libido often return following renal transplantation. Sexual activity may safely be resumed 3 to 4 weeks after transplantation if the wound has healed and the patient has suffered no complications. Positioning and frequency of activity should not result in complications. Because of the placement of the kidney in the iliac fossa, patients often fear harming it and need reassurance that this will not occur.

Issues of personal hygiene and the danger of acquiring sexually transmitted diseases must be discussed with patients. Limiting the number of sexual partners is advisable to minimize the risk of acquiring such infections.

Contraception should be discussed with all patients. Male transplant patients may father a child at any time after resuming sexual activity without fear for the fetus. Female transplant patients should be advised to prevent pregnancy for at least 1 year, and longer if renal function is not stable. The danger is that pregnancy may increase the risks of infection, obstruction to the flow of urine, hypertension, and rejection, all of which may cause serious deterioration of renal function. However, the methods of contraception to be recommended are limited. Oral contraceptives are discouraged because of problems with thrombophlebitis and the fear of oncogenesis. Intrauterine devices are strongly discouraged because of the risk of infection, particularly pelvic inflammatory disease. Condoms, diaphragms, foams, and gels are the preferred methods of contraception, but patient desire to use these methods may be a problem. If a female transplant recipient chooses to become pregnant, she must be very carefully monitored by her obstetrician and nephrologist. Such patients often require hospitalization during the third trimester for problems with toxemia, diabetes mellitus, hypertension, edema, and deterioration of renal function.

Data collected to date in many centers indicate no evidence for an increased risk of birth defects among the children of renal transplant recipients treated with conventional immunosuppresive agents (prednisone and Imuran). Insufficient data are available to comment on those treated with cyclosporine.

REHABILITATION

Return to work, school, or previous activities is certainly the goal for patients who are successfully transplanted. A large percentage of patients are able to do so. Some patients will require vocational counseling to learn new skills to assist them in this process. Employers are sometimes reluctant to hire persons who are chronically ill even though they have been successfully transplanted. Members of the transplant team need to be as helpful as possible in assisting patients in overcoming such obstacles.

A few patients will not be motivated to return to work or school. This may be due to disincentives provided through the disability insurance system or to a long period on dialysis when they were unable to work or attend school regularly. Requests for certification of disability must be objectively examined and all attempts made to assist patients in achieving maximum rehabilitation.

CONCLUSION

Great strides have been made in transplantation in a relatively short period of time. Two major obstacles still confront us. The first is an imperfect understanding of the immune system and immunologic responses. This limits our ability to find the perfect immunosuppressant to prevent rejection of the transplanted organ while preserving the patient's ability to fight infection. We continue to move closer to this goal through the efforts of many scientists and clinicians.

The second obstacle to transplantation is an insufficient number of cadaver organs to transplant. Efforts at federal, state, and local levels are directed to increase public awareness of the need for organs and to encourage professionals to consider organ donation when there is nothing else they can offer brain-dead patients and their families. Only when organ and tissue donation become a normal part of the process of dying will we be able to offer the gift of life or a second chance to all those who need it.

REFERENCES

Brenner, G. M. (1983). Hemodynamically mediated glomerular injury and the progressive nature of kidney disease. *Kidney Internat, 23,* 647–655.

Briggs, J. D. (1984). Preparation of the recipient for transplantation. In P. J. Morris (Ed.), *Kidney transplantation—principles and practice* (2nd ed.). New York; Grune & Stratton.

Goldstein, G., Schindler, J., Sheahan, M., et al. (1985). Orthoclone OKT3 treatment of acute renal allograft rejection. *Transplantation Proceedings, 27,* 129–131.

Hopper, S. A., Sweeney, J. T., & Pierce, P. (1984). The patient receiving a renal transplant. In L. E. Lancaster (Ed.), *The patient with end stage renal disease* (2nd ed.). New York: Wiley.

Klintmalm, G., Brynger, H., Flatmark, A., et al. (1985). The blood transfusion, DR matching, and mixed lymphocyte culture effects are not seen in cyclosporine-treated renal transplant recipients. *Transplantation Proceedings, 25,* 1026–1031.

Morris, P. J. (1984). Results of renal transplantation. In P. J. Morris (Ed.), *Kidney transplantation—principles and practice* (2nd ed.). New York: Grune & Stratton.

Opelz, G. for the Collaborative Transplant Study (1985). Current relevance of the transfusion effect in renal transplantation. *Transplantation Proceedings, 25,* 1015–1022.

Opelz, G., Sengar, D. P. S., Mickey, M. R., & Terasaki, P. I. (1973). Effect of blood transfusion on subsequent kidney transplant. *Transplantation Proceedings, 5,* 253–259.

Salvatierra, O., Jr., et al. (1980). Deliberate donor specific blood transfusions prior to living related renal transplantation: A new approach. *Ann Surg, 192,* 543–552.

Salvatierra, O., Jr., Vincenti, F., Amend, W., Jr., et al. (1983). Four-year experience with donor-specific blood transfusions. *Transplantation Proceedings, 25,* 924–931.

Schoenberg, L. (1984). Clinical results of the use of cyclosporine in renal transplantation. In B. D. Kahan (Ed.), *Cyclosporine: Nursing and paraprofessional aspects.* New York: Grune & Stratton.

Sheil, A. G. R. (1984). Cancer in dialysis and transplant patients. In P. J. Morris (Ed.), *Kidney transplantation—Principles and practice* (2nd ed.). New York: Grune & Stratton.

Spees, E. K., Vaughn, W. K., Williams, G. M., et al. (1980). Effects of blood transfusions on cadaver renal transplantation: The Southeastern Organ Procurement Foundation prospective study 1977–1979. *Transplantation, 30,* 455–463.

Taylor, J. (1981). Thoracic duct drainage. *AANNT Journal, 8,* 42–47. U. S. ESRD Program Selected 1983 Statistics (1984). *Contemporary Dialysis and Nephrology, 5,* 51–58.

Velosa, J. A., Anderson, C. F., Torres, V. E., et al. (1985). Long-term renal status of kidney donors: Calculated small risk of kidney donation. *Transplantation Proceedings, 27,* 100–103.

Winearls, C. G., Lane, D. J., & Kurtz, J. (1984). Infectious complications after renal transplantation. In P. J. Morris (Ed.), *Kidney transplantation—Principles and practice,* (2nd ed.). New York: Grune & Stratton.

The Pediatric Renal Patient*

Sue N. Sauer and Marlys E. Nolander

OBJECTIVES

After reading this chapter on pediatric nephrology, the nurse will be able to:

1. Compare and contrast the various treatment modalities based on pediatric considerations
2. Describe the management problems that can be expected in the pediatric nephrology patient
3. Understand how the stages of growth are affected by the onset and treatment of end-stage renal disease
4. Discuss the nutritional management of infants and children with end-stage renal disease
5. Understand the psychosocial aspects of pediatric nephrology
6. Discuss alternative methods for educating the pediatric nephrology patient and family

Rapid advances in the pediatric nephrology field have set the stage for perhaps the most challenging and adventurous nursing role yet to be encoun-

---

*Note to reader: This chapter is referenced more heavily than the others. This is due to the paucity of generalized nephrology nursing knowledge on this subject, and the specialty nature and source of the references.

tered. Each year more and more children are treated for renal disease. Whether these children are inpatients in a hospital or treated as outpatients in a clinic, the nursing care needed by them requires a special blend of empathy, sensitivity, and emotional support along with an alertness and extra measure of specialized knowledge of complex care.

From the nurses' point of view, there are special frustrations and stresses, along with unique challenges, in caring for the child with renal problems over a long period of time. There is the constant pressure of coping with a patient population that includes a large number of depressed, angry, regressive, and difficult children. Clearly, pediatric nephrology nursing is no place for the faint of heart. Some have likened working in this specialty to riding on an emotional roller coaster. No other member of the health-care team is so relentlessly exposed to the physical problems and emotional vicissitudes of their patients and their families. Some see pediatric nephrology nursing as depressing, but don't appreciate that it is rewarding and enriching to care for children during a very difficult period of their lives.

The myth of doom that surrounds renal disease should be dispelled because thousands of children each year are winning personal victories over their problems. We, as pediatric nephrology nurses, have the privilege of seeing these success stories and experiencing the closeness that develops between the nurse, child, and family, and obtaining a deep sense of fulfillment when the victories are accomplished.

Frustrating problems are also experienced by children, who often encounter a confusing spectrum of health-care facilities and an overwhelming array of professional staff involved in their care. They may experience fragmentation of care on several units—the referring center or hospital, the pediatric ward, the dialysis and transplant unit, and the outpatient clinic. Children may also experience bombardment by the medical team, surgical team, dialysis nurses, general pediatric nursing staff, dietitian, psychiatrist, respiratory therapist, and so on. In the face of heightened anxiety, children and their families often feel confused, stampeded, and overwhelmed. In view of all this, we are then bound to use totally the concept of individualized care. An investment of time and attention is urgently needed to construct and implement a realistic and positive approach to the spectrum of care required for the special needs of these children.

The pediatric patient with renal disease presents a uniqueness of differences, characteristics, and developmental factors that challenge and confront the nurse. Quality care for these children is complex and requires extraordinary knowledge and specific expertise to develop a comprehensive approach to the special needs of the patient. The medical care and treatment of children afflicted with renal disease has changed dramatically over the last 20 years, and current experience and treatment varies nationwide and changes rapidly. All of this has greatly influenced the outcome and outlook for the renal child and demanded that the pediatric renal nurse play a pivotal role in a multidisciplinary approach to plan and execute the best care for the child.

There are many aspects of general renal nursing that are similar between adults and children but the child is not just a little adult. When it comes to treating children, there are unique differences in the treatment of the child with renal disease, differences primarily related to growth, development, body requirements, and psychosocial demands. These concerns will be addressed further in this chapter. Other information will focus on unique components affecting the child with primary renal disease, end-stage renal disease (ESRD), and the treatment methods and modalities. An effort will be made to suggest ways to enhance special care aspects in order to foster optimal care for the child's needs.

PRIMARY RENAL DISEASE IN CHILDREN: INCIDENCE AND OUTCOME

Knowledge concerning the etiology of renal disease and the potential outcome is important because treatment regimens and learning needs of the child and family vary greatly. The incidence of primary renal disease and the general course the disease can take are summarized in Table 10–1.

Available studies lead to the tentative conclusion that more than half of ESRD in children results from congenital or hereditary diseases for which there is no prevention of an inevitable progression to renal failure. On the other hand, early efforts to treat renal disease in children, and our now impressive therapies and modalities, have extended the life afforded these patients and in many ways have enhanced the normalcy of the lives they lead. The situation today is that it is now technically possible to offer many therapeutic options to all children, even the very young infant.

TREATMENT MODALITIES: SPECIFIC PEDIATRIC CONSIDERATIONS

Children have different needs and different responses to treatment than do adult patients. As a result, additional factors must be considered when selecting the best treatment modality for the pediatric patient.

Hemodialysis

The decision to dialyze a child is a complex judgment based on a number of different clinical findings. Laboratory values provide data on the child's degree of uremia, hyperkalemia, and acid-base balance. In addition, fluid imbalance may be severe enough to warrant the initiation of dialysis. Realizing that it is not a procedure without risks, the indications for dialysis must be weighed against the child's ability to tolerate the treatment.

TABLE 10-1. PRIMARY RENAL DISEASE IN CHILDREN

Disease (Most common to least common)	Most Likely Outcome
Young child	
Anomalies of the urinary tract	Variable depending on severity
Obstructive uropathy	May be correctable by surgery
Ureteral reflux	Normal to end stage disease
Maldevelopment of the kidney	
Dysplasia	Renal insufficiency
Hypoplasia	
Cystic disease	
Multicystic kidney	Usually unilateral; excellent outlook
Polycystic kidney	Renal insufficiency; portal hypertension
Hemolytic uremia syndrome	Usually recover in 90% of cases
	Varying degrees of renal insufficiency in remainder
Congenital nephrotic syndrome	Poor prognosis unless transplanted
Familial nephritis	Makes progressive to renal failure, females no problem
Older child	
Recurrent urinary tract infection	Usually excellent. Depends on extent of anomalies
Anomalies of kidney	
Obstructive uropathy	Same as for younger child
Uretral reflux	
Glomerulonephritis	
IGA nephropathy	Generally mild course; slowly progressive disease in 20% of cases
Post streptococcyl glomerulonephritis	Recovery the rule
Membranoproliferative glomerulonephritis	Usually progressive
Membranous glomerulonephritis	In children usually nonprogressive
Idiopathic nephrotic syndrome	95% of cases responsive to steroids; may recur but long term outlook excellent
Lupus glomerulonephritis	Variable depending on severity; stabilized by steroids
Diabetic nephropathy	Clinical onset of nephropathy usually after 19–20 years of diabetes
Renal vascular hypertension	Usually correctable by surgery
Familial nephritis	Same as for younger child

Access. Once the decision to hemodialyze is made, access to the child's vascular space must be obtained. This can be a difficult task in a small child. Scribner shunts can technically be placed, though vessel size may limit the size of shunt tips that can be used. Ideally, large enough tips are used to produce good blood flow, but not so large as to cause obstruction created from the formation of intimal flaps. Complications of shunts include thrombosis, infection, ischemia, accidental disconnection, and hemorrhage.

In the newborn, umbilical catheters used for infusion of fluids and medications can also be used for dialysis if blood flow rates are adequate. Shaldon catheters placed in the femoral vein are too large for use in very small children (less than 10 kg). Instead, smaller, polyethylene percutaneous catheters can be placed over a guidewire (Seldinger technique) in the femoral vessel to serve as a temporary access.

Arteriovenous fistulas have been created in very small children (less than 10 kg) through use of microsurgery with 90 percent success rates when performed by experts; however, long maturation periods of 6 to 8 weeks are required for sufficient development of the fistula for needle insertion (Bourquellot, Wolfelir & Lamy, 1981). Another consideration is the psychological trauma to the child caused by the discomfort and anxiety of venipuncture before each treatment. Usually, dialysis is an immediate need in the small child, so other access methods are employed.

An exciting advance in access devices is the use of the Hickman right atrial catheter. Constructed of polymeric silicone (silastic rubber), the Hickman catheter has a single end hole, with an attached Dacron cuff to anchor the catheter subcutaneously. A leur-adapted external end allows the attachment of a Y connector to the catheter, facilitating unipuncture or single-needle dialysis (Fig. 10–1). The Hickman catheter is available with three internal diameters: 1.6, 2.0, and 2.6 mm. A larger diameter permits a greater blood flow, thereby facilitating more efficient dialysis in larger children (Fowler, Mahan, & Nevins, 1984).

The Hickman right atrial catheter is surgically placed under general anesthesia. Vessels most commonly used for placement are the right internal and external jugulars and the left internal jugular. The catheter is then tunneled subcutaneously to exit over the third or fourth rib. A chest x-ray is taken to verify the position of the catheter tip in the right atrium, and adequate blood flow is assessed by aspirating with a syringe. The catheter may be used for dialysis immediately after placement. Using a Y connector, a unipuncture or "single-needle dialysis" machine is used so that blood can be both removed from the patient and returned to the child through the one Hickman catheter.

At the University of Minnesota Hospitals and Clinics, the Hickman catheter was used to dialyze 57 infants for 1585 dialysis treatments from October 1980 to January 1984 (Fowler, Mahan, Nevins, 1984). Patients were dialyzed 3 times a week for 4 to 6 hours. Blood flow allowed BUN clearances of 3 ml/kg/min. Flow rates of 50 to 60 ml/min were consistently achieved.

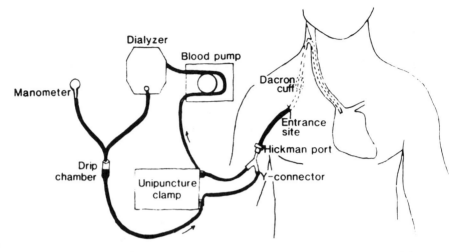

Figure 10-1. Hickman dialysis diagram. (*Fine, R. N., & Gruskin, A. [1984].* Treatment of end stage renal disease in children. *Philadelphia: Saunders.*)

The percentage of recirculation was maintained at less than 15 percent. Fifty-six percent of the catheters were free of complications. Others encountered problems with sepsis, local infection, bleeding, poor blood flow, catheter perforation, or cuff extrusion.

Care of the Hickman catheter involves heparin injection twice daily using 2 cc of 100 U/cc heparin. A resealing injection cap placed on the end of the catheter makes this a simple procedure, handled by the parents at home between dialysis treatments. Exit site care is done every 2 to 3 days using hydrogen peroxide, Betadine, and Opsite transparent dressing. Use of the Hickman catheter for dialysis is increasing, because its advantages are appreciated and its minimal stress on the child is realized to be a valuable attribute.

Dialyzer. A dialyzer with the appropriate blood volume for the small child must be selected in order to achieve safe dialysis. For infants less than 10 kg, a dialyzer with a surface area of 0.23 m^2 and a priming volume of less than 20 ml is desirable. Neonatal blood lines with a volume of approximately 15 ml are used to connect the infant to the blood pump and dialyzer. For a larger child, a dialyzer with a priming volume of less than 30 ml and pediatric blood lines with a volume of about 50 ml are used. In principle, the dialysis circuit should not contain more that 10 percent of the patient's blood volume (Nevins & Mauer, 1984).

Interdialytic Monitoring. The infant or small child must be closely monitored during the dialysis procedure, and vital signs must be taken frequently. Pulse is continuously monitored with a cardiac monitor. Blood pressure is checked at a minimum of every 15 minutes using either a standard pediatric sphygmomanometer, automatic noninvasive arterial pressure monitor, or a direct arterial line for the critically ill patient. A small child is at risk for hypothermia, and a freestanding infrared heater may be required to maintain the child's core temperature at a suitable level. An accurate electronic scale is essential to supply accurate measurement of body weight during the dialysis treatment. The scale can be attached to the bed or crib, and can detect weight changes in the range of 5 to 10 g. Unexpected weight loss leading to hypotension is a real threat to the small child and must be avoided.

Complications. Complications of hemodialysis include chronic anemia, increased ferritin levels due to frequent transfusions, poor nutrition if the child does not tolerate the dialysis procedure and therefore forfeits the feeling of wellness and appetite, growth retardation, hypertension, osteodystrophy, slowed sexual maturation, and dialysis disequilibrium syndrome.

Uremic children are prone to anemia in the predialysis phase, but this condition seems to exacerbate in some children on hemodialysis. Chronic anemia is easily treated while the child is being dialyzed by administering extra blood through the dialysis system. The frequency of transfusions required by some children has led to another complication, increased ferritin levels in the blood and also stores of iron in the liver. The possibility of resultant liver damage has led to switching these children to peritoneal dialysis (PD), and the use of an iron-binding agent, deferoxamine, administered in the PD solution. It is hoped that this drug will decrease these iron stores and limit organ damage. Other problems noted in the child on dialysis—such as nutritional concerns, growth retardation, hypertension, osteodystrophy, slowed sexual maturation, and dialysis disequilibrium syndrome—will be discussed in separate sections.

Continuous Ambulatory Peritoneal Dialysis

When ESRD strikes a child early in life, it usually means that the family will be tied to a center that can dialyze the child if dialysis or transplant therapy is chosen. This upsets the family's life patterns and keeps the child in a hospital environment for hours each week. With the availability of smaller volume and custom-filled bags of peritoneal dialysate, small children can now be maintained with an effective home dialysis program of continuous ambulatory peritoneal dialysis (CAPD).

The first step is to determine if the child has any contraindication to the use of CAPD. The presence of an insufficient peritoneal cavity, due to such conditions as omphalocele or gastroschisis, is the only absolute factor that rules out peritoneal dialysis. CAPD has been used to treat children following major abdominal surgery, children with ureterostomies and other urinary tract diversions, and those with prune-belly syndrome. Blindness, mental retardation, paralysis, major neurological deficits, and psychiatric disorders are considered as relative contraindications to CAPD in adults. However, in pediatric patients, a parent is usually trained to do the dialysis, so these problems can be overcome. If the child does have a major psychiatric problem, this would probably create appreciable difficulties. The presence of a colostomy is also a high-risk condition, but with flawless technique in separating the exit site from the stoma, dialysis can be achieved. Age and size are not considered limiting factors, as the literature describes patients aged 12 days to 26 years, weighing from 2.5 to 77 kg, who have been maintained on CAPD (Alexander & Lubischer, 1982; Salusky, Lucullo, Nelson, & Fine, 1982). Prior ESRD therapy, renal transplant status, and primary renal disease have no apparent influence on CAPD status.

Indications for CAPD in children include small size, prior problems with other modes of dialysis, families that live a long distance from the dialysis center, and patient or family desire to perform dialysis at home. For the younger child, CAPD allows the child to remain in the home, able to take part in family activities and to attend school regularly. Adolescent renal patients can usually be trained to do their own dialyses, and this represents an important opportunity for independence and taking responsibility for themselves. Adolescents are no longer dependent on a machine or a hospital unit, but are able to plan their dialysis around daily or special activities that they like to do. A fairly normal life-style can be maintained including school, exercise, showering or bathing, and working a job. Swimming remains a controversial activity that is allowed by some programs and forbidden by others.

Access. A reliable catheter is the foundation for successful CAPD. It is placed surgically, usually under general anesthesia. Of utmost importance is the creation of a watertight seal at the entry point of the catheter into the peritoneal cavity. This is accomplished by using a permanent peritoneal purse-string suture around the proximal cuff. A straight subcutaneous tunnel to the exit site avoids exit site erosion, as a curved silastic tube will try to straighten itself out. A well-healed exit site should show no redness or drainage. Two cuff catheters, if properly placed, form a double barrier against infection. If, however, the distal cuff is placed too close to the exit site, cuff erosion can occur with complicating exit site infection, and necessitate careful removal of this cuff. This is done by shaving the cuff off of the catheter, a difficult process if the cuff is secured by glue. Single-cuff catheters avoid this problem and are being used successfully in many centers (Fig. 10–2).

Dialysate. Guidelines for the CAPD prescription in children remain largely empiric. Exchange volume is determined by the size and weight of the child, 35 to 50 cc/kg being the guideline used by many pediatric programs. Children sometimes require higher average dextrose concentrations than adults to ultrafilter adequate amounts of water in order to maintain a stable weight. Also, more frequent exchanges, averaging from 5 to 6 per day, are often necessary to control potassium, BUN, and creatinine levels.

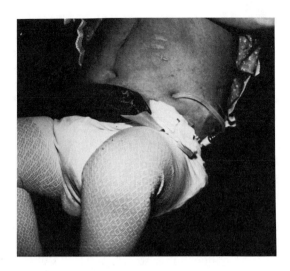

Figure 10-2. Well-healed catheter exit site in a 2½-year-old girl on CCPD.

Complications. Peritonitis remains the chief complication encountered by patients with CAPD. Despite excellent teaching in methods of sterile technique, children are often plagued by infections that can ultimately cause scarring of the peritoneal membrane and loss of the ability to dialyze sufficiently. Innovations by the manufacturers of PD supplies may reduce this problem. The ultraviolet light system treats the spike with bacteria-killing ultraviolet rays before it enters the bag and contacts the dialysate. This device has decreased the number of infections encountered by some patients, especially those prone to having problems maintaining sterile technique during an exchange. Other equipment may also help limit infections by keeping the patient's hands away from the sterile area. Safe-lock and beta cap systems employ Betadine to continuously soak the sterile connection. Incidence of peritonitis in children is similar to the incidence in adults.

Anemia is improved in children on CAPD. Baum and associates (1982) reported that only 0.16 transfusions per month were done in CAPD patients compared to an average of five times this many in children on hemodialysis. Hypertension has been reported to be dramatically improved in CAPD patients, illustrated by the fact that they require much less antihypertensive therapy, sometimes being able to remain off drugs completely (Salusky et al., 1982).

Continuous Cycling Peritoneal Dialysis

Continuous Cycling Peritoneal Dialysis (CCPD) is an alternative to CAPD that employs an automated cycler to do the exchanges, usually at night while the patient sleeps. This method involves fewer connection breaks per day, an advantage in decreasing the peritonitis risk and in not having to keep a young child still while the sterile CAPD exchange procedure is done 4 to 5 times a day. The patient or parent sets up the machine at night, spiking enough bags to accomplish all of the day's dialysis exchanges. A "hook-up" procedure is done to connect the patient's catheter to the cycler tubing. This procedure does not involve a lengthy Betadine scrub and can be accomplished in less than 15 minutes. While the patient sleeps, warmed dialysate flows into and then drains from the peritoneal cavity on a schedule predetermined by settings on the machine. Dwell cycles comparable to CAPD can be used, or shorter cycles can be used to increase the volume of dialysate, achieving better dialysis. In the morning, the "off" procedure is done, leaving from half to a full exchange volume in the patient so that dialysis continues during the day. This method allows the patient freedom from dialysis procedures during the day, a positive feature if both parents of a PD child are working. Subjective comments by parents who have performed both CAPD and CCPD reflect a preference for CCPD, based on the daytime freedom and the increased safety because of fewer breaks in the connection system. Drawbacks of the system include a machine that the child must be hooked to, thereby limiting mobility once the dialysis procedure is started. Also, parents must learn to troubleshoot alarm conditions that may occur anytime during the night's treatment.

Transplantation

Despite the advances made in the field of dialysis, the optimal form of therapy for the child with ESRD remains successful transplantation. This therapy provides the child with the maximum opportunity to grow and develop and to achieve the best quality of life. Children tolerate the transplant surgery very well and are usually up and about within 3 to 4 days. Advances in histocompatibility determinations, surgical techniques, and antirejection therapy make transplantation a very encouraging option for the family facing this situation. Various centers differ on the timing of transplantation, some placing kidneys in children as young as 6 months of age believing the earlier, the better; and others waiting until the child is 3 years or older.

HLA-A and B, and DR typing are tests done beyond ABO compatibility in determining the best donor for a particular renal patient. For children whose siblings are too young to donate, a parent's kidney is preferred over a cadaver because the transplant date can be planned ahead to be done at a time when the child is in optimal condition.

Surgical Procedure. The surgical placement of the kidney in a small child (less than 20 kg) varies from that of an older child or an adult. The kidney is placed on the right side of the retroperitoneum, with the ascending colon being reflected medially (Fig. 10–3). Once the kidney is in place, the bowel is tacked to the upper pole so as to create a "window" to permit a biopsy to be performed. Miller and associates (1983) report that no significant difficulties were encountered in the ability of the child's abdomen to accommodate an

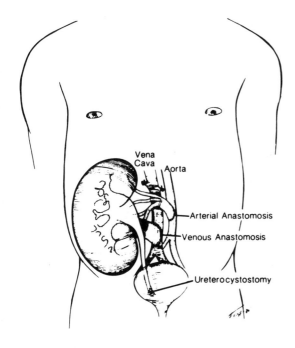

Figure 10-3. Surgical placement of the adult kidney into the small child. (*From Miller, L. C. et al. [1983]. Transplantation of the adult kidney into the very small child. Technical Considerations. American Journal of Surgery, 145, 243–247, with permission.*)

adult kidney. The patients also demonstrated that they had enough cardiac reserve to safely perfuse the adult kidney.

The allograft artery and vein are anastomosed to the child's aorta and vena cava, respectively. A donor kidney with two renal arteries may be preferable, since the vessel size is smaller and they more closely match with the recipient's vessels. The smaller of the donor's two kidneys is selected to maximize the ability to fit the organ into the child's abdomen.

Complications. In Miller's report, minor complications included increase in abdominal girth due to the size of the new kidney, postoperative ileus, and third-space fluid shifts. Respiratory compromise was not a problem. Eighty-three percent of the patients in their report are alive with functioning grafts. This is an encouraging advancement in the treatment of the small child with ESRD, where long-term dialysis has been associated with irreversible central nervous system injury and severely retarded growth and development (Mauer et al., 1985).

Rejection of the allograft remains a problem in pediatric transplantation as in adults. Immunosuppressive therapy consisting of cyclosporine and steroids is the standard approach at most centers. Cyclosporine levels must be closely monitored, because the uptake of the drug varies from child to child more so than in adults.

A final problem facing the pediatric transplant patient is the recurrence of the primary disease in the transplanted kidney. It is believed to occur due to the persistence of the pathological process that led to the original renal disease. Electron microscopy and immunofluorescence are employed to make what is often a difficult diagnosis of recurrence versus a new disease process.

Primary glomerular diseases that have a high rate of recurrence are dense deposit disease (90 percent), IgA nephropathy (58 percent), crescentic, idiopathic glomerulonephritis (GN) (33 percent), membrane-proliferative GN type I (33 percent), and membranous nephropathy (29 percent). Among systemic diseases Henoch-Schonlein purpura has a 40 percent rate of recurrence, with systemic lupus erythematosus at a low 1 percent (Leumann & Briner, 1984). Hemolytic uremic syndrome is considered to have a low risk of recurrence, but recent data on several patients at the University of Minnesota Hospitals suggests this risk to be more significant. The metabolic disorder of primary oxalosis is a very challenging one to deal with, having a recurrence rate of 100 percent in the allograft. New research into posttransplant therapy using drugs that bind oxalates may shed some hope in the treatment of this disease. Therapy to prevent recurrence of other renal diseases is not available. Prolonged dialysis does not prevent recurrence, nor does bilateral nephrectomy in most cases. Pediatric renal diseases that have favorable transplant outcomes are dysplasia, polycystic disease, Wilm's tumor, medullary cystic disease, nail-patella syndrome, Finnish-type congenital nephrotic syndrome, cystinuria, Bartter's syndrome, and Fabry's disease. Recurrence of primary disease may eventually lead to allograft destruction and the initiation of dialysis or retransplantation. The issue of whether or not to retransplant in the face of high-risk recurrence is a problematic one. Emotional strain is high in families who face this devastating situation.

Summary. In summary, renal transplantation is the treatment of choice for the child with ESRD. As advancements in surgical techniques, immunosuppressive therapy, treatment of rejection, and prevention of recurrence of primary disease are made, this area will become an even more promising one for those unfortunate families with this problem.

MANAGEMENT PROBLEMS IN CHILDREN

Managing children with ESRD presents a unique set of problems, regardless of the treatment modality.

Neurological Complications
The association of abnormal renal function and central nervous system problems in children is well documented. Recent studies have shown that infants with chronic renal insufficiency may be more susceptible to the development of neurological abnormalities than older children or adults because of signifi-

cant growth and maturation of the brain that occurs during the first years of life (Rotundo et al., 1982). Typically, infants with chronic renal insufficiency have been found to have varying degrees of central nervous system dysfunction. Decreased head growth, seizures, dyskinesia, hypotonia, and developmental delay have been noted in the infant. Some forms and patterns of neurological dysfunction may be unique to the child's age, uremic state, and the therapeutic modalities used for treatment of ESRD. For example, peripheral neuropathy occurs commonly in adults, but is seen infrequently in children, whereas dialysis dysequilibrium syndrome is seen more often in children. However, the developmental state of the child's nervous system appears to determine susceptibility to uremic effects or neurological insult. Disturbances in function of the central nervous system and peripheral nervous system increase as renal function decreases, and account for a significant portion of the morbidity seen in children. In addition to uremia, hypertension, electrolyte abnormalities, drug-induced therapy, nutritional deficiencies, anemia, and metal intoxication have been shown to be responsible for neurological dysfunctions. The diagnosis of encephalopathy in children may be difficult and is usually based on clinical observation, studies, electroencephalograms, and psychometric testing. A typical infant with chronic renal insufficiency presenting in the first year of life may be noted to have decreased head growth, a marked delay in developmental milestones, and the appearance of seizures, dyskenesia, hypotonia, and an abnormal EEG.

In infants, it is not clear which approach to therapy best protects the developing brain. Dietary therapy with adequate amounts of high biologic value protein and calories, and control of calcium and phosphorus metabolism and acidosis, are important. However, earlier renal transplantation may be necessary to protect the developing brain (Rotundo et al., 1982). As the child grows, other manifestations of encephalopathy may become evident. Subtle disturbances such as a decrease in the child's level of interaction with his or her environment and others may occur. The child may also appear disinterested in surroundings, become preoccupied, and show a decreased ability to concentrate and evidence of a shorter attention span. In addition, early cognitive disturbances may include a diminished capacity for performing the repetitive mental manipulation of symbols and reduced speed of decision making (Ginn, 1975). Progressively poorer performance on testing occurs with increases in serum creatinine. The child's personality alters further and increasing irritability and lack of cooperation are apparent.

In developing uremic encephalopathy, motor disturbances almost always accompany cognitive dysfunctioning. These include myopathy, muscle hyperirritability, cramps, and peripheral weakness. Cramps usually appear first at night but may occur during waking hours as well. They are made worse by movement.

Focal or generalized seizures occur in 35 to 45 percent of children with uremic encephalopathy, and are often attributable to the presence of superimposed hypertension or drug toxicity (Polinsky, 1984). The latter should always be suspected when a child suddenly and unexpectedly develops a psychiatric disorder.

In the last 5 years, a new syndrome has appeared in an increasing number of children with renal insufficiency. It is an unexplained syndrome of progressive neurological deterioration. In young children, it is characterized by a regression from previously achieved developmental milestones. In older children it is characterized by speech disorders, tremor, myoclonus, seizures, and dementia. The pattern of progressive deterioration occurs in three stages. Stage I includes tremors, arrested motor skills, ataxia, hyperreflexia, and positive Babinski's sign. Stage II includes marked ataxia, seizures, myoclonus, regression from previously acquired milestones, and hypotonia. Stage III is a chronic vegetative state with unresponsiveness to visual and auditory stimuli, absence of voluntary movement, and absence of swallowing function. Several causes have been suggested for this progressive deterioration in children. They include congenital renal diseases, metabolic and biochemical derangement, initiation of dialysis, and aluminum and phosphate binder toxicity (Polinsky, 1984).

Neurological Effects of Dialysis. Dialysis, both hemodialysis and peritoneal dialysis, may benefit neurological functioning in children. Many children show improvement in their cognitive functions after dialysis is begun and some adolescents show improvement of peripheral neuropathy.

Dialysis disequalibrium syndrome (DDS) is the most common complication in children undergoing hemodialysis, although it occurs less frequently in children undergoing peritoneal dialysis. DDS tends to develop toward the end of a dialysis treatment or within 8 to 24 hours thereafter. It is observed especially in children beginning dialysis treatment and those with high uremic states, and is associated with high urea clearances. DDS appears to be a consequence of cerebral edema resulting from disproportionate rates of urea clearance from the brain and plasma, causing osmotic disequilibrium in electrolytes, acid-base balance, and glucose concentrations. The symptoms include restlessness, irritability, muscle cramps, headache, drowsiness, nausea, and vomiting. If not corrected, DDS may progress to confusion, disorientation, somulence, hypertension, and twitching. It can further develop to a life-threatening situation that may include seizures, cardiac arrhythmias, and coma. Deaths have occurred in children and adolescents.

The treatment of milder DDS includes reduced blood flow during hemodialysis and mannitol administration. Mannitol should be used prophylactically in children undergoing the first few hemodialysis treatments, especially if the BUN level is very high. Infants especially should receive more frequent dialysis at low clearances for shorter periods of time. Rapid hemodialysis against a mannitol-containing bath or the addition of glycerol to the bath may also prevent cerebral edema and seizures.

Acute copper intoxication from copper tubing bathed by acidic dialysate may also cause neurological problems. Symptoms are similar to those from DDS, and also include diarrhea.

Neurological Effects of Renal Transplantation. Successful transplantation in children usually reverses most of the neurological problems caused by uremia except in the infant where the benefits are less conclusive. Children may improve their performance in intelligence and achievement tests after transplantation.

After transplantation, some children experience a worsening of peripheral neuropathy. This is most likely related to high doses of steroids. Steroids may produce neurological disturbances in several ways. Hypertension, invasion of infection, and induced hypophosphatemia can cause sequelae. Steroids may also cause acute psychosis. This is usually dose related and reversible.

Fluid and Electrolyte Disturbances

Children can manifest sudden and profound fluid and electrolyte changes that may cause severe disturbances. Influencing factors include the age and size of the child in addition to the severity of the renal failure and the kidney disease process. In the normal child, the body maintains homeostatic control of water, solutes, and hydrogen ions. As renal function decreases, disturbances in these parameters are more likely to appear. As a general rule, the problems are more severe and complex in the infant and small child and are also more difficult to correct.

As the population of nephrons falls, the maintenance of the extracellular fluid becomes more difficult to control both in volume and composition of solutes. Children may exhibit problems with either the loss or retention of excess quantities of salt and water. The regulatory mechanisms for salt and water excretion are complex and multifactorial. Salt intake in uremic children often varies widely from day to day. The regulatory capacity for balancing the amount ingested and absorbed with the amount excreted does not exhibit wide variations but may decline at a fairly constant rate over time.

Failures in the regulatory mechanism do occur. In clinical situations that involve inappropriate loss or retention of both salts and water, the balance is not maintained. Some patients manifest a salt-losing tendency with advancing renal failure. If the sodium intake falls concurrently, a negative sodium balance will occur. If the sodium chloride loss is excessive, water loss will also occur and results in a decrease in the total extracellular fluid volume. These losses cause major problems especially for the infant and small child. If negative water balance is proportionately less than negative sodium balance, the child will become both salt depleted and hyponatremic. Water will shift from the extracellular fluid into the intracellular fluid. Treatment of salt depletion consists of expanding the extracellular volume with sodium chloride solution. The child needs careful observation of vital signs and frequent checks to make sure the cardiovascular system is not overloaded.

Salt retention associated with volume expansion is more frequent than salt depletion in children with chronic renal failure. Nephrotic syndrome is one true cause of salt retention in children. Because these children have continuous proteinuria and hypoalbuminuria, they excrete little or no salt. The salt intake must be adjusted for the state of edema present. Other conditions where salt retention may occur include acute glomerulonephritis, renal insufficiency of any cause, and congestive heart failure.

The most common cause of salt retention in children with chronic renal failure is when the amount of salt intake exceeds the amount of excretion. This is treated by lowering the salt intake below the upper limits of excretion. The salt restriction often poses difficult problems in maintaining a dietary regimen for the child. Diuretics are often required.

Hyper- and hyponatremia may result from dialysis treatment. Hyponatremia is most commonly dilutional and due to excess quantities of fluid and the absence of adequate ultrafiltration. The child may exhibit symptoms of weakness, increased fatigue, emotional lability, and neurological signs such as hyperreflexia and seizures. Hypernatremia may also result from dialysis using a dialysate too high in sodium. Hypernatremia may be exhibited by intense thirst, irritability, and restlessness. It may progress to lethargy, stupor, and seizures.

In children, any basic plan of fluid therapy depends upon the condition of the child and must be subject to careful monitoring. The child's metabolic rate, insensible fluid loss, sweating, increases or decreases in urine volume, and enteric losses must all be considered.

Renal Osteodystrophy

Disturbance in vitamin D and calcium metabolism leading to the occurrence of bone disease and skeletal abnormalities is a very complex and troublesome problem for the child.

The pathogenesis of childhood renal osteodystrophy can be best appreciated with an understanding of the four generic morphological functions of osteoblasts and osteoclasts. These functions are: (1) growth, which involves the increase in skeletal mass; (2) modeling, the process by which the small bones of the fetus are shaped into their adult counterparts; (3) remodeling, the process ultimately related to mineral homeostasis; and (4) repair, the prototype of which is fracture healing.

Those processes that are unique to the growing skeleton are growth and modeling. Remodeling, on the other hand, is a process that occurs through life and is abnormal in uremic children. Osseous tissue is continually being deposited and reabsorbed, primarily as a result of the activity of the connective tissue cells covering its surfaces. Changes in the activity of bone depend on the continuous transformation of undifferentiated cells to osteocytes, osteoblasts, and osteoclasts (Avioli & Teitelbaum, 1978). The responsiveness and alterations that occur in growth and remodeling of bone are dependent on vitamin D, calcium, PTH, and calcitonen.

The pathological changes that occur in the bone are secondary to alterations in phosphorus and vitamin D metabolism. Growth retardation is common in children with impaired renal function. The younger the child, the greater the impact on linear growth. At the time of ESRD, the height of about one third of all children is below the third percentile, but the actual growth rate is subnormal in 50 percent of all patients (Mehls, Ritz, Gilli, & Kreusser, 1978). These percentages are higher if renal insufficiency is present in infancy.

Many other factors contribute to the growth retardation, such as anorexia, acidosis, and poor absorption of calcium from the intestine. The clinical manifestations of renal osteodystrophy are multifaceted, making it difficult to manage. Often these are age related. Craniotobes and frontal bossing of the skull may occur in the child under 1 year of age.

Stunted growth is the most common clinical sign of bone disease in uremic children. Young children rarely complain of skeletal pain, but tend to restrict their exercise and physical activity. They may have difficulty climbing stairs or rising from a sitting position, for example. Activity restriction may also be the result of the association of myopathy with renal osteodystrophy, which affects the musculature. If children complain of continuous pain, it may be a sign of a fracture, epiphyseal slippage, or serious orthopedic problems.

In very young children, bone disease resembles vitamin-D-deficient rickets, with enlargement of wrists and ankles, rachetic rosary, knocked knees, and deformities of the tubular bones at the metaphyseal sites. Children over 10 years of age may show signs of ulnar deviation of hands, swelling of the wrists and ankles, pseudo-clubbing of the fingers, and epiphyseal slipping of the femoral head. These children may also walk with a waddling gait. Figure 10–4 illustrates the severe deformities and consequences of osteodystrophy that may occur.

Epiphyseal slipping is the most severe clinical manifestation of renal osteodystrophy in a growing child. This abnormality is associated with severe skeletal deformities and impairment of the child's activity. Epiphyseal slipping tends to occur late in the course of uremia, and is seen more frequently in children with congenital renal disease who have a longer duration of renal failure (Mehls et al., 1975). The pattern of slipping of the epiphyses is age related. Young children present with upper and lower femoral epiphyseal slipping. In contrast, upper femoral, radial, and ulnar epiphyses are involved in school-age children. In adolescents, epiphyseal slipping is coincident with the onset of puberty and may include the involvement of the forearm epiphyses (Dabbagh & Chesney, 1984). Surgical correction is often recommended for epiphyseal slipping, but treatment of the metabolic bone disease must come before any orthopedic attempts are made.

Effects of Hemodialysis on Renal Osteodystrophy. Calcium and vitamin D metabolism is disturbed in children undergoing chronic dialysis. However, the incidence of bone disease manifestations has markedly decreased over the last several years due to improved dialysis techniques and advances in drug therapy that are instituted earlier. Calcium imbalances occur because of the transfer of calcium across the dialysis membrane, which is influenced by blood flow, dialysate flow, and the rate of ultrafiltration (Mehls, 1984).

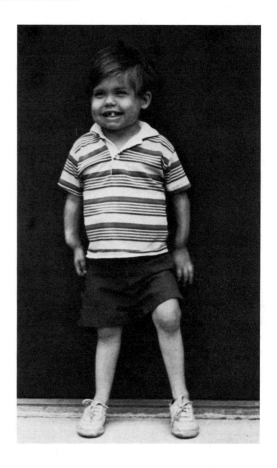

Figure 10-4. Child with severe deformities and consequences of osteodystrophy.

Osteopenia (decreased cell population) is a feature of renal osteodystrophy that occurs during dialysis, and reflects a substantial reduction in the amount of bone mass and the changes that occur because of it, such as bone pain and fractures. Osteomalacia (defective mineralization) may also occur in dialyzed children due to vitamin D deficiency and hypocalcemia.

Effects of Peritoneal Dialysis on Renal Osteodystrophy. Peritoneal dialysis may affect metabolic bone disease in children. Alterations and consequences are dependent upon calcium and phosphorus balance, the loss of PTH in the dialysate, the loss of vitamin D, and the removal of inhibitors of bone mineralization.

Concentrated dextrose solutions can create a negative calcium balance in the peritoneum and result in alterations in calcium and phosphorus balance. Increased protein loss occurs with peritonitis related to peritoneal dialysis. Most of the protein lost is albumin, which influences the loss of protein-bound vitamin D in the dialysate and alters bone metabolism.

Aluminum Intoxication. Aluminum intoxication has been implicated in both osteomalacia and osteopenia. The problem has been appreciated previously in adults and is now beginning to be recognized in children. Encephalopathy and bone fractures have prompted the investigation of high aluminum levels in children. Aluminum osteomalacia is characterized by progressive skeletal pain, proximal muscular weakness, bone pain, and unresponsiveness to vitamin D therapy (Mehls, 1984). It has been proposed that high concentrations of aluminum are toxic to osteoblasts and may explain low alkaline phosphatase levels and loss of bone mass (Alvarez-Ude et al., 1978). Aluminum may enter the body parenterally or by oral absorption, and accumulates on the bone surfaces.

High aluminum levels in dialyzed patients may originate from the presence of aluminum in dialysate water, aluminum in the water supply, chemicals from which the dialysate is produced, and from the ingestion of aluminum-containing phosphate binders (Kaehny, Hegg, & Alfrey, 1977). Tissue accumulation of aluminum occurs because the child cannot excrete it. Aluminum then accumulates in the bone matrix and causes defects in cell production. Aluminum can also accumulate in parathyroid tissue and interfere with the release of PTH, causing further bone problems. Because of the severity of the problem, many centers now recommend that children not be placed on aluminum-containing phosphate binders.

Effect of Transplantation on Renal Osteodystrophy. Preexisting renal osteodystrophy usually resolves with successful renal transplantation. The rate of healing depends on the preexisting hyperparathyroidism. Children treated previously with hemodialysis for more than three years show a slow resolution of the hyperparathyroidism compared with children treated for a shorter period of time (Mehls, 1984).

The administration of corticosteroids to prevent rejection of a transplanted kidney also appears to affect the skeleton in children. However, most researchers have failed to find a consistent correlation between the frequency of bone problems and the daily steroid dosage. Osteoporosis is seen more frequently with high steroid doses. Depleted stores of phosphorus may result from antacids, increased excretion by the kidney due to residual hyperparathyroidism, or steroids. Osteonecrosis usually appears in the first year after transplant, but late occurrence has been reported up to 4 years following transplantation (Mehls, 1984). The femoral head is the most commonly affected site. Pain is the most dominant symptom and may preceed x-ray evidence by several months.

Treatment of Renal Osteodystrophy. Management and treatment of bone and mineral abnormalities in children are difficult, since mineral homeostasis, parathyroid function, and vitamin D metabolism all rely on kidney function. Any decrease in renal function will cause serious disturbances in all these processes. As kidney function decreases there is a progressive elevation of serum phosphorus. Since the kidney is the chief means of phosphate excretion, the decreased glomerular filtration rate of renal failure causes retention of phosphate and an increased serum phosphate. An elevation of the serum phosphate upsets the normal calcium-phosphorus ratio, and to compensate, the serum calcium decreases. The parathyroid glands respond to the decreased calcium by stimulating parathormone (PTH) production. PTH affects the bones by causing a proliferation of osteoclasts and a degeneration of osteoblasts. The net effect is that calcium is pulled from bone tissue in an attempt to increase the serum level, which has profound implications for the growing child. To further complicate the problem, the failing kidneys are unable to convert vitamin D to its active metabolite, and this impairs calcium absorption from the intestines. In addition, acidosis can aggravate this imbalance.

Lowering the serum phosphate is extremely important. However, it is very difficult to accomplish in children. Meat and dairy products are important nutritive sources for growth, but these same foods are responsible for the majority of the dietary intake of phosphorus. Strict adherence to low-protein diets can reduce phosphorus but also restricts the necessary elements for active growth in children. Phosphate-binding gels, therefore, are mandatory. These gels bind phosphorus in the gut. Magnesium-containing antacids are not recommended in children because of potential hypermagnesemia.

Aluminum-containing products are not without consequences for the child. As already mentioned, tissue concentrations of aluminum can cause encephalopathy and renal dystrophy. The child may experience nausea, vomiting, and constipation from the products, and in addition, phosphate-binding agents have a chalky taste and adherence to the prescribed therapeutic regimen becomes a difficult issue. Aluminum hydroxide capsules can be successfully used in older children but are too large for younger children. Children also tend to reject the cookies that contain aluminum hydroxide. Infants and young children should receive a formula low in phosphate or with a high calcium:phosphate ratio.

Vitamin D analogs are used in an attempt to increase the intestinal absorption of calcium. However, vitamin D also increases absorption of phosphorus and raises the phosphate level. When phosphate levels are high, the use of vitamin D is contraindicated because of the danger of producing metastatic calcifications.

The administration of vitamin D_2 (of plant origin), vitamin D_3 (of mammalian origin), or the synthetic vitamin D analog, dihydrotachysterol (DHT) may be given to improve calcium absorption and thus decrease the reduction in mineral content in the bone. Several of the analogs are difficult to give to infants or small children because of difficulty in swallowing the capsule. The capsule can be opened and the medication dissolved in milk, but the exact dose is hard to measure and may lead to hypercalcemia. DHT liquid form can be used for infants and children. Another problem is the short half-life of these products, and children may have complications of vitamin D deficiency. Because of this, the analog usually used for children who do not always act in accordance with prescribed medications should have a longer half-life.

The aim of therapy in childhood renal osteodystrophy is to provide sufficient doses of whatever vitamin D analog is chosen to overcome the resistance to the actions of vitamin D that typify uremia, and yet still be safe. Clearly, hypercalcemia, hypercalcuria, and the consequent reduction in renal function must be avoided. No analog of vitamin D is safe if the potential for hypercalcemia is forgotten and if serum calcium levels are infrequently evaluated. The therapeutic use of vitamin D in children is very controversial. Most studies in children are short-term studies and are difficult to interpret and evaluate.

The overall therapeutic approach to renal osteodystrophy in children must be individualized. Calcium intake should be adequately adjusted and supplemental oral calcium may be necessary. The phosphate binder and vitamin D analog chosen must fit the needs of the patient with consideration of age, growth needs, serum levels, and willingness to take medications. The aim is to improve calcium absorption and assist bone mineralization. Phosphate intake and levels must be corrected and acidosis and PTH secretion controlled. Early recognition and treatment along with an individualized approach and plan is the key to controlling renal osteodystrophy in the child.

Acid-base Imbalances

Many disorders of volume and composition are associated with acid-base imbalances. The body attempts homeostatic control by balancing the production and excretion of hydrogen ions so that the pH of the extracellular fluid remains constant.

The acidosis of renal failure is caused by the kidney's inability to excrete excess hydrogen ions. As these ions are retained in the body, the increasing pH must be neutralized and buffered. The body is then maintained by a major portion of buffers extracellularly and cannot conserve them, thus creating a state of acidosis.

Acid retention is particularly detrimental in children because of their metabolic requirements for growth. Disturbances in pH of body fluids may have profound effects on the biochemical processes responsible for energy production and utilization. As renal failure progresses, calcium salts of bone are metabolized to buffer the acid that is retained. This interferes with growth of the bone and alterations in the bone structure. Attempts at correction of acidosis are therefore of considerable importance in maintaining growth. By correcting acidosis, the aim is to create a positive calcium balance so that new bone formation can occur. Specific correction therapy for acidosis in children is controversial. Many times, more problems can be created by attempting to correct acid-base abnormalities than if the condition is left untreated. The metabolic acidosis associated with acute renal failure is generally not treated in children. The acidosis is usually mild and does not cause a problem for the child. Thus, the controversy solely concerns children with chronic renal failure.

For severe acidosis, dialysis may be the mode of treatment if it is perceived that the administration of sodium bicarbonate may cause problems with hypertension, congestive heart failure, or neurological effects for the child. However, rapid correction of acidosis with dialysis has produced complications of cerebral edema and death in children. In addition, attempts to lower acidosis with dialysis may result in hypocalcemia and cause tetany and convulsions.

Hypertension

Hypertension is often a problem in children with all forms of renal disease, whether early in the course, in the process of renal failure, or following transplantation.

Cardiac output and the peripheral vascular resistance determine the blood pressure. When the child's kidneys fail, the blood pressure is affected by fluid volume changes, cardiovascular influences, hormonal factors, and autonomic nervous system control. For example, a child with renal failure usually has an expanded extracellular volume. This increases the cardiac output and compensating autoregulation may cause a rise in the resistance of the peripheral vessels, producing hypertension. This leads to an increase in the ventricular workload and function. Renin and hormonal substances such as aldosterone and angiotension may affect the reactivity of the vessels. In addition, the autonomic nervous system may play a role in hypertension.

In the differential diagnosis of hypertension in the child, it is important to distinguish acute hypertension (often reversible) from chronic hypertension. Often the child's history and other clinical clues will suggest a cause. The most common causes of hypertension secondary to acute renal disorders are acute glomerulonephritis, anaphylactoid purpura, nephritis, and hemolytic uremic syndrome. Chronic hypertension may be caused by renovascular or renal parenchymal disease.

Most children with chronic renal disease develop hypertension as they progress into renal failure. As children approach end-stage disease, there appear to be two distinct groups of patients, those with previous hypertension who have had glomerular disease, and those with renal dysplasia, hypoplasia, or a structural defect in whom hypertension is less common. The Children's Hospital Medical Center in Boston reported 98 percent of children with glomerular diseases had predialysis hypertension whereas only 23 percent of those with structural lesions had hypertension (Ingelfinger, 1982).

Once children begin dialysis, most have problems with periods of hypertension. Ultrafiltration controls blood pressure. However, in children, ultrafiltration to dry weight often produces hypotension. The major cause of dialysis-related hypertension is intravascular volume expansion. Thus, reducing the intravascular volume will control blood pressure unless the hypertension is renin dependent. Because vascular volume is so fragile in the child, special importance is given to the child's weight.

When peritoneal dialysis is first initiated in children, hypertension is seen as frequently as it is in children on hemodialysis. As the course of peritoneal dialysis progresses, these children have far better blood pressure control than children on hemodialysis. The reason may be better fluid control or less frequent fluid shifts.

If the child's kidneys are removed, blood pressure changes may occur, but these reflect changes in vascular volume. Volume depletion during dialysis becomes an important consideration since hypotension may result.

Posttransplant hypertension is common in children. In fact, almost all will be hypertensive during the first week after transplant. The hypertension appears to be due to either volume expansion or the effects of renin. Electrolytes, water, and colloid solutions can produce fluid overload and hypertension in the immediate postoperative period. The smaller the child, the more frequently this occurs. In addition, steroids used to prevent rejection may also induce hypertension by currently unknown mechanisms. The small size of the renal arteries in the child's transplanted kidney may also lead to an increase in blood pressure. The circumstances where renin appears to influence hypertension are hypoperfusion of the transplanted kidney, nephritis, or rejection episodes. In transplanted children who have kept their own kidneys, renin may be released from either of the kidneys, thus creating or contributing to hypertension.

Treatment of Hypertension. Control of hypertension during the course of renal disease is extremely important in preventing complications and problems with other organs (heart and brain) and in decreasing morbidity. Good blood pressure control can also slow the progression of the renal failure and improve the quality of life for the child. Many pharmacological agents are used in children. The agents used depend upon the response to the medication, the status of renal function, and the special problems of the child. The processes in children that determine drug absorption, distribution, metabolism, and excretion undergo considerable change between birth and adolescence. The most dramatic changes occur in the first few months of life and extend to about 1 year. Changes coincide with functional and developmental maturity and can affect the use and effectiveness of pharmacological agents.

As failure progresses, the effect of absorption, metabolism, and the elimination of these drugs becomes increasingly important. Medications for the hypertensive anephric patient carry further implications.

The effect of dialysis on the blood levels of medications varies greatly. Some agents are removed and are dialyzable and others are not. The effect of vasodilating agents can present special problems for the child on dialysis.

The immediate posttransplant control of hypertension involves careful attention to regulation of fluid volume. Colloid and fluid administration, urine output, and the cardiovascular status should be monitored very closely. Most children respond to diuresis and fluid restriction. Some children have volume expansion in association with acute tubular necrosis (ATN); on the other hand, hypotension in the early posttransplant days can lead to prerenal azotemia and acute renal failure. Because of this, diuretics and fluid administration must be monitored carefully.

Sometimes postoperative hypertension may require specific drug therapy for management. If the transplanted kidney has normal function, no special precautions regarding drug therapy are necessary. If the transplanted kidney is showing signs of insufficiency or if the child has hypertension, then dosage and metabolism concerns surface, and adjustment may be needed. Drug implications are always more tenuous and difficult to manage in the child than in the adult.

It is vital to enlist the help of the child and family in monitoring the blood pressure. Frequent blood pressure readings are important especially if the child is receiving multiple medications. Objective information supplied by the child and family will also aid medication adjustment.

Other factors are also important in controlling blood pressure in the child. Dietary restrictions can provide control of fluids and electrolytes. Exercise, relaxation techniques, and biofeedback may also be useful in the control of hypertension in children, but in general are of limited value.

System Dysfunction
Dysfunction of systems other than the renal system are often observed in children with ESRD.

Liver Dysfunction.   Liver dysfunction has been associated with renal disease in children and can cause significant problems and severe damage. Many times the children are asymptomatic and often the etiology of the problem remains difficult to pinpoint. Viral infection is the most common cause of liver dysfunction in children. The specific viruses will be discussed later in this chapter.

The liver is a prime target for drug toxity in children with poor renal function because it is the other major site where metabolism and the degradation of drugs occur. Liver damage from drugs may include a spectrum of changes including hepatitis, necrosis, and cirrhosis. The injurious agent may be difficult to determine even with careful investigation. If a drug is suspect, it should be eliminated and further monitoring of liver function continued.

Pulmonary Dysfunction.   Changes in the pulmonary function may also cause problems for the child with renal insufficiency. Dysfunction may occur from viral and bacterial infections, calcium deposition, and as a result of congestive heart failure or muscle weakness. Pulmonary changes have been appreciated in adults for a long time but are just beginning to be studied in children. Any condition that causes a decrease in the lung volume may present problems for the child. Again, the smaller the child, the greater the problem.

Accumulation of fluid in the lung causes a loss of elastic recoil of the lung. This produces a decrease in the perfusion of the lung as well as decreased ventilation and impaired gas exchange. These changes may become severe and irreversible. Dialysis may correct and improve this condition as fluid balance is achieved and lung edema decreases, permitting greater air flow. In some instances, children show patterns of irreversible changes in the lung interstitum and dialysis does not improve their disease. As renal insufficiency progresses in children, pulmonary parenchymal changes may occur, creating fibrosis or calcifications.

Cardiovascular Dysfunction. The cardiovascular status of the child with renal failure is an important determinant of survival. The cardiac changes that occur are an adaption to the changes produced by renal failure—anemia, electrolyte, and acid-base problems, and volume changes. Echocardiography in some children has demonstrated left ventricular changes and deterioration of function, but in ESRD disease the most striking cardiovascular finding is the presence of heart murmurs. These may be a consequence of anemia, overhydration, hypertension, or aortic changes. Severe uremia in children has been linked with cardiomyopathy and greatly decreased left ventricular function due to the effect of "toxins" on the ventricle (O'Regan, 1984). Other factors associated with renal failure, such as hyperkalemia and acidosis, also may depress the contractility of the heart.

Pericarditis does occur in children with renal disease. The incidence may be as high as 50 percent of untreated children with uremia and as high as 15 to 20 percent in children on dialysis (O'Regan, 1984). After transplantation, when the anemia, fluid, and electrolyte problems resolve and the uremic toxins are eliminated, the effects on the cardiac muscle may resolve. It may take up to a year or more for cardiac function to improve. Until the time of transplantation, the mainstay of treatment includes management of the many factors affecting the cardiovascular system and administration of red blood cell transfusions. Transfusion needs in the child are highly variable but may be required for such symptoms as fatigue, chest pain, exercise intolerance, anorexia, or evidence of heart failure. Children need close monitoring for signs of hypertension, overload, and heart failure to insure safe transfusion.

Hematologic Dysfunction. Anemia is more severe in children than adults and is a major cause of increased cardiac output. The degree of anemia is directly proportional to the degree of renal failure. Children also experience accelerated red cell destruction on dialysis, but in addition, a greater amount of blood may be lost because of a relatively greater amount of blood left in the tubing dialyzer.

Anemia reduces the capacity for oxygen delivery to the tissues. In renal insufficiency, the oxygen consumption by the heart muscle and the workload of the heart are increased. Therefore, if the child has significant anemia, the oxygen demand may not be met and will contribute to decreased cardiac function and decreased oxygenation of tissues. When anemia is severe in children, it causes fatigue, limits exercise tolerance, and may affect the growth rate.

When arteriovenous shunts for hemodialysis are constructed in children, there appears to be similar cardiovascular hemodynamic changes as seen in the adult. However, in children, cardiac failure attributable to arteriovenous shunts has rarely been reported.

Infection

Urinary tract infection (UTI) is one of the major bacterial diseases of childhood. The occurrence of UTI is influenced by the age and sex of the child, the presence of anatomic abnormalities of the urinary tract, and the site and frequency of infection. In children, a febrile state often indicates renal infection. Urinary tract infections due to obstruction are more common in boys, and infections due to bacteria ascending the urinary tract are more prevalent in girls.

The immune response of the child is diminished and altered in both acute and chronic renal failure and infection is a frequent complication. Both cellular and humoral immunity are affected. Splenectomy, urologic and vascular surgical procedures, anemia coagulation alterations, malnutrition, and immunosuppression with drugs, make the child susceptible to an opportunistic infection.

The incidence of vascular access site infections appears to be similar to that of adults. These infections involve mostly *Staphylococcus aureus,* but *streptococci* and gram-negative organisms are also observed. The incidence of local infections has been reported from one to three episodes per year (Potter et al., 1970). Hemodialysis access complications in children will be discussed later in the chapter.

Hepatitis. Hepatitis B virus infection is the most common infectious complication of children on long-term dialysis and may pose a significant risk to the child. Children with hepatitis B antigen in their serum should be considered infectious and precautions observed. Because of the prevalence of hepatitis B in hemodialysis units, immunization or prophylaxis is often considered. The goal of the immunization is the production of antibody to hepatitis B antigen and protection from the virus infection. Readers are referred to specific guidelines established in their institutions regarding the use of immune serum globulins and hepatitis B virus vaccine for the prophylaxis protection.

Posttransplant Infections. The immunosuppressant therapy used to prevent rejection decreases the immune response of children to infection. The T-lymphocytes and the phagocytic system that are critical for the defense against organisms are affected. Therefore, opportunistic pathogens may readily invade the body due to a weakened defense system. Bacteria, fungi, protozoa, and viruses have been shown to complicate the child's posttransplant course. Bacterial infections usually respond well to antibiotic therapy. Fungi and protozoa infections, of course, make the child more seriously ill. Temperatures of 101F or greater and the time and the height of fever are important. Viral infections are responsible for half of the posttransplant fevers that may persist for long periods of time (Peterson et al., 1981). Except for fever, these children are often asymptomatic.

Other infections also may pose a hazard to the transplant child. Bacteria may invade the wound, urinary tract, blood, or lungs. The urinary tract is the most common site for bacterial infections posttransplant and an incidence as high as 58 percent has been reported in the pediatric population. The outcome and course depends on the time of onset and the association with surgical complications. Those infections occurring in the first 3 months after transplant are often severe, as opposed to relatively benign infections after 6 months. Significant concerns include septicemia, pyelonephritis, and the graft dysfunction. Avoidance of surgical complications and institution of antibiotic therapy have greatly reduced these threats. However, bowel perforation associated with CMV infection or steroid therapy and resulting gram-negative septicemia still remain a significant threat for the child.

Fungal infection in renal transplant children occurs with a reported incidence of 13 percent (Leone & McEnery, 1984). Sites of infection include lungs, gastrointestinal tract, genitourinary system, and central nervous system. The cryptococcus organism is the most frequent complication. Other opportunistic organisms include *Candida, Aspergillus,* and *Coccidiodes.* Concurrent infections with viruses, bacteria, and protozoa are often present.

Cytomegalovirus (CMV) is the most frequent serious infectious complication following transplantation. Usually the child will have a fever for longer than 7 days, which most often occurs during the first 4 months after transplant. The clinical course may be severe and significant morbidity may occur.

Varicella-zoster virus in children with renal transplant is either primary (chicken pox) or secondary (shingles). In children who have had a documented infection, reinfection may lead to a second episode of chicken pox. The incidence of primary infection (chicken pox) in the pediatric transplant population is reported to be 12 percent (Feldhoff, Balfour, & Najarian, 1981). Because of the virulence of this organism, children who have been exposed should receive zoster immune globulin or plasma within 72 hours of exposure. Children who develop varicella may need to be admitted to the hospital for careful observation. If the child is already in the hospital, isolation procedures should be instituted for a period of up to 28 days following the exposure. The incubation period in the transplant child may be prolonged, and isolation of children potentially incubating chicken pox from other susceptible patients is necessary.

Dental Abnormalities

Abnormal teeth are a common finding in children with chronic renal failure. Formation of organic tooth matrix, calcification, and enamel formation may be adversely affected in the child from the fourth fetal month until age 8 years. Any systemic insult such as calcium imbalances, vitamin D deficiencies, and elevated serum phosphorus and parathormone levels may produce teeth deformities. Bone growth and mineralization are disrupted by the metabolic abnormalities of chronic renal failure and result in hypoplasia of the enamel formation of permanent teeth. This appears to correspond with the age of onset of advanced renal failure (Woodhead & Nowak, 1982). The disfiguring effects of enamel hypoplasia must be recognized. The burden of chronic illness is made worse by visible signs and effects on the child's personal appearance. Parents and children need to know that there are procedures and treatment that can restore the enamel and appearance of the teeth.

GROWTH AND DEVELOPMENT OF CHILDREN WITH RENAL DISEASE

Delayed growth and development due to chronic renal insufficiency (CRI) can have a marked effect on a child's ability to cope with life. This can be very stressful, especially when it is added to the child's already formidable physical health problems. Chronic renal insufficiency can be defined as the state of decreased renal function due to disease or injury. Growth retardation is multifactorial and may involve protein malnutrition, acidosis, hyperparathyroidism, inadequate caloric intake, renal osteodystrophy, and hormonal alterations, in varying degrees. It is therefore very important to make careful study of these areas and to adjust therapy to minimize these problems.

Stages of Growth

During the first year of life, a baby is expected to grow from a birth length of 20 to 22 inches to 30 to 32 inches at the end of the year. This is considered a period of high growth rate. The infant who is born with dysplastic kidneys, obstructive uropathy, or other congenital renal problems is at increased risk of having growth depression begin earlier and be more severe than in children with acquired kidney disease (Scharer & Gilli, 1984). In addition, infants with congenital renal abnormalities are likely to suffer loss of statural growth and also loss of increase in occipital-frontal circumference (OFC) during this first critical year. Concern surrounds the lack of head growth in these children, as it may mean severe learning disabilities and other central nervous system problems in the future.

The rapid growth rate declines in the normal child over the first 3 to 4 years after infancy. This is followed by a period with steady growth of 6 to 7 cm/year until the onset of puberty. In children with known renal disease, this growth velocity varies depending on their degree of renal insufficiency and their loss of glomerular function. Body growth may be markedly retarded, even early in their course of renal insufficiency when loss of glomerular function is minimal.

This growth retardation is seen most often in children with congenital metabolic disorders such as cystinosis or with diseases causing severe protein losses. Overall it is observed that the most significant factor influencing growth retardation is the duration rather than the type of primary renal disease (Scharer & Gilli, 1984).

Final growth occurs in the pubertal period, beginning in girls at a mean age of 11 years and in boys at age 13. A growth spurt with peak height velocities reaching 7 to 9 cm/year can be expected during this stage.

The child with renal insufficiency is very likely to experience delayed pubertal development. In a 1980 study, Ferraris and colleagues evaluated 31 adolescent males with CRI. The subjects were divided into three groups: those presently on hemodialysis, those not on any form of dialysis, and those who were postrenal transplant. Bone growth and secondary sexual characteristic development was delayed in the majority of children in all groups. Adrenal androgens were reduced in the nontransplanted adolescents. Serum testosterone levels were normal relative to pubertal stage. The patients requiring dialysis or transplantation showed more severe bone age and sexual maturation delay than did the nondialyzed CRI patients.

Assessment of Growth

Anthropometric measurements should be obtained every 6 months in the child with CRI. Notation should be made of any changes in treatment since the previous measurement. Measurements should include height, weight, OFC, midarm circumference, and triceps skinfold thickness. Midarm circumference should be measured at the site halfway between acromian and olecranon when the child's right arm is bent at the elbow (Fig. 10-5). The measurement should be obtained with the child's arm hanging relaxed at the side. Figure 10-6 demonstrates how tricep skinfold thickness may be obtained in this same position and at the same site on the arm using a Lange skinfold caliper manufactured by Cambridge Scientific Industries (Cambridge, Maryland). These data are used to estimate body fat and muscle mass.

Bone age films are useful in assessing skeletal maturity, and some sources feel should also be obtained every 6 months. Included are radiographs of the left hand and wrist and the left knee. Score and range for bone age can be found in methods developed by Tanner and associates (1975) and Greulich and Pyle (1959). Reference data for measurements of height and weight can be found in the standards of the National Center for Health Statistics (Hamill, 1977).

Tanner's maturity ratings based on testicular size and amount of pubic hair in the male, and breast size and amount of pubic hair in the female, are widely accepted as a method for the staging of puberty (Tanner, 1962). Tes-

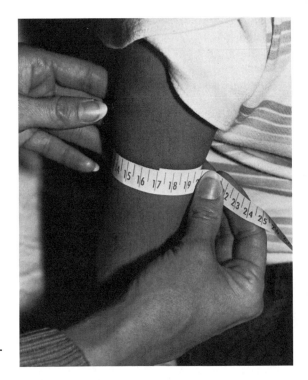

Figure 10-5. Midarm circumference measurement.

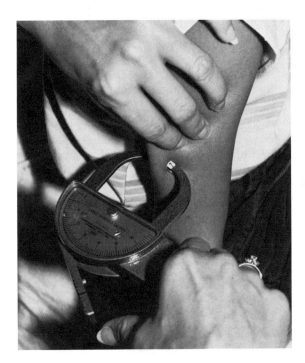

Figure 10-6. Tricep skinfold.

ticular size should be measured and the first signs of puberty should be recorded so that the initiation of the growth spurt can be documented. In females, the date of menarche should also be noted.

Possible Causes of Decreased Growth
Growth retardation is a descriptive phrase using body height and chronological age and thus determining that the child is 2 or more standard deviations below the normal mean or below the third percentile. Catch-up growth is a phenomenon observed when, after the removal of the problematic, growth-disturbing conditions, the child who had been following a retarded pattern of growth has a restoration of the growth deficit. It is usually characterized by an increase in growth velocity and then a deceleration until the child levels off at his or her normal curve (Scharer & Gilli, 1984). Many theories exist as to why children with CRI do not grow normally. Calorie and protein malnutrition, poor bone growth due to renal osteodystrophy, hormonal alterations, electrolyte imbalances and acidosis, and chronic uremia and its toxins will be discussed here.

Caloric Malnutrition. Lack of appetite in the child with CRI has been attributed to several possible factors including changes in taste perception, hypertension, polydipsia, and psychological stress of chronic illness. The child whose intake falls below normal requirements goes into a state of negative nitrogen balance. It appears that with uremia, the caloric and protein requirements for growth are increased over normal standards. Thus, a uremic child may need to consume above-normal amounts of calories to try to avoid growth retardation and stay in positive nitrogen balance.

Controversy surrounds the role of caloric supplementation and its influence on growth. Betts, McGrath, & White (1977) attempted to supplement the caloric intake of children with CRF and did not observe an increase in growth rate. What was observed was the difficulty of maintaining a high energy intake in the CRF patient. Scharer and Gilli (1984) observed that growth in their population did not increase even when nasogastric hyperalimentation was given. Rather, the increase occurred in the amount of adipose tissue and the weight-height ratio. Other groups report more encouraging data.

Despite the controversy in the area of supplementation, it appears to be advantageous to prescribe a diet containing at least 90 to 110 percent of the RDA for calories to maximize a CRI child's growth potential. Nasogastric tube feeding may be necessary to deliver this number of calories to the child whose appetite is abnormal.

Protein. Protein intake is considered an important factor in growth of children with CRI. Children at risk of having low levels of protein are those with increased loss of protein as in nephrotic syndrome and children on peritoneal dialysis. It is not clear what level of protein intake is most beneficial for growth. A study by Kleinknecht and associates (1980) of 76 pediatric patients on long-term hemodialysis showed better growth occurred when protein intake was modified to allow only 75 percent of RDA. In a multicenter study reported by the European Dialysis Transplant Association, the growth rate of children taking in 100 percent of RDA of protein was 4.3 cm/year; next best was the growth rate of children with protein restriction, who grew 3.2 cm/year; and the slowest growth was in the group on unrestricted protein diets (Donckerwolcke et al., 1982).

When considering altering the level of protein intake, effect on the kidney function must be considered. It appears that a protein intake similar to that of a normal child (100 percent of RDA) is optimal for growth of the child with CRI. The protein should be of high biologic value, containing a high proportion of essential amino acids. This type is most abundant in meats. Too much protein will lead to high BUN measurements and too little, to protein malnutrition. If a child is taking in adequate calories, the goal would be to have the diet include 2 g protein/100 kcal.

Renal Osteodystrophy. Renal osteodystrophy refers to the bone disease that results from the disturbed calcium and phosphorus metabolism and biochemical bone abnormalities seen in CRI. Two mechanisms play roles in causing this problem: abnormal vitamin D metabolism and secondary hyperparathyroidism. Administration of vitamin D analogues may hold hope for limiting the progress of bone disease and thereby minimizing growth failure. The effect of therapy causes either improvement in bone deformities or actual increase in bone mass and length. Secondary hyperparathyroidism results from altered calcium and phosphate absorption. After parathyroidectomy some children with CRI have accelerated growth, but usually very short-term.

Hormonal Alterations. There are several hormones that are altered in children with CRI that may be linked to growth retardation. Uremic patients have been found to have increased levels of immunoreactive plasma growth hormones (Rauh & Oertel, 1984). Somatomedin levels are found to be significantly diminished in children with chronic renal disease (Pennisi et al., 1979). This hormone is measured by several different assays and reflects the level of growth hormone. Uremic patients may have decreased levels due to an inhibitor present in their bodies. Hemodialysis increases somatomedin levels and transplantation returns plasma levels to normal, and this normalization has been correlated with some increase in growth rate.

Normal thyroid function is necessary for maintaining growth rates. Some abnormalities of thyroid function, which may contribute to growth problems in children with CRI, have been reported (Rauh & Oertel, 1984). It is not simply that levels of thyroid are low, although this is seen in children with cystinosis. Patients usually are not hypothyroid and often have normal TSH levels. Whether administering thyroid hormone would stimulate growth in uremic children has not been determined.

Testosterone levels have been found to be below normal prior to and during puberty in CRI patients (Scharer et al., 1980). Because it is the rapid increase in testosterone level that leads to the increase in growth velocity during puberty, boys with CRI fail to experience this very significant growth spurt. As mentioned previously, androgen levels are usually low in most of these children. Speculation exists as to whether estrogen levels may be altered in CRI and thereby produce growth failure in girls.

Electrolyte Imbalance and Acidosis. The abnormal loss of increased amounts of electrolytes from the body may be another factor leading to growth retardation in CRI. Tubular loss of water, electrolytes, and bicarbonate disturb the homeostasis of the body and may decrease the growth potential. These factors come into importance most often in the long-term, more slowly progressing congenital nephropathies such as dysplastic or polycystic kidneys.

Calcium. Calcium may be chronically low in the child with CRI due to hypercalcuria and may lead to decreased growth rates, especially if it contributes to the development of renal osteodystrophy. The problem is often due to decreased calcium absorption from the gut. Calcium supplementation may partially alleviate this problem, but it remains a therapeutic challenge in many children with renal disease.

Phosphorus. Phosphorus appears to be another important electroyte to keep in balance to potentiate growth. This hypothesis is based on the observation of patients suffering from vitamin-D-resistant rickets, who experience an increased growth rate when supplemented with phosphate. Low phosphorus may be a problem in patients on dialysis due to overuse of phosphate binders or dietary deficiency.

Potassium. Increased potassium loss is seen in patients with congenital tubular disorders, as in Bartter's syndrome. It is possible that this increased loss of potassium may play a part in the renal patient's growth problem.

    Hyposthenuria, the secretion of urine of low specific gravity, causes the blood to become hyperosmolar and may be responsible for growth failure in renal patients. Those at greatest risk are patients with diabetes insipidus. When this condition is corrected by administering fluids, improvement in growth is seen.

Sodium. Sodium chloride levels may be low in patients with renal disorders that cause them to be salt wasters. This chemical is employed during the growth of connective tissue and cartilage, and thus may play a role in the growth process.

Acidosis. West and Smith (1956) noted that metabolic acidosis was an important factor in causing growth retardation in azotemic children. They reported that 76 percent of growth-stunted children had acidosis. This thought is exemplified by children with renal tubular acidosis who, when corrected with bicarbonate, demonstrate catch-up growth (McShary & Morris, 1978). The role of acidosis is difficult to measure, but it does appear to perhaps lead to hypophosphatemia, which may influence growth and also may deplete the body of cations and inhibit 1, 25 $(OH)_2D_3$ production (Kleinknecht, Broyer, Huot, Marti-Henneberg, & Dartois, 1983). This vitamin D analog is thought to be essential for bone growth.

Toxins. Uremic toxins that build up in the blood and are not removed by the diseased kidney may lead to growth failure. In a study by Kleinknecht and associates (1983) of nondialyzed children, where GFR was greater than 25 ml/min/1.73 m^2, the children were less growth retarded than those with GFR less that 12 ml/min/1.73 m^2, although the difference was not statistically significant. In dialyzed children, growth was less if predialysis levels of BUN and creatinine were high.

Other factors being considered as possibly affecting growth are anemia, hypertension, chronic hypertonicity from nitrogen retention, and chronic infection. In summary, many causes of growth failure in uremic children are being investigated with hopes of limiting their deleterious effects.

Specific recommendations to maximize growth appear to be the following:

1. Supplement calories to provide 100 to 110 percent of the RDA
2. Supplement protein to provide 100 percent of the RDA
3. Follow vigorous therapy to prevent renal osteodystrophy
4. Monitor and supplement if hormone imbalances exist
5. Correct electrolyte imbalances
6. Correct acidosis
7. Control uremia with diet or dialysis

Growth on Hemodialysis

Most available data comes from the European Dialysis and Transplant Association, where long-term hemodialysis in children is a common mode of therapy. Data collected for over 10 years show that 39 percent of all patients below 15 years of age had a body height below the third percentile for chronological age when dialysis was initiated. The mean growth rate for prepubertal children who had been hemodialyzed for at least 3 years was 2.8 cm/year (Scharer et al., 1976) as compared to an expected growth of 6 to 7 cm/year. Growth-rate data is commonly expressed in standard deviations (SD) above or below the mean. In prepuberty children on dialysis, the annual loss of height for chronological age was 0.43 SD (Donckerwolcke et al., 1978). Accepted limit for maximal loss is less than 0.2 SD/year.

On long-term dialysis, the growth velocity of European children remained reduced at a fairly constant rate, which produced a progressive decrease in height percentile. An average height loss of 2.4 SD was seen in prepubertal children who had been dialyzed for more than 5 years (Chantler et al., 1978). Dialyzed children do show some potential for improved growth during puberty (Donckerwolcke et al., 1982). Kleinknecht and associates (1980) reported a height gain of 3 cm/year, which still falls short of the normal child's peak velocity of 7 to 9 cm/year. The pubertal growth spurt seems to occur later in dialyzed children and may last up until they are 20 years old or more. The late growth does not usually compensate for height previously lost.

Varying hemodialysis techniques do not appear to alter growth (Scharer & Gilli, 1984). No significant difference has been noted with different hours on dialysis per week, different types of dialyzers, or variable efficiency of dialysis expressed as dialyzer surface area per body surface area. The child with residual renal function does not experience any better growth while on dialysis.

Although hemodialysis does an effective job in fluid waste removal, it apparently is not able to correct the problems that lead to growth failure in CRI patients. These children are usually several standard deviations below the mean for height and are growing at a rate much below the accepted range of normal. Despite aggressive therapy, they are often sentenced to a life of short stature, which can have widespread emotional and psychological effects.

Growth on Peritoneal Dialysis

Peritoneal dialysis offers several theoretical advantages over other dialysis techniques that may lead to improved growth in children. Patients on peritoneal dialysis have a largely unlimited diet, especially in terms of protein intake, and a constant source of carbohydrate calories from their dialysate. Peritoneal dialysis provides a more stable internal body environment and, as a result, BUN, creatinine, and potassium levels may never reach the peaks observed with hemodialysis.

Kohaut (1982) studied children on CAPD for 12 to 26 months (mean 14.7 months). Expected statural growth was defined as the increment in height expected of a normal child of the same sex and bone age who was growing along the 50th percentile curve on standard growth charts. Out of 11 children aged 3 months to 16 years, 5 grew at rates over 100 percent of that expected, exhibiting definite catch-up growth. Three others grew at rates of 88 percent to 95 percent of that expected. The final 3 children grew at rates of 28 percent, 67 percent, and 75 percent of expected growth. Aggressive supplementation of diet was employed using glucose and medium chain triglycerides. Protein supplements were not usually used. Nasogastric feeding was used when the child was ill with peritonitis or other acute illnesses. Renal osteodystrophy was monitored closely with x-rays periodically and treated with phosphate binders and calcium supplements. Possible factors influencing this improved growth were control of hyperparathyroidism and daily energy and protein intake. All 5 children who grew 100 percent of the expected growth had serum PTH levels no greater than twice normal, and 4 of the 5 children had daily protein intakes in excess of 2 g/kg and energy intakes greater than 100 percent of the RDA for normal children of the same sex and height. Growth rates did not correlate with residual renal function.

This study showed impressive results of improved growth with good nutrition and control of bone disease and efficient dialysis using CAPD. Not all programs report these encouraging results, and thus growth remains a concern on this form of dialysis as in hemodialysis and intermittent peritoneal dialysis, where growth in these two forms occurs at a similar, slow rate.

Growth After Transplantation

Growth appears to be better following transplantation than that experienced on dialysis. Optimal growth rates are achieved when the duration of CRI prior to transplant is the shortest, because during this period children experience decreased growth velocity and may fall below their previously established growth curve. Very young children show the most promising growth rates followed by prepubertal children and then those in and beyond puberty. In children transplanted below the age of 7 years, Ingelfinger and associates (1981) showed a growth rate above the 50th percentile. In contrast, only 1 of 16 patients over 7 years showed this impressive growth rate.

When the function of the allograft decreases, the growth rate also usually decreases. Pennisi and associates (1977) state that the critical level of GFR associated with the reduction of growth is approximately 60 ml/min/1.73 m². When a child's growth rate starts to severely decline, some centers believe it is time to start looking for a new allograft to transplant to try to limit time lost and maximize growth before puberty.

Fine and colleagues (1978) observed that when skeletal maturation is advanced (the child having bone age of 12 years or more with fusion of epiphyses) prior to transplantation, growth after transplant will be minimal. Conversely, Donckerwolcke and associates (1978) found that some adolescents with advanced skeletal maturation had a high growth rate following transplantation.

The amount of steroids used for immunosuppression has a marked effect on the child's growth rate. Steroids are known to have several negative effects on the growth process, such as inhibition of growth hormone secretion, depression of growth activity of cartilage and bone cells, reduction of somatomedin activity, and limitation of calcium absorption from the gut (Scharer & Gilli, 1984). A child's individual ability to metabolize and eliminate the steroids from the body may explain the wide range of growth rates seen following transplantation.

Controversy surrounds the issue of daily versus alternate-day steroid therapy. When the daily dose exceeds 0.5 mg/kg/day, the growth rate is seen to decrease. Doses of 0.2 to 0.3 mg/kg/day allow growth to remain at normal rates in transplanted children. Alternate-day therapy may allow a child to experience some increase in growth rate but there are also risks of increased incidence of rejection. Further study in this area is necessary to determine the steroid therapy schedule that is safest yet the most beneficial for growth rate.

Pediatric patients on long-term hemodialysis or who have been transplanted continue to show growth at an age when normal children have stopped. This continued later growth may partially compensate for the slowed growth rate of CRI. Despite this, in a study of 34 patients with CRI, their final adult heights were mostly in the lower percentile and 23 percent had a final height below the third percentile. Female patients reached their final height at 16.9 years; males at 18 years (Gilli et al., 1980).

NUTRITIONAL MANAGEMENT IN CHILDREN WITH ESRD

Adequate nutritional assessment and intervention can influence the course of a child's battle with renal disease. With good dietary review and counseling, the pitfalls of malnutrition, growth retardation, hypertension, and bone disease can often be limited. Active involvement of a dietitian as a valuable member of the health team can provide necessary, ongoing evaluation of the CRI child's nutrition and the intense teaching vital to attaining maximum well-being for these patients.

Nutritional Assessment

A comprehensive nutritional assessment establishes the child's current status and determines the most pressing needs. A 3-day diet history provides an account of all foods taken in over that period of time. It allows the dietitian to calculate caloric, protein, vitamin, carbohydrate, sodium, calcium and phosphorus, potassium, fat, and fluid intake. It helps identify problem areas that can then be modified in the child's individual diet plan. This information is obtained by interviews and from food records kept by the child or parents. The interview should seek out knowledge about the child's appetite, eating habits, recent weight changes, level of activity, past surgical procedures, transplant and dialysis status, bowel habits, likes and dislikes in the four food groups, and where the child usually eats his or her meals. Getting to know the family and their economic and social status may shed some light on their eating habits and their potential for adhering to the prescribed diet plan. The diet history should be as detailed as possible, including weights of foods, measurements of fluids, and brand names of convenience foods. This allows the dietitian to make the most accurate assessment of the child's intake and to see where improvements can be made.

It is important to note which medications the child is presently taking. Some medications interact with food intake to bind certain elements in the foods. Others contain substances that may add to the child's problems, such as those containing sodium. For example, Kayexalate, the medication used to maintain a normal serum potassium level, contains sodium (100 mg Na/g Kayexalate), and this amount needs to be considered in a sodium-restricted child's intake. Medications may have an effect on the child's appetite or elimination. Phosphate binders often cause constipation so that a stool softener may need to be used prophylactically. Kayexalate, if mixed with Sorbitol, can cause diarrhea.

Frequent review of the child's medications by the dietitian can avoid the oversight of their effects on diet and may also shed light on whether or not the child takes the prescribed medications.

Close monitoring of serum lab values aids in the total assessment of the child's nutrition. Electrolytes, BUN, creatinine, calcium, phosphorus, total protein, albumin, glucose, magnesium, cholesterol, and triglycerides should be checked on a monthly basis. BUN, total protein, and albumin reflect the child's protein intake and help to evaluate actual protein intake. Protein recommendations are given in Table 10-2.

Anthropometric measurements provide data on how the dietary regimen is affecting the child's growth and development of muscles and fat stores. Height, weight, occipital frontal circumference (OFC), midarm circumference (MAC), and tricep skin fold (TSF) thickness should be measured monthly to allow graphing of the child's progress and determination of lack of expected development. Growth charts developed by the National Center for Health Statistics (1977) provide standardized percentiles for comparison. Accuracy is enhanced if the same individual obtains the measurements following the standard protocol (method of MAC and TSF), as described in "Growth and Development" earlier in this chapter.

To teach nutrition to children and to parents, it helps to establish some rapport with them first. After several visits to gather information, the dietitian may sit down with the family and explain what the dietary plan is for the child. Covering only what is necessary at that point will give the family a basic outline without overwhelming them with details. Frequent reviewing of materials is essential to discover points that the family may not understand. This area of teaching can be enhanced by any creative approach that makes the information easier to remember. Charts, games, and pictures as well as written materials will aid the patient and family in retaining the information shared with them. Nutritional plans must be flexible and should try to accommodate some favorite foods and eating habits. Equally necessary is the es-

TABLE 10-2. PROTEIN RECOMMENDATIONS

Weight	Restricted Protein Diet (g/kg/day)	Increased Protein Diet (g/kg/day)
10–20 kg	2.0	2.0–3.0
20–30 kg	1.5	1.5–2.0
30–40 kg	1.5	1.5–2.0
>40 kg	1.0	1.0–1.5

tablishment of consistent guidelines by the parents to govern their child's eating behavior at home.

Infant Nutrition

When renal disease presents in infancy, it represents a severe threat of growth retardation due to malnutrition, rickets, and acidosis. Infants with renal insufficiency require prompt assessment of nutritional status and early implementation of a dietary prescription that supplies the high energy and increased protein needs of this age group for growth.

Special formulas are available that are low in renal solutes, such as sodium, potassium, phosphorus, and magnesium, and resemble the mineral content of human milk. These formulas can be fortified with additives to increase calories and protein. The need for high value feedings makes formula feedings preferable to breast-feeding. Many CRI infants are poor feeders and require nasogastric supplementation at night or after each bottle attempt during the day. The poor feeders often demonstrate slow weight gain and growth retardation. Children malnourished during infancy are less likely to recover intellectual deficits caused by poor brain growth than those malnourished later in life.

To increase the calories per ounce of a formula, it is best to add one of the available carbohydrate and fat supplements rather than concentrating the formula. By adding less water, the calories would be increased but the solute load and osmolality would also increase. Corn syrup may be used as a carbohydrate supplement in the older infant, the advantages being its availability and low cost.

Increasing the caloric value of the formula should be done gradually, allowing the child's gastrointestinal tract to adjust to the changes. Vomiting and diarrhea may indicate that the infant isn't tolerating the increase in osmolality of the formula. Starting with 20 kcal/oz formula, the formula can be enriched to provide 24 to 30 kcal/oz. Older infants may tolerate strengths as high as 40 to 45 kcal/oz without adverse effects. Osmolality should not exceed 300 to 400 Osm/kg water (Hetrick & Shah, 1982). Caloric needs are based on recommended dietary allowances, with an intake goal of between 100 and 200 kcal per kg body weight (Food and Nutrition Board, 1980). More calories are necessary if the child shows evidence of failure to thrive or has severe renal disease. To achieve maximum calories, it is recommended that the child receive only formula for the first 12 months. Fluid limitations usually are not required in infants until their renal function declines to a GFR of 8 to 10 percent of normal. If an infant requires dialysis, this plan may need to be altered as fluids will be restricted. Baby foods may be added to the diet, but it must be noted that they contain a high percentage of water, which must be calculated into the fluid limits. The daily sodium requirement for an infant is 2 to 3 mEq/kg/day. This is supplied by the formulas mentioned previously (6 to 7 mEq/L). The introduction of baby foods should not cause problems in infants requiring sodium restrictions because manufacturers normally do not add salt to commercial infant foods. Package labels should be checked for sodium content because some junior foods (for example, meat sticks) do contain sodium.

Infants on peritoneal dialysis may require sodium supplementation if their serum levels are low or they demonstrate hypotensive problems. Sodium may be lost in the urine in some infants with renal dysplasia or obstructive uropathy, referred to as "salt wasters." The amount can be determined from a 24-hour urine sample, and then supplementation, using sodium chloride or sodium bicarbonate, can be added to compensate for this loss.

Serum potassium levels need to be followed in the infant with chronic renal disease. As GFR decreases, potassium levels may become a concern. Levels of 5.0 to 5.5 mEq/L are acceptable but higher levels may need to be treated by adding Kayexalate to the child's formula. This ion exchange resin will bind the potassium in the formula and thus reduce the amount to which the infant is exposed. If tube feedings are being employed, care must be taken not to allow the Kayexalate to plug the gavage tubing. This problem can be partially alleviated by adding the Kayexalate to the formula and then letting it stand until it settles out to the bottom. When the top solution is poured off, most of the Kayexalate will be left in the container, having already done the desired task of binding the potassium and removing it from the formula.

Maintaining serum levels of calcium and phosphorus within the normal range is important for early bone development in the infant. Other blood values to monitor are alkaline phosphatase, serum parathyroid hormone, and N-terminal PTH. Calcium supplements and vitamin D analogues can be given to decrease the chances of renal osteodystrophy. Phosphorus levels usually run somewhat higher in the neonate when rapid bone mineralization is taking place. Phosphate binders containing aluminum are perhaps best avoided. Calcium carbonate (Titralac) is a good substitute, because it both binds phosphorus and is a source of calcium. Phosphorus levels are less of a problem to maintain if the infant is on peritoneal dialysis. Low phosphorus formulas may not be necessary for these children.

If formula intake is not adequate, a multivitamin may be used to assure the intake of the RDA of vitamins. Also, folic acid in the amount of 1 mg/day should be given to the infant undergoing dialysis therapy, because it is a water-soluble vitamin that is lost during dialysis.

Infants on hemodialysis who require frequent blood transfusions are at risk of building up large stores of iron in their bodies. The infant formulas previously mentioned and many infant cereals are fortified with iron. Intake of these should be monitored and if iron levels start to rise, the nonfortified formulas should be used.

The amount of protein required for an infant depends on what stage of renal insufficiency the child is in. This can be determined by the GFR during the predialysis stage. If the GFR is 15 percent or greater, the infant can probably tolerate a normal RDA protein intake of 2.0 to 2.2 g/kg/day during the first year of life (Food and Nutrition Board, 1980). Most formulas will supply this amount of protein, so the infant will have the best chance of experiencing normal growth and development.

To prevent azotemia in infants with more severe renal dysfunction, the amount of protein intake should be limited to approximately 1.5 mg/kg/day. If high BUN becomes a problem, peritoneal dialysis or hemodialysis may need to be initiated. Some infants may experience proteinuria and, due to the increased protein loss, require increased protein intake. This can be achieved by adding one of the commercially available products. Infants on peritoneal dialysis also have increased protein loss in their dialysate and usually benefit from the addition of a protein supplement to their formula.

Older Children

The goal of the nutritionist working with the older uremic child (over 1 year old) is to provide adequate caloric intake and other necessary substances so that the child will attain optimal growth and development. This can often be a challenge, because older children have more established likes and dislikes and may not adhere to the recommended dietary regimen. The alteration in the taste sensation that uremic patients experience creates a serious problem. When severe, this can lead to the child becoming almost anorectic. It is then difficult to achieve the desired caloric intake, which should be at least that stipulated by the RDA for normal children of the same height age, or 38 to 100 kcal/kg/day (Food and Nutrition Board, 1980).

Creative methods of augmenting the child's diet should be employed to increase energy food intake. The problem of maintaining adequate intake is made more difficult when protein, mineral, and fluid restrictions are required. High-calorie carbohydrate supplements are expensive and sometimes not accepted as palatable by the child. Calorie-containing fluids such as sodas and fruit juices, ice cream, or fruit ice should make up the largest part of the child's fluid allowance. Increasing the fat content of the child's diet can be accomplished by the use of margarine on foods such as rice, noodles, toast, and vegetables. Sweets are often most palatable and provide concentrated calories for the child. Basically, it takes a very individualized plan to promote adequate caloric intake in the child with CRI.

With the ready availability of salty snack foods and fast foods, it becomes increasingly difficult to enforce a sodium restriction in an older child. To be effective, the nutritionist must work closely with the child to help identify which foods are highest in sodium and how to allow some intake of these foods without causing severe problems with edema and hypertension. Pizza, hotdogs, pickles, canned soups, luncheon meats, and salty snacks can be allowed in small quantities that will keep the child satisfied and aid in overall adherence to the dietary plan. A palatable diet is the only diet that will ultimately provide the necessary caloric intake. When hospitalized, renal patients are usually placed on a sodium-restricted diet that is often very tasteless. The dietitian must work with the child to allow for some regular items in the diet such as a hotdog or some corn chips so that the child will not become anorectic in the hospital. Definite limits, must be set, however, and the salty food should come as a reward after other foods have been eaten. Recommended maintenance amount of sodium for the older child is 1.0 to 3.0 mEq/100 kcal expended per day.

Potassium restriction is not usually necessary until the GFR falls to less than 10 percent of normal. The diseased kidney continues to eliminate potassium and, when stimulated by Lasix, eliminates increased amounts of potassium. Some of this mineral is eliminated by the bowel also. If the amount of potassium loss becomes excessive, potassium-rich foods such as leafy green vegetables, fruits and fruit juices, and potatoes and tomatoes may be required. If restriction is needed, a child is usually placed on a 1000 to 2000 mg/day potassium diet. This is equal to 25 to 50 mEq. Requirements are summarized in Table 10–3. By eliminating high-potassium foods, the potassium restriction can usually be maintained. If not, Kayexalate can be prescribed to bind the potassium in the diet.

As in the infant, maintenance of normal calcium (10.5 mg/dl) and phosphorus (3.5 to 4.75 mg/dl) levels is important to permit normal growth and to limit bone disease. Calcium levels should be monitored and an adequate intake of calcium along with vitamin D analogues should be maintained. This therapy becomes necessary when the GFR drops below 50 percent of normal (Wassner, 1982). Calcium-rich foods, however, are also high in phosphorus, so they must be limited to prevent high phosphorus levels. Phosphate binders are commonly used to decrease phosphorus levels. These need to be taken at meal and snack times in order to be most effective. Concern surrounding the use of aluminum-containing phosphate binders makes limiting phosphorus intake the preferable choice. Protein restriction lowers phosphorus intake, because protein-rich foods such as dairy products, meats, and eggs are also high in phosphorus. Milk is usually limited to 240 cc or less in the CRI child. A phosphorus intake of 500 to 600 mg daily is acceptable in the small child (less than 20 kg) and 600 to 1000 mg daily in the older child (Nelson & Stover, 1984).

CRI patients sometimes are found to be deficient in zinc (the normal level is 55 to 150 mg/dl). A number of problems are associated with this

TABLE 10–3. POTASSIUM AND FLUID RESTRICTION BY WEIGHT OF CHILD

Weight	Potassium Allowance (mEq/kg/day)	Fluid Volume Allowance (ml/kg + urine output)
< 6 kg	——	25
6–10 kg	——	22–24
10 kg	1.5–1.7	——
10–20 kg	1.3–1.5	20–22
20–30 kg	1.1–1.3	18–20
30–40 kg	1.0–1.2	16–18

deficiency, such as anorexia, impaired taste acuity, hair loss, ataxia, and poor growth. Zinc supplementation has produced improvement in patient's appetite and taste acuity (Chantler, 1984). It is therefore important to insure adequate intake of this element. Foods rich in zinc are oysters, crab, organ meats, and other meats.

Vitamin intake from the child's diet should be followed to assure that it is adequate. A multivitamin supplement is usually prescribed to assure minimal intake of vitamins on a daily basis, because diet intake may fluctuate as restrictions are placed on food and fluids. Most sources agree that iron supplementation is not usually required in predialysis children or children who are currently being dialyzed.

Serum levels of copper may be low in predialysis children. This can be treated by encouraging foods high in this element such as nuts, shellfish, raisins, and organ meats.

Predialysis children are usually not protein restricted—that is, they are allowed to have the RDA for normal children. Current research suggests that ingestion of protein may result in reducing glomerular function in the diseased kidney (Brenner, Meyer & Hostetter, 1982). It is now suggested that protein be limited to 50 to 60 percent of the RDA when GFR falls below 50 percent. It should be stressed to the patient that the protein allowed should be of high biologic value—that is, animal protein.

During the predialysis period, fluid intake may be limited or, as in the case of "salt wasters," it may need to be increased. When restricted, it must be remembered that foods such as fruits and vegetables are high in fluid content. Processed baby foods contain a large percentage of water. When the renal child is hospitalized, the nurse should record all foods that are fluid at body temperature on the intake sheet. Diuretics may be useful during the predialysis period to help with fluid control. It is important to weigh the child twice daily on the same scale to evaluate the effects of therapy.

In summary, an individualized care plan for each child, allowing for favorite foods, adequate vitamin and mineral content, and an appropriate amount of calories, is necessary to promote the best chance for the CRI child to attain maximal growth and development and minimize problems such as hypertension and bone disease.

The Child on Hemodialysis

Hemodialysis therapy is initiated when the child's level of uremia begins to interfere seriously with his or her life-style or when serum levels of BUN or potassium become too high to be controlled by diet or medication. A child usually requires hemodialysis between 12 and 18 hours per week. Inherent in this schedule is a significant amount of fluctuation in the body's state of health. On hemodialysis days, the child experiences significant alterations in body chemistries. Even though this is a beneficial alteration, it occurs over such a short period of time (4 to 5 hours) that it stresses the child and limits appetite. On days off dialysis, the child may feel better and eat better, but the body is already building up waste products. Some children feel relatively well on dialysis and nondialysis days and are able to maintain adequate caloric intakes. Others lack this feeling of well-being and their nutritional status suffers.

Because hemodialysis has limitations in the amounts of water and solutes that can be removed in a single treatment, some restrictions need to be made on the child's diet. Limits are commonly placed on protein, potassium, sodium, phosphorus, and fluid intakes. Predialysis BUN levels greater than 100 mg/dl may indicate the need to restrict meats, fish, and other high protein foods. Low predialysis BUN may signal inadequate protein intake, which may also mean that insufficient calories are being consumed. A diet history should be obtained and counseling done to correct these nutritional problems.

Sodium intake on dialysis should be similar to that taken predialysis. "Salt wasters," however, may need to scale down their sodium replacement when urine output begins to decrease due to hemodialysis. Dialysis patient sodium recommendations are 40 mEq/m^2 or: for a 20-kg child, 2 mEq/kg/day; for a 20 to 40-kg child, 1.5 mEq/kg/day. A 2000-mg sodium diet equals 90 points or 90 mEq/day.

High potassium levels (greater than 6) due to decreased GFR present a risk to the renal patient's life and must be monitored and treated promptly. It is best to prescribe a diet limited in potassium to prevent the risk of hyperkalemia, a condition that can cause irritability of the heart muscle seen as elevated T-waves on the ECG. A level less than 5.5 mEq/L is accepted as safe. Diets prescribed usually limit the intake of potassium to 1000 to 2000 mg (25 to 50 mEq) per day. Complete teaching by the dietitian covering which foods are highest in potassium allows the renal patient or the child's parents to select a safe daily diet. Orange juice, tomatoes, potatoes, chocolate, and other fruits and vegetables are the foods to be avoided. These foods must especially be withheld during the weekend or whenever the child's longest period without dialysis occurs. If levels are repeatedly elevated, Kayexalate may be prescribed. As a powder, it can be added to Kool-Aid. It is often mixed with Sorbitol, which causes diarrhea and mild potassium loss. Diarrhea also minimizes the risk of impaction of the resin.

Calcium and phosphorus requirements are the same for dialysis patients as for predialysis children. They remain important elements to be followed by serum levels in order to promote maximum growth and healthy bones.

Supplemental multivitamins and folic acid should be prescribed for children on hemodialysis. Dietary restrictions can cause limited intake of vitamins, and water soluble vitamins are removed by dialysis. Chewable vitamins are usually well accepted by children.

Fluid limits are calculated by taking 500 ml/m^2 and adding urine output, or by the scale in Table 10–3.

Children on Peritoneal Dialysis

Caloric intake requirements for children on various forms of peritoneal dialysis (PD) vary on an individual basis. After dialysis begins, some patients seem to experience an improvement in their general feeling of health, and usually have improved dietary intake. An increased activity level also helps increase the desire for food. Other children on PD have poorer intakes, perhaps due to a feeling of fullness when they have dialysate dwelling in their abdomen or from the glucose in the dialysate, which provides calories and may decrease the desire for food. In the small child who has marginal caloric intake, the additional calories gained from the dialysate are of positive benefit. Small, frequent meals are useful to maintain adequate calories when the child is being dialyzed. If calorie supplements are necessary, prepackaged products are available but become expensive for long-term therapy. Insurance companies rarely reimburse patients for foods.

Hyperlipidemia is a common complication of peritoneal dialysis. Elevated cholesterol and triglyceride levels result from the constant exposure to dextrose and the increased protein losses of the PD patient. Products containing unsaturated fats, such as corn or safflower oils, should be encouraged. Concentrated sweets should be limited and carbohydrates encouraged as a better source of calories.

As much as 4 g of protein may be lost in the dialysate of a child on PD. Even higher losses may be observed in younger children whose peritoneal surface area is proportionately larger (Salusky et al., 1982). Providing a protein intake to replace these losses and allow for growth is often a challenge to the nutritionist and the parents. It is recommended that most of the child's protein intake be of high biologic value, emphasizing meats, poultry, and fish. Egg yolks are usually limited to one a day and milk to 240 cc/day because of the high phosphorus content.

Protein intake for children with height ages of 3 to 5 years is 3.0 g/kg/day; ages 5 to 10 years, 2.5 g/kg/day; and 2.0 g/kg/day for pubertal children. These values are based on the RDA for the patient's height age adding on extra amounts to replace protein loss (Nelson & Stover, 1984). Intermittent peritoneal dialysis (IPD) patients may have lower requirements for protein based on less protein loss because they spend fewer hours on dialysis.

Water and sodium allowances are more liberal on CAPD and continuous cycling peritoneal dialysis (CCPD) than on hemodialysis because the child is constantly having fluid removed. As a result, the risk of edema and hypertension is lessened. IPD patients who are only dialyzed 12 to 15 hours 3 times a week are more likely to require a sodium-restricted diet. Diets restricted to less than 2 g sodium/day are hard to enforce because of their lack of palatable taste. In order to achieve good caloric intake, the maximum, safe amount of sodium should be prescribed for the patient's dietary regimen. Caloric supplements may be required.

Potassium allowances can be more liberal on CAPD or CCPD than on hemodialysis. The child is constantly exposed to dialysate containing no potassium, thus producing a gradient for continual removal of this electrolyte. It seems prudent to evaluate each child individually and not to assume that unlimited potassium intake is going to be safe for every child. A persistent serum potassium value greater than 5.5 mEq/L may indicate that some avoidance of high-potassium foods may be necessary.

Many foods rich in protein are, unfortunately, also rich in phosphorus. In order to meet the CAPD or CCPD child's protein needs, an increased amount of phosphorus may be ingested. Phosphate binders may be required to treat this problem. Milk is limited to one cup (8 oz)/day or an equivalent amount of phosphorus in the form of milk products.

Calcium is usually low in the child's diet due to other dietary restrictions; thus a calcium supplement and a vitamin D analogue are usually necessary. Serum calcium should be monitored frequently and the vitamin D dose adjusted to try to achieve a normal level. Multivitamins and folic acid are necessary for PD patients to supplement their dietary intake.

If the child on CAPD or CCPD has normal ability to ultrafiltrate or remove fluid, strict fluid restriction should not be necessary. Some patients, after bouts of peritonitis, experience decreased ultrafiltration and, if hypertension or edema are present, may need to balance their intake with the amount of fluid that they are able to remove in a 24-hour period (urine + ultrafiltrate + insensible loss of 400 cc/m^2).

The Child with a Renal Transplant

Nutritional recommendations after transplantation surround the known effects of the immunosuppressive therapy on the child's body. Corticosteroids cause increased protein catabolism, including DNA and RNA, decreased protein anabolism due to decreased uptake of amino acids in muscle tissue, and increased uptake of amino acids by the liver. These alterations cause increased urea production and gluconeogenesis. Sodium retention occurs and potassium excretion is enhanced by alterations of cation exchange in the renal tubule.

Steroids affect carbohydrate metabolism, causing elevated glucose uptake by fat cells, glycosuria, impaired glucose tolerance, and relative resistance to insulin. Protein wasting affects the integrity of bones and may, if severe, lead to aseptic necrosis. Altered calcium absorption from the intestine also puts bones at risk. Elevated cholesterol, triglyceride, and lipid levels have been observed in the posttransplant patient. The sooner that the dose of steroids can be tapered, the less the risk of severe consequences of this therapy. Protein intake should be at least 2 to 3 g/kg/day to help counteract the altered protein metabolism caused by the steroids (Nelson & Stover, 1984).

Because of the impaired glucose tolerance, intake of simple sugar should be limited following transplantation, with emphasis placed on increased carbohydrate foods. Calorie intake should be sufficient to maintain the patient's weight but limited enough to avoid rapid, excessive gains that would add to problems of hypertension and cause increased stress on bones and joints.

Moderate limitation of sodium (3 to 4 g/day) will help decrease the fluid retention caused by steroids. Sodium intake, if not limited prophylactically, can lead to increased weight gain and hypertension.

Vitamin D supplementation may be continued following transplantation in children to aid in maintaining normal serum calcium levels. Levels should be monitored closely and therapy may be discontinued when it appears that the new kidney is providing normal vitamin D metabolism. Calcium intake is encouraged and need not be limited. Phosphate levels may drop below normal with increased urinary losses and may need to be supplemented by use of Phosphagel and increased dietary phosphorus.

Azathioprine has been observed to inhibit RNA and DNA synthesis, adding to the problems caused by steroids (Gradus & Ettenger, 1982). The nutritional effects of ALG (antilymphocyte globulin) are not described in the available literature.

When problems of acute tubular necrosis or rejection occur, the patient needs to be reevaluated as to necessary nutritional requirements and restrictions. Adequate caloric intake is an advantage if it can be maintained during these periods of increased metabolic stress.

It is an ongoing challenge for the involved dietitian and nurse to work with the child with renal disease from infancy, through childhood including times on dialysis, and following transplantation. Frequent reevaluation is necessary in order to optimize therapy and decrease the risk of complications that may be severe and long-term. Creativity is very useful in designing a dietary regimen that will be acceptable to the child, parent, and health-care personnel. The goal is to provide optimal nutrition to promote maximal growth and development, maximal rehabilitation, and minimal complications.

PSYCHOSOCIAL ASPECTS OF PEDIATRIC NEPHROLOGY

Like the physical aspects of pediatric nephrology, there are psychosocial aspects of renal disease that are specific to the pediatric population.

Emotional Development

Emotional development during the period of infancy is critical, and is greatly affected by the parents' ability to interact with the infant. When parents are worried, anxious, depressed, and stressed due to the illness of their child, their emotional input and interactions with the child are affected and this can severely alter the child's emotional development. Several stages of measurable emotional development have been identified (Greenspan, 1985).

The first stage, birth to 2 months, is the child's introduction to the world through his or her senses. It is a homeostasis stage where children learn to calm themselves.

The second stage from 2 to 4 months, is the attachment stage. The child prefers the animate world (parents), as opposed to the inanimate (blue ball). The child must have the spark of interest and love from his parents in order for trust formation to occur. If the parents are depressed, the baby may miss this interaction. Parents must find something to take pleasure in with the child so that the pleasure-joy experience can be found. This interaction is vital for the formation of an emotional foundation and trust to occur.

The 4-to-8-month stage is the stage of purposeful communication of cause and effect. The child expects his or her signals to be heard and a response given. Through this children learn to distinguish their own needs. Feedback at this point from parents is necessary. If parents are overwhelmed, two sets of responses may occur: the first is overprotectiveness, by not letting the child try new things; the second state is the depressed parent, who cannot pick up signals from the child.

In the 9-to-12-month stage, the child acquires behavioral organization. This is the time when the child pieces together a series of behaviors, organizes them, and learns to use the distal communication mode. For example, they use their eyes and ears to communicate distally or from further away. This stimulates independence and initiative. Children expect parents to respond and give approval from across a room or at a distance.

At 18 to 24 months, the child gains the ability to create mental symbols or images. The child also uses language development functionally and will symbolically express phases of his or her life. Themes of assertiveness and curiosity are positive features of this stage. The child needs emotional play on the floor and parents need to involve themselves in this play. Parents have to shift from a concrete world to the abstract and enjoy the child's imagination and play. This stage helps the child to internalize rules and develop a foundation for empathy and love as he or she gets older. It sets the basis for concentrations, attention span, and future learning.

Parents who are coping with the needs of a sick child plus their own emotional turmoil need to be cognizant of the critical emotional tasks that need to be developed in the child and the role that they must culture. They must recognize their stresses and behavior and recognize the critical influence their interaction will have on the emotional development of their child.

Stress

The stresses created as a result of renal disease are numerous and sometimes tax the child and his or her family beyond their capacity to adjust. First, the child must deal with what is happening physically as a result of the disease process. The child may feel ill or poorly much of the time. Fatigue, apathy, drowsiness, and generalized weakness may be present. Irritability and mood vascillation are common, leading to regression.

Because of the debilitating nature of the illness, the child faces alterations in body image and self-concept. Evidence of the disease process is omnipresent. Weight loss and changes in skin color are examples. Because of the chronicity of the disease the child may not grow well and short stature is a constant reminder of the difference from other children. Needless to say, items such as arteriovenous shunts are outward visible signs and constant reminders of the child's uniqueness. At times the child may experience emotional conflicts over self-image. These conflicts are enhanced by necessary procedures such as dialysis treatment.

Renal children face many basic frustrations and conflicts surrounding food and fluid. Certain dietary regimens that are necessary are a huge source of frustration. Very few children cope well with dietary or fluid restriction. Food holds a very personal meaning for everyone but it becomes even more significant for the renal child. All children need to have a certain control over their environment, especially the older child. Restricting diet and especially restricting fad foods strips the child of independence and control.

Family Relationships

The family's structure and usual patterns of functioning may be significantly altered by the illness of the child. The family structure as well as all the variables affecting the family must be considered in order to assist the family to cope with the situations. Relationships within the family constellation may change as attempts are made to adapt to the needs of the child. Many times parents change their attitudes toward the afflicted child by automatically assuming lowered expectations of the child. Children are often aware of subtle changes in relationships within the family and changes in behavior may be brought about by their perceptions and the stressed family interplay.

Behavior Problems

Behavior problems created by chronic illness can greatly alter the child's self-concept. Motivation, adjustment, and how self-worth are demonstrated are greatly affected by the child's self-perception. Quite often the child is confronted with the dependence–independence conflict. The health team and the parents constantly give the child the message that independence must be maintained and normal functions accomplished. They stress that the child must not become dependent on others, but the fact is that often others must be relied on for treatment and constant necessary care. This dependence–independence conflict creates a negativity in the child that may be reflected in behavior toward the family and nursing staff. The child may feel anger and hostility and become uncooperative. Behavior is a way of acting out.

Most often, acceptance of these feelings along with a loving attitude and limit-setting in a consistent environment, quickly tempers the problem. Personalized care—which gives the child options and alternatives, a measure of control, and ways to meet uniquely individualized needs—will greatly affect motivation and well being. The nursing goal should be to foster care that is designed to optimize the child's positive response to illness and minimize the limitations imposed by medical regimens and nursing measures. Nursing care should reflect an emphasis on the child's physical and psychosocial development. Nurses must urge the child toward normalcy and growth and development tasks with a sensitive understanding and appropriate expectations.

The child should be urged to participate in and assume responsibility for health care when possible. When the child participates in the care and helps design the treatment program, the response is usually a more positive adjustment and outcome. The primary goal should be to maintain the integrity and individuality of each child as we attempt to teach and guide their growth through adaptive responses.

EDUCATION

Increased understanding and knowledge can reduce anxiety for the child and family. The basic methodology for planning care should include assessment, planning, intervention, and evaluation. The methods used for educating the child and family and the information given will be guided by the child's developmental stage, stresses, coping abilities, and readiness to assimilate information. Nurses must be cognizant of all developmental tasks for each age group as they tailor an approach to each individual child and family.

Teaching should be simple, accurate, and in a language the child can understand. Various teaching materials may be designed and used with the child for each age group. A teaching doll such as "Kelly Kidney" (Fig. 10–7) can be a very effective tool for children of all ages. The doll has the various dialysis accesses shown, scars indicating surgery for transplant, and organs that can be removed and snapped back in place. With the aid of the doll, the very young child can easily comprehend several aspects of renal care and modality measures. The doll may be used in a more sophisticated manner when teaching the older child. Expressions of feelings and anxieties may be demonstrated through play therapy with the doll (Dory, 1982).

Other visual teaching aids such as teaching storybooks or coloring books can also be very effective. The story about Mike, *Someone Special* (Fig. 10–8), for example, states his frustration with diet regimens, collecting urine, curtailed sports activities, and feeling different from other boys. Books such as these can help renal children to relate their own anger, fears, and anxieties and serve as a stimulus to discuss these feelings with health professionals or family.

Other books can be designed to prepare the children for procedures or surgery. *Special Care for Special Needs* (Fig. 10–9) explains the care required for surgery. This book has perforated pages that can be removed if a specific care regimen is not going to be required by the child. Therefore, the teaching

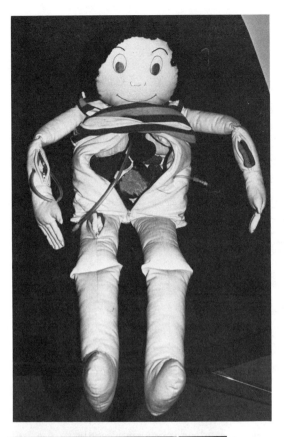

Figure 10-7. Kelly Kidney teaching Doll. (*Designed and created by Janice McCormick, Tulane University Medical Center, New Orleans, Louisiana, with permission*).

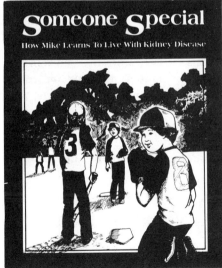

nuisance. I had to collect all of my urine, each time I went to the bathroom for twenty-four hours before my appointment. The nephrologist understood that I wouldn't want to haul the big plastic collection jug around in school. Instead, I collected the urine on Sunday. Mom dropped the container off at the clinic the next day. The urine collection is really important because certain chemicals in the urine give the doctor clues about how well the kidneys are working.

After the nephrologist finished the exam and studied the lab reports on the blood and urine, she told us that she had a few more clues about what was wrong. She told us that there were still blood and protein in the

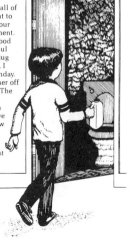

Figure 10-8. Teaching storybook, Someone Special: How Mike Learns to Live With Kidney Disease. (*University of Minnesota Department of Pediatric Nephrology, with permission.*)

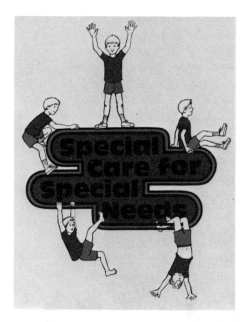

N.G. Tube

While you are on the CSCU your stomach will need to rest so you will have a tube that goes in your nose and down into your stomach. This will allow your stomach to stay empty so it won't feel upset. This is called a naso-gastric tube or an n.g. tube. While the n.g. is in, your throat may feel a little sore and you may not want to talk very much; this is normal. You will also notice tape around the tube and on your nose. This keeps the tube from sliding out. In a few days when your stomach is rested, your nurse will remove the tape on your nose and gently slide the tube out. You will feel a funny tickle in your throat but it will not hurt.

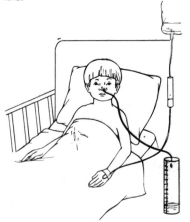

Figure 10-9. Teaching storybook, *Special Care for Special Needs. (From Sauer, S., et al., University of Minnesota, Department of Pediatric Nephrology, with permission.)*

tool can be very individually tailored and adapted specifically to the individual child and his or her situation.

The teaching process with the child and family is not only a way to disseminate information but is also a unique opportunity to foster esteem in the child. Appropriate encouragement and praise fosters a positive sense of accomplishment and sense of pride as the child masters bits and pieces of knowledge that affect well-being. A positive environment conveys support and is of value in addressing psychological needs. Involvement of the child and parents in the care and teaching can reduce separation anxiety, lessen parental guilt and feelings of helplessness, and provide the opportunity for the nurse to assess the family's understanding, adjustment, and parent–child relationship.

CARE PLANNING FOR THE PEDIATRIC RENAL PATIENT

It has been stated previously that care planning must be individualized and developmentally appropriate. The plan should reflect the following goals:

- The child's participation in self-care activities
- Encouragement of appropriate developmental tasks
- Encouragement of child's independence

TABLE 10-4. SAMPLE NURSING CARE PLAN FOR CRF CHILD INCLUDING NURSING DIAGNOSIS, NURSING INTERVENTIONS, AND PATIENT OUTCOME CRITERIA

Patient Problems	Nursing Orders and Interventions	Expected Patient Outcomes
Potential failure of health management due to: Failure to meet care objectives Lack of information about disease and care regimen	Identify knowledge deficits Assess child's need and ability to understand Teach child and parents about renal function, disease, dialysis, medication, and diet Encourage child to participate in treatment, dialysis, and other Allow choice in care regimen when possible Encourage sharing, teaching, and demonstration among patients Provide comfort measures Provide diversional activities Communicate with parents on a regular basis to identify problems Evaluate compliance with therapeutic regimen	Describes normal kidney functions as urinary output—able to verbalize what "kidneys do" Describes ESRD disease as inability to excrete wastes—"kidneys are sick" Discusses personal prognosis—"make body better"; parents discuss donating kidney Describes dialysis purpose and procedure—describes machine as "kidney" Demonstrates and states reasons for shunt care (need to protect) Family describes symptoms of dialysis complications: headache, hemorrhage, clotting, infection Keeps scheduled appointment for dialysis Participates in dialysis procedure: weighs self, takes temperature, prepares (helps), plans menus, chooses diversional activities, applies dressing to shunt after dialysis, repeats weight Complies with medication regimen: identifies medications, identifies dosage and frequency, explains why drugs are taken, explains appropriate action to take when question arises, takes medications prescribed, assumes primary responsibility for medication administration Complies with diet regimen: defines purpose, explains allowances, explains restrictions, follows prescribed diet

(continued)

TABLE 10-4. (*CONTINUED*)

Patient Problems	Nursing Orders and Interventions	Expected Patient Outcomes
Alteration in role relationship pattern due to renal disease and its treatment	Interact with child on a level appropriate for age Encourage child to assume age-appropriate responsibilities Schedule dialysis to allow school attendance or make arrangements for a tutor Provide counseling for parents regarding psychosocial development of child Encourage activities with peers Encourage independence and self-expression	Demonstrates age-appropriate behavior Attends school Participates in peer group activities Participated in family activities

Data from Southby, J., & Moore, J. (1983). Nursing diagnosis for a child with end stage renal disease. J AANNT, 10, 23–27.

- Therapeutic use of time to allow for school and recreation
- Appropriate peer interactions
- Aspects to foster normalcy of life-style
- Parent involvement in therapeutic treatment measures and medical parameters

Nursing diagnosis, nursing intervention, and patient outcome criteria encompass all the goals of care and give specific measurable parameters to assess the effectiveness of implementation of planned care. Some specific examples of care planned for the pediatric renal child are given in Table 10–4. The nurse is responsible for not only implementing the specific care but should constantly reevaluate and adjust the plan to meet the changing needs of the child and family.

SUMMARY

The child with renal disease presents a unique challenge. It is often overwhelming for the nurse to deal with the complexities of the care that is required. In addition, the nurse must also effectively manage a complex child and family with many psychosocial forces influencing their coping behavior. In addition to these issues, the pediatric renal nurse must deal with his or her attitudes, beliefs and values. This very special challenge provides a tremendous opportunity for personal growth as the nurse supports and enhances the child's and family's well-being. The pediatric nephrology nurse must have a high level of technical and interpersonal skills to assist these highly stressed families in need of care, competence, support, and love.

REFERENCES

Alexander, S. R., & Lubischer, J. T. (1982). Continuous ambulatory peritoneal dialysis in pediatrics: Three years' experience at one center. *Nefrologia* (Madrid), 2, 53.

Alvarez-Ude, F., Feest, T. G., Ward, M. K., et al. (1978). Hemodialysis bone disease: Correlations between clinical, histological, and other findings. *Kidney Int., 14,* 68.

Avioli, L. E., & Teitelbaum, S. (1978). Renal osteodystrophy. In C. Edelman, Jr. (Ed.), *Pediatric kidney disease* (p. 366). Boston: Little, Brown.

Baum, M., Powell, D., Calvin, S., et al. (1982). Continuous ambulatory peritoneal dialysis in children: Comparison with hemodialysis. *N Engl J Med, 30,* 1537.

Betts, P. R., McGrath, G., & White, R. H. (1977). Role of dietary energy supplementation in growth of children with chronic renal insufficiency. *Br Med J, 1,* 416.

Bourquellot, P., Wolfelir, L., & Lamy, L. (1981). Microsurgery for hemodialysis distal arteriovenous fistulae in children weighing less than 10 kg. *Proc Eur Dial Transplant Assoc, 18,* 537–541.

Brenner, B. M., Meyer, T. W., & Hostetter, T. H. (1982). Dietary protein intake and the progressive nature of kidney disease: The role of hemodynamically mediated glomerular injury in the pathogenesis of progressive glomerular sclerosis in aging, renal ablation, and intrinsis renal disease. *N Engl J Med, 307,* 652–659.

Chantler, C. (1984). Nutritional assessment and management of children with renal insufficiency. In R. N. Fine & A. B. Gruskin (Eds.), *End stage renal disease in children* (pp. 193–208). Philadelphia: Saunders.

Chantler, C., Donckerwolcke, R. A., Brunner, F. P., et al. (1978). Combined report on regular dialysis and transplantation of children in Europe. *Proc Eur Dial Transplant Assoc, 16,* 74.

Dabbagh, S., & Chesney, R. W. (1984). Treatment of renal osteodystrophy during childhood. In R. N. Fine & A. B. Gruskin (Eds.), *End stage renal disease in children* (pp. 251–270). Philadelphia; Saunders.

Donckerwolcke, R. A., Broyer, M., Brunner, F. P., et al. (1982). Combined report on regular dialysis and transplantation of children in Europe, XI, 1981. *Proc Eur Dial Transplant Assoc, 19,* 60–94.

Donckerwolcke, R. A., Chantler, C., Brunner, F. P., et al. (1978). Combined report on regular dialysis and transplantation of children in Europe, 1977. *Proc Eur Dial Transplant Assoc, 15,* 77–116.

Dory, J. M. (1982). Teaching the young child nephrology care. *Nephrology Nurse, 4,* 50–52.

Feldhoff, C., Balfour, H., & Najarian, J. (1981). Varicella in children with end stage renal transplants. *J Pediatr, 98,* 25–31.

Ferraris, J., Saenger, P., Levine, L., et al. (1980). Delayed puberty in males with chronic renal failure. *Kidney Int, 18,* 344–350.

Fine, R. N., Malekzaeh, M. H., Pennisi, A. J., et al. (1978). Long-term results of renal transplantation in children. *Pediatrics, 61,* 641–650.

Food and Nutrition Board, National Academy of Sciences, National Research Council (1980). *Recommended dietary allowances.* Washington, D. C.: Food and Nutrition Board.

Fowler, A., Mahan, J., & Nevins, T. (1984). The Hickman catheter—Today's vascular access for pediatric hemodialysis. *ANNA J, 11,* 36–38.

Gilli, G., Mehls, O., Fischer, W., & Scharer, K. (1980). Final height of children with chronic renal failure. *Pediatr Res, 14,* 1015.

Ginn, H. E. (1975). Neurobehavioral dysfunction in uremia. *Kidney Int, 7,* 5217.

Gradus, D., & Ettenger, R. B. (1982). Renal transplantation in children. *Pediatr Clin North Am, 29,* 1013–1038.

Greenspan, S. (1985). Mental health center study, Adelphi, Maryland. *Proceedings of Third International Workshop on Renal Failure in Children.*

Greulich, W. W., & Pyle, S. I. (1959). *Radiographic atlas of skeletal development of the hand and wrist* (2nd ed.). Stanford: Stanford University Press.

Hamill, P. V. (1977). *NCHS growth curves for children, birth–18 years.* United States Department of Health, Education, and Welfare publication no. (PHS) 78-1960. Hyattsville, Md.: U.S. D. H. E. W.

Hetrick, A. R., & Shah, R. V. (1982). Dietary management of infants on CAPD. *J AANNT, 9,* 46–48.

Ingelfinger, J. R., Grupe, W. E., Harmon, W. E., et al. (1981). Growth acceleration following renal transplantation in children less than seven years of age. *Pediatrics, 68,* 255–259.

Ingelfinger, J. R. (1982). Hypertension in end stage renal disease and renal transplantation. In J. R. Ingelfinger (Ed.), *Pediatric hypertension* (p. 252). Philadelphia: Saunders.

Kaehny, W. D., Hegg, A. P., & Alfrey, A. C. (1977). Gastrointestinal absorption of aluminum from aluminum-containing antacids. *N Engl J Med, 296,* 1389–1390.

Kleinknecht, C., Broyer, M., Gagnadoux, M. F., et al. (1980). Growth in children treated with long-term hemodialysis: A study of 76 patients. *Adv Nephrol, 9,* 133–163.

Kleinknecht, C., Broyer, M., Huot, D., et al. (1983). Growth and development of non-dialyzed children with chronic renal failure. *Kidney Int, 24* (Suppl. 15), S15–S40.

Kohaut, E. C. (1982). Growth in children with end stage renal disease treated with CAPD for at least one year. *Periton Dial Bul, 2,* 159.

Leone, M. R., & McEnery, P. T. (1984). Infection in the child receiving therapy for ESRD. In R. N. Fine & A. B. Gruskin (Eds.), *End stage renal disease in children* (pp. 416–423). Philadelphia: Saunders.

Leumann, E. P., & Briner, J. (1984). Recurrence of the primary disease in the transplanted kidney. In R. N. Fine & A. B. Gruskin (Eds.), *End stage renal disease in children* (pp. 528–540). Philadelphia: Saunders.

Mauer, S. M. & Vernier, R. L. (1985). Renal transplantation in children aged 1–5 years: Review of the University of Minnesota experience. In *Chronic renal disease— causes, complications, and treatment* (pp. 334–360). New York: Plenum.

McShary, E., & Morris, R. C., Jr. (1978). Attainment and maintenance of normal stature with alkali therapy in infants and children with classic renal tubular acidosis. *J Clin Invest, 61,* 509.

Mehls, O. (1984). Renal osteodystrophy in children: Etiology and clinical aspects. In R. N. Fine & A. B. Gruskin (Eds.), *End stage renal disease in children* (pp. 227–245). Philadelphia: Saunders.

Mehls, O., Ritz, E., Gilli, G., & Kreusser, W. (1978). Growth in renal failure. *Nephron, 21,* 237–247.

Mehls, O., Ritz, E., Krempien, B., et al. (1975). Slipped epiphyses in renal osteodystrophy. *Arch Dis Child, 50,* 545–554.

Miller, L. C., Lum, C. T., Bock, G., et al. (1983). Transplantation of the adult kidney into the very small child. *Am J Surg, 145,* 243–247.

National Center for Health Statistics (1977). *NCHS growth curves for children 0–18 years.* (United States Vital and Health Statistics, series 11, no. 165.) Washington, D.C.: U.S. Government Printing Office.

Nelson, P., & Stover, J. (1984). Principles of nutritional assessment and management of the child with ESRD. In R. N. Fine & A. B. Gruskin (Eds.), *End stage renal disease in children* (pp. 209–226). Philadelphia: Saunders.

Nevins, T. E., & Mauer, S. M. (1984). Infant hemodialysis. In R. N. Fine & A. B. Gruskin (Eds.), *End stage renal disease in children* (pp. 39–53). Philadelphia: Saunders.

O'Regan, S. (1984). Cardiovascular abnormalities in pediatric patients with ESRD. In R. N. Fine & A. B. Gruskin (Eds.), *End stage renal disease in children* (pp. 359–374). Philadelphia: Saunders.

Pennisi, A. J., Costrin, C., Phillips, L. S., et al. (1979). Somatomedin and growth hormone studies in pediatric renal allograft recipients who receive daily prednisone. *Am J Dis Childr, 133,* 950.

Peterson, P. K., Balfour, H., Fryd, D., et al. (1981). Fever in renal transplant recipients: Causes, prognostic significance, and changing patterns at the University of Minnesota Hospital. *Am J Med, 71,* 345.

Polinsky, M. S. (1984). Neurologic complications of ESRD, dialysis, and transplantation. In R. N. Fine & A. B. Gruskin (Eds.), *End stage renal disease in children* (pp.

307–339). Philadelphia: Saunders.

Potter D., Larson, D., Lumen, E., et al. (1970). Treatment of chronic uremia in childhood: II. Hemodyalysis. *Pediatr, 46,* 678.

Rauh, W., & Oertel, P. J. (1984). Endocrine functions in children with ESRD. In R. N. Fine & A. B. Gruskin (Eds.), *End stage renal disease in children* (pp. 296–306). Philadelphia: Saunders.

Rotundo, A., Nevins, T. E., Lipton, M., et al. (1982). Progressive encephalopathy in children with chronic renal insufficiency in infancy. *Kidney Int, 21,* 486–491.

Salusky, I. B., Lucullo, L., Nelson, P., & Fine, R. N. (1982). Continuous ambulatory dialysis in children. *Pediatr Clin North Am, 29,* 1005–1012.

Scharer, K., Broyer, M., Vecsli, P, et al. (1980). Damage to testicular function in chronic renal failure of children. *Proc Eur Dial Transplant Assoc, 17,* 725.

Scharer, K., Chantler, C., Brunner, F. P., et al. (1976). Combined report on regular dialysis and transplantation of children in Europe, 1975. *Proc Eur Dial Transplant Assoc, 13,* 59–105.

Scharer, K., & Gilli, G. (1984). Growth in children with chronic renal insufficiency. In R. N. Fine & A. B. Gruskin (Eds.), *End stage renal disease in children* (pp. 271–290). Philadelphia: Saunders.

Southby, J., & Moore, J. (1983). Nursing diagnosis for a child with end stage renal disease. *J AANNT, 10,* 23–27.

Tanner, J. M. (1962). *Growth at adolescence.* Oxford: Blackwell.

Tanner, J. M., Whitehouse, R. H., Marshall, W. A., et al. (1975). *Assessment of skeletal maturity and prediction of adult height (TW2 Method).* London: Academic Press.

Wassner, S. J. (1982). The role of nutrition in the care of children with renal insufficiency. *Pediatr Clin North Am, 29,* 985–1004.

West, C. D., & Smith, W. C. (1956). An attempt to elucidate the cause of growth retardation in renal disease. *Am J Dis Childr, 91,* 460–476.

Woodhead, J. C., & Novak, A. J. (1982) Dental abnormalities in children with chronic renal failure. *Pediatr Dent 4,* 281–285.

Psychological Aspects of Nephrology Nursing

Beth Tamplet Ulrich

OBJECTIVES

After reading this chapter on psychological aspects of nephrology nursing, the nurse will be able to:

1. Identify the psychological issues associated with renal disease
2. Differentiate among the defense mechanisms that may be used to deal with the psychological issues associated with renal disease
3. Understand the adaptive process with regard to end-stage renal disease
4. Establish therapeutic relationships with nephrology patients

Patients with end-stage renal disease (ESRD) present a unique psychosocial picture as they struggle to regain and maintain equilibrium. In the process, many issues may surface that require the support and intervention of the nursing staff.

PSYCHOLOGICAL ISSUES

It is generally agreed that the independence–dependence conflict is a major psychological issue with ESRD patients. Role change, loss of status, lack of control, and a frustration of basic drives such as sexuality are issues with which the individual with ESRD and the significant others must deal.

Independence–Dependence

The independence–dependence conflict begins with the determination that dialysis is necessary. Without a transplant, the patient faces lifelong dependence on machines (in the case of hemodialysis or CCPD) or a daily exchange routine (CAPD). Regardless of the modality, there is dependence on the dialysis staff, who either performs the procedures or trains and provides backup assistance for the patient who dialyzes at home. The dialysis staff stresses independence on the one hand and cooperation and adherence to the treatment regimen on the other. The result is a set of psychologically conflicting messages that the patient often has difficulty sorting out.

There appear to be two patient groups who enter the dialysis treatment phase of ESRD: individuals who have been independent prior to the onset of symptoms and individuals who have been basically dependent. The dependent patient may deal better with the initial stages of dialysis, when the sick role is emphasized. The patient feels sick or nauseated, tired, and so forth, and at least one hospital visit is necessary to establish the access. The dependent patient usually has little trouble accepting this sick role.

In contrast, the independent patient often reacts negatively to the dependent, sick role. Denial of the symptoms is often seen along with acting out in the form of nonadherence to the medical regimen and anger towards the staff and significant others. It is important for the nursing staff to work with the patient who is adjusting to this dramatic life change. The independent patient often most needs the very support and understanding that he or she tends to reject. In the later stages of dialysis treatment, when rehabilitation becomes the goal, the independent patient seems more likely to do well.

Locus of Control

Locus of control is the concept that refers to the belief that an individual's life is under the control of that individual (termed *internal locus of control*) or that occurrences in the individual's life are the result of outside forces such as chance, fate, or powerful others (termed *external locus of control*). Ulrich (1981) found that in contrast to healthy adults, dialysis patients tended to score high in both internal and powerful others loci of control. These data are consistent with the composite data reported by Wallston and Wallston (1982) for subjects characterized as chronic patients. The results of these studies indicate a realistic viewing of the life situation. The tendency of dialysis patients, as indicated by high internal scores, was to believe that they control what happens to their lives. The patients also, however, appeared to recognize their dependence on dialysis equipment and personnel.

Nephrology nursing personnel have long advocated a patient-centered approach, which promotes independence and decision-making by the patient. Patients are often seen in control of their lives whether they believe that philosophy or not. It is necessary for the nephrology nurse to assess each patient's belief about his or her own locus of control before initiating a plan of care or a teaching strategy.

For example, individuals who see themselves as being in control of their lives (internal locus of control) would tend to respond better if given detailed explanations of their alternatives. For these individuals, the nurse assumes the role of a health consultant and works in a partnership with the client. On the other hand, those who see others (nurses, doctors, the government, and so on) or fate as controlling their lives (external locus of control) would tend to desire less detailed explanations. To these people, the nurse is an authority figure; and they will tend to respond better if he or she fills that role. It should also be noted that a client's locus of control can change, especially in crisis situations; for example, a normally internally oriented individual may become more externally oriented in the initial stages of dialysis treatment. The nursing approach must then be altered in response to the changes.

Patient education must be individualized to meet these needs with regard to the issue of control. To achieve this, nephrology practitioners must be aware of patient differences as well as similarities and be prepared to individualize approaches based on these differences.

Role Change and Loss of Status

Role changes frequently accompany the integration of the ESRD medical regimen into the client's life-style. As the symptoms become more pronounced, the individual tires more easily and may not be able to participate in work situations or relationships in the usual manner. The individual who was once the breadwinner and decision-maker may have to relinquish that role to another family member, at least through the initial treatment period. A sudden, unwanted role change requires a great deal of energy—energy that the ESRD client may not have.

American culture tends to promote the concept that an individual's worth is based on his or her ability to perform. The dialysis client who is not able to work or play extensive sports with friends may feel a *loss of status.* Even if the individual wants to work, the federal and state financial bureaucracies may eliminate the possibility. Often clients find that they make more money by not working than by working. The dilemma then becomes to work and make less money or to feel a loss of status by not working. Neither alternative is very attractive.

The issue of role change may also be seen in the transplant patient. This is more often the case when the patient has been on dialysis for a prolonged period of time. Dialysis patients who have grown accustomed to the sick role may find it difficult to adjust to the role of "well person" after the transplant. They may also miss the socialization opportunities offered at the dialysis unit which they no longer have access to upon posttransplant release from the hospital. The increasing incidence of primary transplantation may decrease these role-change issues.

Frustrations of Basic Drives

The basic drives of food, water, and sex are, to one degree or another, unmet in the general dialysis population. In addition, the coping methods used by many people become virtually unavailable to the dialysis client.

Food and water are both restricted in some manner. Discipline takes the place of spontaneity and flexibility. Going on food binges or drowning sorrows are no longer coping options for the dialysis patient. Eating, once a pleasant social experience, becomes a time-consuming task of restricting electrolytes while pushing calories. Eating outside the home becomes like Russian roulette or, at the very least, an accounting game where payback will be extracted later.

Role change, dependence, and physiological changes result in varying levels of sexual dysfunction.

Defense Mechanisms

Given the psychological issues of the independence–dependence conflict, role change, loss of status, and frustration of basic drives, it is little wonder that ESRD patients may resort to defense mechanisms in their adaptive process. DeNour and associates (1968) note that ESRD patients use defense mechanisms especially during periods of depression, when the defense mechanisms protect the patient from experiencing an even more intense feeling of helplessness; and during periods of contentment to help preserve the client's well-being.

Denial.   Denial is the simplest of the defense mechanisms and the one most used by ESRD patients. In one study, Glassman and Sugal (1970) looked at a group of ESRD patients using the Shipman Anxiety Depression Scale. Little or no anxiety was found despite the fact that many of the individuals looked lethargic and depressed. Glassman and Sugal concluded that patients cope with the stress of the ESRD lifestyle by the massive use of denial as an adaptive mechanism.

The adaptive value of denial is frequently debated. One school of thought holds that denial is negative, constructs a fantasy world for the patient, and should be dissuaded. In contrast, others are of the opinion that denial in moderate degree helps the patient adapt to his or her drastically altered lifestyle. DeNour (1972) feels that removal of the denial defense mechanism as an option would make the patient more compliant but less adjusted to the other aspects of his or her life. Flannery (1978) believes that resolution of such coping defenses may not always be helpful, unless the defenses have become counterproductive.

Regression.   Regression is the adoption of previous behaviors that in the past have resulted in a feeling of well-being. An example of this is a move toward increased dependency. Moore (1976) notes that dialysis may recreate early mother–child dependency. The patient is forced to rely on an external life support system that functions, in a placenta-like manner, to clean the blood. If the patient experienced some conflict and anxiety with the mother–child relationship before, this symbolic representation may lead to a reexpression of anxiety.

Displacement. Displacement can be defined as the discharging of pent-up feelings, generally of hostility, on an object less dangerous than the object that aroused the feelings (Wilson & Kneisl, 1979). This defense mechanism can be seen, for example, when the client discharges pent-up feelings about being on dialysis or having diet restrictions by yelling at a family member. Since patients literally place their lives in the hands of the staff each dialysis, they may be fearful of showing hostile feelings to staff members.

Projection. Projection occurs when the individual unconsciously attributes his or her own feelings to others. For example, a client may note that his family is angry about his being sick or that people don't like to see his needle marks. By attributing these feelings to others, the patient spares himself the pain of his own feelings.

Reaction Formation. The ESRD patient may manifest the use of reaction formation in several ways. Feelings of dislike of dialysis may be overtly expressed as excitement about the treatment or affection for the staff. The patient who fears the actual dialysis may instead express extreme independence. An inappropriate intensity of feeling and an inability to consider alternate points of view are clues that reaction formation is occurring.

Intellectualism. In the use of intellectualism, the painful emotion is avoided by means of a rational explanation that divorces the event from any personal significance. The patient who discusses the theory of the dialysis treatment or transplant process often and in depth may be using this defense mechanism. It may be difficult to determine whether the patient has a real need to know about the minute details or whether he or she is avoiding uncomfortable feelings or fears. The determination is made more difficult due to the fact that because the staff stresses patient knowledge and responsibility, they may unwittingly buy into this mechanism and reinforce it.

PSYCHOLOGICAL ADAPTATION TO ESRD

It is clear that each patient adapts to the ESRD life-style in some way, be it positive or negative. Greenburg and associates (1975) offer three factors that may contribute to positive adaptation:

1. The use of defense mechanisms, especially the use of denial, but also the use of displacement, isolation, projection, and reaction formation

2. The patient's ability to cope with the dependency of the dialysis procedure
3. The presence of a functional family support system

Foster, Cohn, and McKegney (1973) compared demographic patient-identifying characteristics for survivors and nonsurvivors in a dialysis center. The study revealed that 79 percent of the survivors had established and maintained nuclear families while only 42 percent of the nonsurvivors had done so. In addition, 50 percent of the survivors' natural parents were deceased at the time of the study, while 80 percent of the nonsurvivors' parents were deceased.

A similar study by Moore (1976) found that the individual who had negatively adapted to the ESRD life-style was more likely to have lost a parent before age 18 and was more likely to describe the parental relationship as poor. This patient also tended to have had unhappy or unsuccessful school and vocational experiences. These two studies would tend to support Greenburg's third factor.

Terry Oberly, an ESRD patient and a physician, and his wife who serves as his home dialysis partner, have identified three essential factors for a successful adaptation (Oberly & Oberly, 1979):

1. Stable physical and mental health
2. The opportunity to pursue one's most cherished goals
3. Hope for the future

The Oberlys also support the family as an important factor in successful adaptation. As Edith Oberly (Oberly & Oberly, 1979) phrases it, "A family's love, commitment, and dedication to the success of the dialysis venture is a heartening, invigorating presence in a patient's life" (p. 89).

Stages of Adaptation

In 1968, Abram outlined four stages in the adaptation to dialysis. These stages were:

1. The uremic syndrome
2. The shift to physiologic equilibrium
3. Convalescence—the return to living
4. The struggle for normalcy

In 1972, Reichsman and Levy described adaptation to dialysis in three stages:

1. The honeymoon phase, which occurs with the initial physiological improvement that dialysis brings
2. Disenchantment and discouragement, which occur when the client begins to struggle with the idea of being "on the machine" for life
3. Long-term adaptation

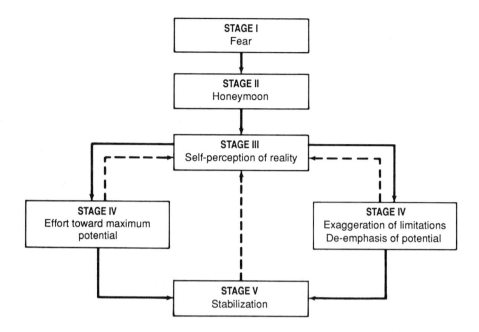

Figure 11-1. Stages of psychological adaptation to end-stage renal disease.

Ulrich (1980) proposed an adaptation model that further detailed the psychological adaptation to ESRD (Fig. 11-1). The Ulrich model is composed of the five stages described in the following sections.

Stage I: Fear. The initial reaction to the ESRD life-style in general and to the dialysis procedure in particular is fear, confusion, and a sense of being overwhelmed by it all. It would appear that even the most "stable" patient goes through this stage and that this reaction is quite appropriate. Stage I may last from a few days to a few weeks depending on the severity the illness has reached and the problems encountered in performing the initial procedures.

Stage II: Honeymoon. As Reichsman and Levy (1972) have noted, a honeymoon period exists when the effects of the dialysis take hold and the patient experiences an increased feeling of well-being. The length of this stage may vary from a few weeks to several months.

Stage III: Self-perception of Reality. The end of the honeymoon stage begins when patients start to look at themselves in a more realistic manner. It is important to note that it is the patient's self-perception of his or her own reality rather than the perceptions of the health-care team or significant others that form the basis for movement into the next stage. Certainly the opinions of others are of interest to the patient, but ultimately, patients make their own choice on how they perceive their potential and limitations.

Stage IV: Effort Toward Maximum Potential or Exaggeration of Limitations and Deemphasis of Potential. The patient, based on self-perception of reality, moves into one area of this stage or the other. Some patients aim toward maximum potential, taking into account their limitations but not being overwhelmed by them. Other patients appear to emphasize their limitations rather than their potential. It is unclear what factors, or combinations of factors, either internal or external to the patient, significantly influence which area of stage IV the patient moves towards. Several studies concerning adaptation predictors have been discussed earlier, but none appears to be conclusive. This is certainly an area where further research is indicated.

Stage V: Stabilization. Despite the patient's position in stage IV, stabilization in that position tends to occur. Patients mold a role for themselves and, barring crisis events, tend to stay within the boundaries of that role. When crisis events such as access failure or transplantation occur, the patient may move through all or part of the adaptation process once again. In this sense, the model is a dynamic one.

Following the Doctors' and Nurses' Orders
Much discussion and research has centered on whether patients do what is prescribed by nephrology physicians and nurses. While this is often referred to as "compliance," the use of the term compliance should be questioned. Compliance denotes subjugation and a deference to a higher power. Some researchers have even described noncompliance as a type of deviant behavior, thereby appearing to imply that normal people would comply (Ferraro, Dixon, & Kinlaw, 1986). The principle of autonomy, discussed in detail in chapter 13, precludes the use of such a term to describe decisions made by competent nephrology patients whether or not nephrology personnel concur with the decisions. Compliance literature, therefore, may be most useful in identifying those patients who are more likely to go along with the orders or prescriptions of nephrology personnel and those patients who are more likely to question such orders and test stated limits.

Another major problem encountered when labeling patients as noncompliant is the subjective nature of the term. Ferraro, Dixon, and Kinlaw (1986) reviewed the compliance literature and found little agreement about the definition of compliance or the instruments or measurements used to determine it.

Kasch and Knutson (1987) studied the compliance-gaining strategies of nephrology personnel and found that role and rule power are heavily relied on. Strategies which symbolize and dramatize the role boundaries between nurses and patients, which cast patients into a passive role, and which focus on the patients' role obligations are often used rather than a strategy of encouraging collaborative decision making. This is particularly true with LPNs and technicians.

Kasch and Knutson note that asking patients to change their behavior and comply or account for their noncompliance can threaten the patient's identities and self-esteem, especially if the strategies used are those previously described. The goal, rather than using strategies which can threaten the identity, should be to use strategies which can enhance the identity. These strategies include encouraging patient autonomy and freedom of choice and positively reinforcing the patient as one who is capable of making difficult choices and doing what must be done to accomplish goals.

Nursing Implications

The implications for nursing are varied. Support is indicated in stage I, as are some education endeavors. It should be noted, however, that these education efforts are being used to decrease the patient's immediate fear of the unknown. It is highly unlikely that the patient in stage I will remember or integrate most of what he or she is told at that time.

In stage II, the patient will be more receptive to learning about the disease process and its treatment. Patients will also require support and some degree of reality testing at this time. The nurse need not subvert patient feelings of increased wellness, but neither should the nurse allow the patient to fantasize a life-style that is beyond reality.

Nursing implications in stage III include the clarification of alternatives and the provision of information as well as support and continued education. The patient is in the process of determining his or her ESRD life-style. To make this decision, the patient may well need more information and the nurse serves as a primary resource.

Stages IV and V nursing interventions must be highly individualized to patient needs and desires. Certainly support is indicated throughout for the patient and significant others. Psychological reassessment is a continuing effort, as is response to assessment findings.

THERAPEUTIC COMMUNICATION

Assisting the patient in his adaptation to ESRD requires the nurse to understand and utilize therapeutic communication skills. Communication is defined by Wilson and Kneisl (1979) as an "ongoing, dynamic, and ever-changing series of events in which one event affects all the others" (p. 101). There is a difference, however, between socially superficial communication and therapeutic communication. In socially superficial communication, exchanges between nurses and patients are not goal-oriented, focus on the past and future, discourage and inhibit expression of feelings, and do not acknowledge individual worth. Therapeutic communication, on the other hand, is characterized by goal-directed and purposeful exchanges, a focus on the present, the encouragement and nurturing of the expression of feelings, the acknowledgement of individual worth, and the clarity of roles (Ulrich, 1980).

Therapeutic Relationships

The therapeutic relationship is a planned series of therapeutic communications between the nurse and patient. It is a mutually defined, mutually collaborative, goal-directed professional relationship for the purpose of counseling or crisis intervention.

Both the nurse and patient voluntarily enter a therapeutic relationship. Commitment from both individuals is important to the maintenance and the ultimate success of the relationship. Each participant brings personal abilities, capabilities, and power to the relationship. Each is accountable for his or her own behavior and assumes no responsibility for the behavior of the other. The relationship is goal-directed. The patient is expected to identify and achieve specific goals (physical, emotional, social) within the context of the relationship. Often, the client's initial goal is to solve an immediate problem, and this serves as a basis for establishing more extensive psychosocial goals.

The final characteristic of a therapeutic relationship is that it is a professional rather than a social relationship. The focus of the relationship is on the patient's identifying, developing, and assessing ways to meet needs effectively, rather than on meeting personal needs of the nurse (Wilson & Kneisl, 1979).

Philosophical Framework. A humanistic philosophy forms the basis of the therapeutic relationship. Openness and honesty are stressed. The experience is one of shared dignity, with the participants respecting the worth of themselves and each other. The patient is seen as an active decision-maker.

Commitment is based on a therapeutic contract between the nurse and the patient (to be discussed). Problems can arise in this area if the nurse is under- or overcommitted. If the nurse is undercommitted to this being a therapeutic relationship, beneficial confrontations may be avoided. This protects the nurse from having to address the patient's dysfunctional behavior, thereby allowing the patient's dysfunction to continue or worsen. The overcommitted nurse, on the other hand, may assume an omnipotent role; this robs the patient of active decision-making and self-accountability. The nurse's degree of commitment will be tested at some point in the relationship, and must be dealt with explicitly by both the nurse and patient.

Phases. The therapeutic relationship consists of three phases: the beginning or *orientation phase,* the middle or *working phase,* and the end or *resolution phase.* The beginning phase involves the formation of a working relationship. During this phase, the purpose of the relationship is discussed, as are the roles and responsibilities of both nurse and patient. The nurse directly addresses the patient's situation and offers to work with the patient. Concerns about trust and confidentiality tend to surface at this time. Both concerns must be discussed openly.

The final task in the beginning phase is the establishment of a therapeutic contract. This is most often a verbal contract, and an initial definition of the patient's goals and the nurse's professional responsibilities forms the basis of the contract. The time and place for meeting are also included (for example, "We will meet once a week for 30 minutes while the dialysis treatment is being performed").

The middle phase of the therapeutic relationship is the working phase. The first objective of this phase is to mutually determine the dynamics of the patient's behavioral patterns. This is accomplished through the identification and detailed exploration of the behavioral patterns. Patient self-assessment is then facilitated and encouraged.

The second objective of the middle phase involves the initiation of behavioral change. Several therapeutic tasks are involved in achieving this objective. The first task is to address the forces that inhibit the change. The patient's personal resistance to change may well be the major inhibiting force. The second task involves the creation of an atmosphere conducive to the testing of new behaviors. Permission to try out new behaviors includes the freedom to make mistakes.

Behavioral changes do, however, create some degree of anxiety, and the third task is to facilitate the development of the coping skills needed to deal effectively with the anxiety created. It should be noted that this middle phase can take weeks, months, or years, especially in the ever-changing environment of the ESRD patient.

Termination is the last phase of the therapeutic relationship. In the dialysis center, it occurs most often when the goals of the relationship have been reached or when the nurse or client leaves the center. The objective of this phase is to terminate the therapeutic relationship in a manner that is mutually planned and mutually satisfying. An important task in this phase is the patient's evaluation of the contract and the experience in general. If the goals of the relationship have not yet been reached, the patient should be encouraged to form a therapeutic relationship with another nurse.

Termination is an important phase that is often overlooked or avoided. Omitting this phase, however, leaves both the nurse and the patient with a feeling of incompleteness. The effectiveness of future therapeutic relationships may well be determined by the manner in which this relationship is terminated (Wilson & Kneisl, 1979).

Practicing Therapeutic Communication

Peplau (1952) sees three processes in therapeutic communication:

- Observation—feedback to the patient about what is seen
- Description—encouraging the patient to give specific examples
- Analysis—the patient makes connections between events

Communication is centered on the present, with references to past events or feelings when there is a direct connection to the current situation. Discussions of the future are avoided since the future is seen as only speculation, not contributing data.

In therapeutic communication, the nurse provides careful and deliberate guidance. This is done by asking clarifying questions: "Who?" "When?" "Where?" "What happened?" At appropriate times, further guidance is supplied by way of sequential questions: "What were your thoughts?" "What were your feelings?" "What did you do at that time?"

"Why" and "how" questions are avoided. They tend to put the patient on the spot, because he or she often does not have the answers. Questions that can be answered "yes" or "no" are kept to a minimum and asked only where exact clarification is needed.

Several behaviors form easy traps for the nurse. Giving premature approval or praise often ends the problem-solving rather than encouraging it. Patients benefit only when they make the evaluation for themselves. Changing the subject is often the result of the nurse's not hearing what the patient is really saying. This may come from inexperience or from the nurse's own uncomfortable feelings with the topic at hand. Advice-giving may be acceptable in a short-term crisis intervention session, but not in a long-range therapeutic relationship. The questions "Could you . . . ?" "Can you . . . ?" "Will you . . . ?" should be replaced with statements such as "Tell me . . . " and "Talk about that some more."

Often, silence traps nurses in therapeutic communication. Many times when the patient is silent, the nurse feels uncomfortable and comes to the rescue by changing the subject. Sometimes a patient's silence is a test to determine whether the nurse will stay and complete the session. Silence is all right. If the period of silence is prolonged, it is often helpful to confront it directly.

Being where you say you will be when you say you will be there is of prime importance in the therapeutic relationship. If the patient says, "I don't want to talk today," it might be easier to say, "Okay, we'll meet next week." Unfortunately, the patient loses trust in the nurse who responds to this test of trust by leaving, and the whole therapeutic relationship suffers as a result. A more appropriate response would be, "This is our time to talk. I'll be here for the next 30 minutes." The nurse then remains visible to the patient for the agreed-upon time. In another setting, the nurse would stay at the agreed meeting place and the patient would have the option of returning if he or she chose. In the dialysis setting where the patient is not free to come and go at will, it seems appropriate for the nurse to remain visible so that the patient can easily resume the session.

SUMMARY

Therapeutic communication and the formation of therapeutic relationships offer the nephrology nurse a means of caring for the psychosocial needs of the

ESRD patient. These needs may include the resolution of dependent–independent feelings, adjustment to role changes, and coping with crisis events such as access problems. Therapeutic communication requires the commitment of the participating nurse. Establishing therapeutic relationships with patients requires the commitment of the whole nephrology team.

In dialysis centers where primary nursing is practiced, participation in therapeutic relationships can easily be added to the role of the primary nurse. In other centers, each nurse may be assigned to a group of patients. It is more difficult to form a therapeutic relationship with the renal patient who is hospitalized because of the short length of the hospitalization. Therapeutic communication, however, can and should be practiced.

It should be noted here that every nurse cannot form a therapeutic relationship with every patient. Provision must be made for nurses to switch patients when the need arises. These efforts require coordination and working with the total nursing staff to promote confidence and increase communication skills.

The results can be well worth the efforts put forth. Time currently spent communicating with patients on a social level or monitoring patients from the nursing station can be converted into time used to provide psychosocial care for the patients. The holistic, preventative approach nurses preach can be the holistic, preventative approach nurses deliver.

REFERENCES

Abram, H. (1968). The psychiatrist, the treatment of chronic renal failure, and the prolongation of life, I. *Am J Psychiatry, 124,* 1351.

DeNour, A. et al. (1968). Emotional reactions of patients on chronic hemodialysis. *Psychosom Med, 30,* 521.

DeNour, A. (1972). Personality factors in chronic hemodialysis patients causing noncompliance with medical regimen. *Psychosom Med, 34,* 333–344.

Ferraro, K. F., Dixon, R. D., & Kinlaw, B. J. (1986). Measuring compliance among incenter hemodialysis patients. *Dialysis and Transplantation, 15,* 226–236, 266.

Flannery, J. (1978). Adaptation to chronic renal failure. *Psychosomatics, 19,* 784.

Foster, F., Cohn, G., & McKegney, F. (1973). Psychobiologic factors and individual survival on chronic renal hemodialysis—A two-year follow-up: Part I. *Psychosom Med, 35,* 64.

Glassman, B., & Sugal, A. (1970). Personality correlates of survival in a long term hemodialysis program. *Arch of Gen Psychiatry, 22,* 566.

Greenburg, I., et al. (1975). Factors of adjustment in chronic hemodialysis patients. *Psychosomatics, 16,* 178.

Kasch, C. R., & Knutson, K. (1987). A descriptive analysis of caregivers' compliance-gaining strategies, Part II. *Dialysis and Transplantation, 16,* 129–131.

Moore, G. (1976). Psychiatric aspects of chronic renal disease. *Postgrad Med, 60,* 140.

Oberly, T., & Oberly, E. (1979). Learning to live with dialysis: A personal perspective. In L. E. Lancaster (ed.): *The patient with end stage renal disease* (pp. 82–93). New York: Wiley.

Peplau, H. (1952). *Interpersonal relations in nursing.* New York: Putnams.

Reichsman, F., & Levy, N. (1972). Problems in adaptation to maintenance hemodialysis. *Arch of Intern Med, 130,* 859.

Ulrich, B. (1980). Therapeutic communication: The key to a holistic approach with the ESRD client. *Dialysis and Transplantation, 9,* 787–793.

Ulrich, B. (1981). Adherence to the prescribed therapy for chronic renal failure. *Nephrology Nurse, 3,* 14–21.

Wallston, K., & Wallston, B. (1982). Health locus of control scales. In Lecourt, N. (Ed.), *Advances and innovations in locus of control research.* New York: Academic Press.

Wilson, H., & Kneisl, C. (1979). *Psychiatric nursing.* Menlo Park: Addison-Wesley.

12

Educating Nephrology Staff and Patients

Beth Tamplet Ulrich

OBJECTIVES

After reading this chapter on educating the nephrology patient and staff, the nurse will be able to:

1. Perform a learner assessment
1. Construct goals and objectives for the education of nephrology nurses and patients
3. Compare audiovisual aids for education
4. Compare teaching methods
5. Evaluate learning

Education in the field of nephrology is generally divided into patient education and staff education. Although the recipient of the educational effort is different, many of the educational principles are the same.

DEFINING THE CONTENT

In planning an educational effort, the initial step is to determine the content. Education should occur when the learner has a knowledge deficit. In nephrology, this is usually due to a lack of exposure to the subject. Few nursing schools teach nephrology nursing to the level required to practice in the specialty. The nephrology patient is seldom exposed to nephrology prior to diagnosis. As a result, both enter the world of nephrology needing to be educated in various aspects of the specialty.

Practitioners currently in the field also have knowledge deficits. Advances in technology and successful research in the clinical setting lead to new knowledge, which must then be taught to practicing nephrology nurses. This type of education comes under the heading of continuing education.

Content
The initial question to the educator is "What needs to be taught?" At this time, the educator is looking only at the concepts. How and when to teach the material will be determined later.

Nephrology Nursing Education. The nurse who has chosen the specialty of nephrology must be educated about all aspects of the specialty. It is not enough for the nurse in hemodialysis to know only about hemodialysis or for the transplant nurse to know only about transplants. The professional nurse in nephrology must have a broad base of nephrology knowledge as well as an intensive knowledge of the subspecialty chosen.

Basic nephrology nursing education has a theoretical and a clinical component. This book provides the theoretical knowledge needed in the specialty. It cannot, however, provide the "hands on" knowledge that must be gained in the clinical setting. The essential knowledge and skills recommended for nephrology nurses by the American Nephrology Nurses' Association (1986) are detailed in Table 12–1.

TABLE 12–1. ESSENTIAL KNOWLEDGE AND SKILLS

All nephrology nurses must have a common knowledge base relevant to all aspects of care for adult and pediatric renal patients and their families. This knowledge base includes, but is not limited to, the following:

Anatomy, physiology, and pathophysiology relevant to the care of renal patients

The nursing process as applied to nephrology nursing

Pharmacology

Nutritional aspects of renal impairment

Growth and development

Teaching and learning theory

Counseling and interviewing skills

Interdisciplinary team skills

Research processing

Rehabilitation principles

Concepts related to death and dying

From the American Nephrology Nurses' Association (1986). Scope of practice for nephrology nursing. Pitman, N.J.: ANNA, with permission.

Nephrology Patient Education. Nephrology patient education begins as soon as the diagnosis is made, and never ends. The patient must be educated in general about ESRD and its treatment, and specifically about the chosen treatment modality. The level of education will depend on the involvement level of the patient. The patient selecting home or self-care dialysis, for example, will need to learn exactly how to perform the dialysis procedure, whereas the patient selecting staff-assisted dialysis will only need to understand the concepts.

According to Ulrich (1980, p. 744), nephrology patient education is based on five beliefs:

1. The diagnosis of ESRD is a major life crisis that the individual needs to accept.
2. The individual with ESRD, although suffering from a chronic illness, is rarely an invalid and can adapt to his or her altered state of being.
3. Such an adaptation is facilitated by using the resources of the nephrology health-care team.
4. Education of the ESRD patient, if presented at an appropriate time, increases the individual's adaptation to the life-style imposed by ESRD and its treatment.
5. An established framework for instruction provides consistency in the teaching approach to these individuals and also provides consistency in the material presented.

Patient teaching occurs for one of three reasons: to promote health, to prevent illness, or to cope with illness. The nurse practice acts of most states identify patient teaching as a function of the professional nurse. The ANNA (1986) notes that "Nephrology nurses play a vital role in providing the education patients need to make informed choices" (p. 6).

The patient and the family have the right to acquire the necessary knowledge and technical skills for the patient to function at an optimal level of wellness. Narrow (1979) notes that there are at least six major areas that concern most patients and on which they should be knowledgeable. These areas are language and terminology, anatomy and physiology, diagnosis, prognosis, treatment, and predictable events.

THE LEARNER

Education must meet the individual needs of each learner. It must also be designed to assure the efficient use of resources.

Learner Assessment
Assessing the knowledge level, abilities, motivation, and experience of each learner and individualizing the educational effort based on that assessment

TABLE 12-2. LEARNER ASSESSMENT

Knowledge

What does the learner already know about the subject?

What knowledge does the learner possess about related subjects that would be applicable?

Ability

Does the learner know how to perform the task?

Does the learner know how to perform any part of the task?

Does the learner know how to perform a similar task?

Capability

Is the learner capable of learning the material or performing the task?

Patterns

How does the learner learn best? Alone? In a group? Guided? Independent?

What style of learning has been successful in similar situations in the past?

Motivation

Does the learner see a reason to learn the material?

Where is the learner in relation to the hierarchy of needs?

Is the learner willing to participate?

---

are critical to the success of the education. The main points in learner assessment are described in the following sections and summarized in Table 12-2.

Learner Knowledge Level. What does the learner already know? It cannot be assumed that the experienced professional nurse knows the principles of dialysis, nor can it be assumed that he or she does not. It is equally unsafe to make assumptions about patients. The length of time patients have been on dialysis, for example, has not been shown to correlate with their knowledge of dialysis. Learner knowledge level can be assessed through a written or oral assessment.

Learner Abilities. An individual can know the theory behind a procedure and yet not have the ability to perform the procedure. Ability assessment seeks to determine what the learner already knows how to do. It is best accomplished through actual demonstrations. The nurse who has demonstrated theoretical knowledge of patient assessment should be asked to demonstrate an assessment. If it is done correctly, then the learner progresses to the next content area. If the procedure is not performed correctly, a knowledge deficit has been identified and education must occur. The transplant patient who has demonstrated a knowledge of cyclosporine must also demonstrate an ability to administer the drug. A learner who possesses the knowledge but not the ability will be no more successful in the final outcome than the learner who knew neither.

Learner Capabilities. The terms *ability* and *capability* are often incorrectly used synonymously. Ability refers to whether or not the learner performs a task correctly. Capability refers to whether or not the learner has the resources within himself or herself to do the task at all. Many dialysis procedures require a certain amount of manual dexterity. Without that dexterity, the learner is not capable of learning the procedure. This is not to say that an alternative cannot be found, but the initial question is "Is the learner capable of performing the procedure as it is now designed?"

Patterns of Learning. People learn in different ways and at different speeds. Some people learn best if they hear the information. Others want to read the material. Some learn best in a group, while other learners prefer individualized instruction. Some learn best if guided step-by-step; others want to do it on their own. It is vital that the teacher assess the pattern and style of learning that best meets the needs of the learner. General discussion with the learner about past learning experiences can elicit preferences and dislikes for teaching methods.

Learner Motivation. Motivation is very important to the achievement of educational goals. Abraham Maslow (1954) related human motivation to a hierarchy of needs; the lower-level needs must be met before the higher-level needs can be pursued. It is usually possible to determine whether a person's physiological needs have been met, but the determination of a higher-level of need attainment is more difficult because the higher-level needs are interrelated. A single need may be manifested through multiple behaviors, or several needs may contribute to a single behavior. For example, a highly anxious patient may block out any information until sufficient optimism is gained to counterbalance the fear. Some degree of anxiety can be an important source of motivation for learning. By directing and linking the anxiety to the patient's need for information, the anxiety can have a positive effect.

In assessing learner motivation, the teacher must determine what meaning the content to be learned has for the learner. The teacher may know why the information is important, but the learner may not. The challenge becomes having the learner incorporate the need as his or her own.

THE PROGRAM

Efficient and effective education programs are the direct result of careful planning. The teacher must develop skills in program planning that are built upon the best principles of learning and education. Planning of this nature will help assure a positive outcome.

Goals and Objectives
Mager (1975) clearly described the reason for planning and setting goals and objectives: "If you're not sure where you're going, you're liable to end up

some place else" (p. ii). The teacher must decide, before the teaching begins, what information is to be taught and how the teacher will know that the information has been learned. Although it is preferable to have a formal, written teaching plan, it is not absolutely necessary so long as the teacher conscientiously sets learning goals and objectives as well as criteria for determining if learning has occurred.

Goals form a frame of reference for directing the educational effort. Objectives are the means used to achieve the goals. Objectives are observable and measurable statements that outline the steps for goal achievement. The establishment of clear objectives diminishes the chance for subjective interpretation of the learner's progress and allows for immediate assessment of progress towards the desired goal.

Taxonomy of Objectives. Objectives are planned according to the degree of difficulty. By beginning with simple, easily attainable objectives, and progressing towards those more complex and difficult, the learner can gain confidence and increase motivation towards achieving the more difficult objectives. The end result is goal attainment.

There are three major domains of learning. The affective domain is concerned with feelings, values, and attitudes. As a result, it is the most difficult domain to measure. The cognitive domain entails the development of knowledge. The psychomotor domain includes the learning of skills.

In each domain, there is a hierarchy of learning levels. Verbs that are often used to describe each of these levels are detailed in Figure 12-1.

The cognitive domain includes six levels of intellectual activity: knowledge, comprehension, application, analysis, synthesis, and evaluation.

If the learner can perform at the highest level, then it can be assumed that he or she can perform at all lower levels. For example, if the learner can evaluate nephrology treatment modalities, he or she must have knowledge of each modality and be able to analyze and synthesize the knowledge.

The affective domain consists of five levels: receiving (attracting the learner's attention), responding, valuing, organizing, (making decisions based on the value), and characterizing of a value complex (integrating the value or attitude into a total philosophy). The levels of the psychomotor domain progress from gross bodily movements to well integrated, precise movements and techniques.

Establishing the Objectives. To be complete, an objective must include the performance that must be accomplished, the conditions under which performance must occur, and the criteria for determining that learning has occurred. In addition, the objective must be measurable and clear to anyone who reads it.

The performance aspect of the objective details what the learner will be able to do. This might include performing a skill or comparing vascular access options. The conditions refer to how the performance must be done. For ex-

EVALUATE

Appraise
Argue
Assess
Attach
Choose
Compare
Defend
Estimate
Evaluate
Judge
Predict
Rate
Score
Select
Support
Value

SYNTHESIS

Arrange
Assemble
Collect
Compose
Construct
Create
Design
Formulate
Manage
Organize
Plan
Prepare
Propose
Set-up
Write

ANALYSIS

Analyze
Appraise
Calculate
Categorize
Compare
Contrast
Criticize
Diagram
Differentiate
Discriminate
Distinguish
Examine
Experiment
Inventory
Question
Test

APPLICATION

Apply
Choose
Demonstrate
Dramatize
Employ
Illustrate
Interpret
Operate
Practice
Schedule
Sketch
Solve
Use

COMPREHENSION

Classify
Describe
Discuss
Explain
Express
Identify
Indicate
Locate
Recognize
Report
Restate
Review
Select
Tell
Translate

KNOWLEDGE

Arrange
Define
Duplicate
Label
List
Memorize
Name
Order
Recognize
Relate
Recall
Repeat
Reproduce

Figure 12-1. Verbs used to create objectives at all levels of cognitive domain.

285

ample, a patient or nurse might have to demonstrate independent performance of a procedure rather than performance with assistance.

The criteria specify the level of acceptability. Is being correct 9 out of 10
times acceptable, or must the learner be correct every time to meet the objective? Is there one correct answer, or is any answer within a certain range acceptable? For example, in teaching the nurse or patient how to calculate fluid
removal on dialysis, the criteria portion of the objective could specify that at
the end of dialysis the patient should be within 1 pound of the target weight 9
out of 10 times. This would allow for the variation in dialyzers and other problems for which adjustments could not be made. On the other hand, when
teaching sterile technique, the objective might well require accuracy in performing the procedure 10 out of 10 times, because sterility cannot be maintained partially.

There is also a difference between teacher and learner objectives. The
teacher objectives state what the teacher will do. The learner objectives state
what the learner must do to successfully complete the educational effort.

Finally, the ideal goal or objective is one that anyone, whether a nephrology nurse or not, can understand without clarification from the teacher. It
must stand on its own. The goal in establishing goals and objectives is to be
clear enough that the goal or objective can be given to an objective individual
who can, based solely on the goal or objective and the learner performance,
determine if the goal or objective is met.

Conditions of Learning

Robert Gagné (1970), a psychologist, developed a hierarchy to describe the
kinds of learning in the cognitive and psychomotor domains. This hierarchy
ranges from simple to complex learning, and includes

- Signal learning: Involuntary learning of a conditioned response to a
  signal
- Stimulus–response learning: Voluntary learning of a specific response
  to a specific stimulus
- Chaining: Learning to connect two or more previously learned stimulus–response situations in sequence
- Verbal association: Chaining learned on the verbal level
- Multiple discrimination: Learning an extensive series of simple
  chains
- Concept learning: Learning to make a common response to a number
  of apparently different stimuli
- Principle learning: Learning a chain of two or more previously and
  separately learned concepts
- Problem solving: Learning to create a response based on two or more
  previously learned principles

The first four levels are generally only necessary in teaching young
children. Most learning in nephrology facilities will occur at the higher
four levels.

Both the nephrology nurse and the patient must learn at the problem solving level. To effectively teach at this level, the educator must teach from simple to complex, through at least the top four conditions described by Gagné.

Adult Learning

Most of the learners that the nephrology nurse teaches are adults. Pediatric teaching is addressed in Chapter 10. There are certain characteristics of adult learners that must be considered when educating that population.

Adults are independent. Compared to the child, adult learners are, in general, resistant to the learner role. They also possess a background of experience and knowledge. This requires a more in-depth learner assessment to understand how previously gained knowledge and experience can relate to current learning needs. The adult learner has a variety of motivations that must be incorporated into the education program. Finally, the adult learner has definite expectations about the teaching, the system, and the need to learn the materials. These expectations are not readily changed.

Audiovisual Aids

In addition to choosing the methods of teaching, the teacher must also select the audiovisual aids. Although larger facilities may have virtually everything in audiovisual aids, smaller units usually must work with far less. Creativity, however, can often take the place of money.

Written Materials. Written materials range from one-page handouts to books such as this one, and can be effective in reinforcing learning. A handout given to the postransplant patient reviewing signs and symptoms of rejections can be very useful, as can the step-by-step procedure book designed for the home dialysis patient. Nurses have demonstrated extensive creativity in developing written material for patients and other nurses. Key resources for written material include the American Nephrology Nurses' Association (ANNA), the National Kidney Foundation, the National Association of Patients on Hemodialysis and Transplantation, and corporations in the field of nephrology.

Slides. Slides are useful in lectures or when they can be combined with a tape in an audio–slide projector. Slides require a fair amount of preparation, and can become costly if photographed by professionals. On the other hand, picture slides can be taken by the teacher and developed inexpensively. If the slides are shown using a regular projector in a large room, the room must be darkened.

Overheads. Overheads are quick to produce, and can be effective in small groups. The overhead projector works well in a semidark room, allowing adequate light for notetaking. Overheads can be produced from typed copy or with colored markers.

Audio–Slide Projectors. Audio–slide projectors are very useful in self-instruction or one-on-one teaching. The audio–slide projector is a small slide projector cassette tape player combination that is no bigger than a small television. It is perfect for use in patient rooms or in small conference areas. A major advantage is that once a set of slides has been developed and a script written, the tape can be done in several languages.

Videotape. Video is a very effective method of demonstrating procedures and offering longer teaching programs. The learner can view the procedure in motion, which is often necessary to understand the exact movements necessary to accomplish the task. Video is expensive to produce, but the number of available tapes is increasing. In hospitals with an internal television channel, the video can be shown intermittently for patient teaching. Small video machines have been developed that are no bigger than carramate projectors.

Laser Disk. The laser disk is the newest addition to the audiovisual aids available to the educator. A laser disk works very much like a video, in that the image is shown on a television screen. The difference is that with a laser disk, the teacher can almost instantly access an item anywhere on the disk without viewing everything ahead of that item. The disk also stores a large number of images.

Other Audiovisual Teaching Aids. There are many other audiovisual aids that can be used to teach nephrology nurses and patients. In the pediatric units, dolls are frequently used to demonstrate catheter placement, the transplant surgery, and organ locations. Catheters and other pieces of equipment are also audiovisual aids when used to teach. Models of organs can be helpful when teaching anatomy. Imitation food and posters showing the actual amount of salt in foods are usually much more effective in teaching dietary restrictions than just a lecture from the teacher.

Computers. The power of computers in education has only just begun to be tapped. Computer-assisted instruction is the simplest method of computer education. Interactive video takes the process one step further. Computers can now be programmed to teach assessment, diagnosis, and treatment choices. The options for future uses are endless.

Evaluation

One of the most important aspects of teaching is the evaluation. Regardless of what the teacher tries to teach, the only way to assure that learning has occurred is to evaluate the teaching. The basic rule of evaluation is to never assume anything. A patient may nod his or her head as the nurse demonstrates peritoneal dialysate exchanges, and say "yes" when the nurse asks if he or she understands; but if the nurse does not have the patient perform a return demonstration and explain the reason behind each step, the nurse has no way of knowing that learning has occurred.

If the goals and objectives are clear, evaluation should be easy. The key question the teacher must ask is "How will I know that learning has taken place?"

Teaching Methods

Once the teacher has performed a learner assessment and established the goals and objectives, the teaching methods must be selected. There are many ways to teach. The effective teacher matches the method with the objective and the learner.

Lecture/Didactic Method. The most common method of teaching is the lecture method. This is a form of one-way communication in which the teacher presents the material and the learner listens. Lectures usually take place in classrooms, but many occur one-on-one, though not necessarily with success. Lectures are useful when a large amount of information needs to be covered, when the basic level of knowledge about the subject is relatively the same in all of the learners, when skills are not involved, and when the learners are already motivated.

Question and Answer Sessions. Questions and answers are useful in clarifying information. They may be used by the teacher to assess student learning, or by the learner to better understand what the teacher is trying to teach. Teacher-initiated questions and answers help evaluate student knowledge either prior to or after the teaching. They may be in written or oral form.

Demonstrations. Demonstrations are effective in teaching skills, especially if the learner does a return demonstration so the learning can be assessed. The demonstrations usually accompany or follow a lecture that explains the procedure. It is often helpful to prepare written material that can serve as a reference.

Role Playing. Role playing is especially useful in teaching interactive skills such as interviewing or teaching. For example, in a session on patient assessment, the nurse might be asked to take a patient history from another nurse who is "playing" a patient. Both nurses learn from the procedure. One learns how to phrase questions to get the information needed, and the other learns how the patient feels during an assessment.

Self-instruction. Self-instruction is effective when the learner prefers to learn on his or her own, and when the learner has time to learn but the teacher does not have time to teach. The latter is often the case in the hospital setting. A well-designed self-instruction module allows the learner to attempt to learn the material at his or her own pace. The teacher steps in when the self-instruction module is not effective.

SUMMARY

The education of nephrology nurses and patients is the job of every professional nephrology nurse. The ability to teach must be learned just as any other skill. Teaching is the process of facilitating learning. It is a two-way communication involving the commitment of both the teacher and the learner. Through attention to the needs of the individual learner and a knowledge of the ultimate knowledge and skill level the learner must possess, the teacher can create a successful education program.

REFERENCES

American Nephrology Nurses' Association. (1986). *Scope of practice for nephrology nursing.* Pitman, N.J.: ANNA.
Gagné, R. M. (1970). The *conditions of learning.* New York: Holt, Rinehart & Winston.
Mager, R. F. (1975). *Preparing instructional objectives.* Belmont, Calif.: Fearon.
Maslow, A. (1954). *Motivation and personality.* New York: Harper & Row.
Narrow, B. W. (1979). *Patient teaching in nursing practice.* New York: Wiley.
Ulrich, B. (1980). Teaching the teachers to teach. *Dialysis and Transplantation, 8,* 744–748.

13

Legal and Ethical Issues in Nephrology Nursing

Beth Tamplet Ulrich

OBJECTIVES

After reading this chapter on legal and ethical issues, the nurse will be able to:

1. Discuss national legislation related to nephrology care
2. Discuss state legislation that affects the field of nephrology
3. Discuss legal precedents that have an impact on the practice of nephrology nursing
4. Integrate the four major ethical principles into the decision-making process

There are a number of legal and ethical issues that must be considered by the nurse who chooses to specialize in nephrology. Those issues range from the legal questions of malpractice and negligence to the ethical question of who shall live and who shall die.

LEGAL ISSUES

The key legal issues in nephrology nursing are the enabling and constraining legislation for the ESRD population, the overall health-care community, and the practice of nursing; and the case law and criminal law precedents in the areas of informed consent, malpractice and negligence, and the practice of nursing.

Legislative Issues

National Legislation. There are numerous federal legislative actions each year in the health-care industry. Only those having significant impact on the nephrology community will be covered in this chapter.

Medicare. The Medicare system is very important to patients with ESRD. As will be explained in more detail in the following section, almost all ESRD patients are now covered under the Medicare system.

The Social Security Act of 1965 established a national health-care program for the elderly called Medicare (Title XVIII). The program was divided into Part A and Part B. Part A, or Hospital Insurance, pays primarily for inpatient services; Part B, or Supplemental Medical Insurance, pays for physician care and other related health services. In its original design, Medicare reimbursed the provider for the lesser amount of cost or charges on a line-item by line-item basis. Therefore, if a hospital could show that it cost more to provide a service than the charge that had been set, the hospital could receive more money. It is easy to see that such a method did not reward efficiency and, in fact, discouraged it, creating an environment that encouraged doing more and getting paid more.

Between 1979 and 1982, the annual growth rate of Medicare spending exceeded 19 percent (Davis, 1983), and controlling program costs became a top priority. The Tax Equity and Fiscal Responsibility Act (TEFRA) of 1982 imposed limits on the total inpatient operating costs of hospitals. The limits were calculated on a per-discharge basis, and were adjusted for differences in each hospital's caseload. Inherent in the TEFRA legislation were financial incentives for controlling costs and financial disincentives for exceeding target costs. The TEFRA legislation was seen as an interim solution while a long-term answer to rising Medicare costs could be developed.

The Social Security Amendments Act of 1983 (Public Law [PL] 98-21) was signed into law on April 20, 1983. The act contained a total revision of the inpatient Medicare hospital reimbursement method based on a prospective payment system (PPS). Under PPS, Medicare pays a predetermined rate for each discharge. On the basis of the patient's principal diagnosis and certain other factors, each discharge is assigned to one of over 470 diagnostic-related groups (DRGs) for payment. Each DRG is assigned a relative weight. Based on certain formulas, which are subject to modification by the legislature, a dollar amount per relative weight unit is determined. The weight is multiplied by the dollar amount, resulting in the reimbursement for that DRG. The top five DRGs with regard to weight, and therefore reimbursement, are cardiovascular-related. The DRG for a kidney transplant is DRG 302 and the weight 4.6267, the sixth highest DRG weight. With only minimal variations, the reimbursement for each patient hospitalized for a kidney transplant is virtually the same regardless of the actual cost. As a comparison, DRG 316, Renal Failure, is weighted at 1.3210; and DRG 317, Admit for Renal Dialysis, is weighted at .4907 (Prospective Payment Assessment Commission, 1986). This reimbursement methodology applies to any Medicare admission.

The changes that have resulted from the implementation of the PPS are numerous. Most obvious is an increased pressure to shorten the patient's hospital stay and a reluctance of certain hospitals to admit Medicare patients who will clearly result in financial losses. Chronic patients, such as those with ESRD, tend to fall into this category.

ESRD Legislation. The first national ESRD legislation (PL 92-603) was signed into law on October 30, 1972, with an effective implementation date of July 1, 1973. As one of the Social Security amendments included in PL 92-603, section 299I "extended Medicare protection to any individual who has end-stage renal disease requiring dialysis or transplantation provided that such individual: (1) is fully or currently insured or entitled to monthly benefits under Title II of the Social Security Act; or (2) is the spouse or dependent child of an individual so insured or entitled to such monthly benefits."

This legislation had been eagerly anticipated by the patient and provider members of the nephrology community. Prior to PL 92-603, the cost of treating ESRD was beyond the means of most individuals. Indigent care facilities could only afford to provide minimal services. This scenario had necessitated the formation of selection committees charged with the responsibility of determining the "best" candidates to receive the available treatments. Those selected lived; those not selected died. PL 92-603 guaranteed that treatment options for ESRD would be available to the vast majority of Americans.

The regulations formulated to implement this legislation were also important. Basic interim regulations developed in 1973 gave way to what were termed final regulations on June 3, 1976. The highlights of those final regulations included:

- Limiting reimbursement to facilities meeting regulatory requirements
- Developing ESRD Network Coordinating Councils to serve as liaisons between the facilities and the federal government, and, through their Medical Review Boards, to review the appropriateness of ESRD patient care and service
- Establishing minimum use requirements
- Setting standards for the basic composition, qualifications, and practice of facility personnel
- Setting standards for patient care planning and the existence of policies to assure safe patient care
- Establishing patient rights and responsibilities, as well as a grievance mechanism

To ensure that these requirements were met, a system of surveying facilities was developed under the auspices of the Medicare survey teams already in existence.

The initial legislation was amended in 1978, with the passage of PL 95-292. This law provided incentives for lower cost self-dialysis, eliminated the financial disincentives for transplantation and lengthened the transplant benefits to 3 years, and expended the role of the ESRD Network Coordinating Council.

In 1981, PL 97-35, the Omnibus Budget Reconciliation Act, changed the reimbursement mechanism for dialysis to a *prospective payment model* and made private insurers, rather than Medicare, the primary payor during the first year of chronic dialysis therapy. This change became effective on August 1, 1983, following the publication of the regulations on May 11, 1983, and heralded many changes for the nephrology community.

Under the original method of payment, the facility was paid the lesser of costs or charges. If a facility could show significant costs over the established charges, an exemption could be made and the facility reimbursement increased. Many facilities took advantage of exemptions. The result of this original payment system was a lack of incentives to cut costs. Facilities, physicians, and vendors providing supplies and equipment flourished.

Under the prospective payment method, one reimbursement rate would be paid for any dialysis procedure, regardless of the type or cost of the procedure. Exemptions were the rarity rather than the norm. In addition, the regulations developed for PL 97-35 changed physician payment to one capitated rate without discrimination as to the treatment modality. In the past, physicians had received much less income from home dialysis patients than from those dialyzed in a center. A major goal of these changes was to encourage less costly home dialysis, which the federal government felt was better for the patients.

One immediate result was a decrease in reimbursement for many facilities. A study by the American Nephrology Nurses' Association (Brennan, 1984) investigated the change in nephrology practice after just 6 months of lower facility reimbursement. The findings indicated that referrals to home dialysis had increased. Nephrology nurses were being required to be more productive, often assuming what had been social worker and dietician responsibilities because the availability of these two types of professionals was decreased. The reprocessing of disposables, while practiced in a number of facilities prior to reimbursement declines, was estimated to expand significantly. In addition, many units discontinued or severely curtailed patient items such as food snacks and linens. The reaction of the nephrology nurses to these changes was not totally negative, because some of the results, such as increased home dialysis, appeared to benefit the patients.

In 1987, the reimbursement rates were decreased further. Despite federal government concern over the total cost of the ESRD program, inflation-adjusted per-treatment costs have declined significantly since the original legislation was passed in 1972.

As a result of legislative reimbursement and practice changes, the nephrology business has become very competitive over the last few years. Instead of decreasing patient items, facilities now actively market their services to the patient population. Few facilities are unaware of accurate costs for each aspect of the treatment process. Dialysis has become big business.

Organ Procurement and Transplantation Act. In 1984, the Organ Procurement and Transplantation Act (PL 98-507) became law. This legislation established the National Task Force on Organ Transplantation to study transplant-related issues, provided financial assistance for organ procurement organizations, funded a national organ-matching network, and prohibited the buying and selling of human organs for transplantation.

State Legislation

Certificate of Need. State-legislated certificate of need (CON) processes have also contributed to the changes in nephrology. In the past, facilities wanting to open or significantly expand their services were required to go through a certificate of need process. This involved demonstrating that the services the facility wanted to provide were, in fact, needed by the community it served. Facilities already in the community were given the opportunity to challenge the request of the new or expanding facility. The goal was the efficient use of resources. The result was a method to limit competition. In 1986, states began to eliminate the CON process, based on the economic philosophy that increased competition results in better and less expensive services for the consumer. In states where the CON process has been eliminated, the number of dialysis facilities has proliferated and existing facilities have increasingly become a part of multifacility corporations.

Reimbursement. While the Medicaid program began as a federal-state matching program under the same legislative package that produced Medicare, the trend in the early 1980s toward returning more responsibility to the states resulted in significant individualization of state Medicaid programs. As a result, there are numerous differences in Medicaid regulations and reimbursement. Some states provide ESRD patients with reimbursement for medications and other treatment-related items. Other states do not. It is necessary for the nephrology nurse to understand the provisions that apply to patients within the specific state in order to serve as a resource for ESRD patients.

Nursing Practice. State legislation also affects nephrology nursing practice. Each state, through legislative action, regulates the practice of professional nurses, practical nurses, and, increasingly, technicians through licensing laws. As with state reimbursement, it is clearly beyond the scope of this book to discuss practice regulations throughout each of the states; however, there is one central theme nationwide: *The Registered Nurse is in charge of nursing care.* Although certain aspects of that care may be delegated, the R.N. remains legally responsible. In 1986, the American Nephrology Nurses' Association developed a position statement on the use of unlicensed personnel in dialysis facilities (Figure 13-1). This position statement reflects current state regulations, and will no doubt be used by the states in formulating future licensure requirements not only for the R.N. but for other nephrology personnel as well.

Legal Precedents

The body of law stemming from court decisions is called case law. Although case law is continually evolving, it is influenced by the doctrine of precedent, which holds that when a similar case has been previously decided, the same legal rules and principles will be applied to the current case. The exception is when social conditions or values have changed since the prior cases were decided. Legal precedents, then, reflect past court decisions that would likely be applicable in the current setting.

The Nurse–Patient Relationship. The primary consideration for nephrology nurses is the precedent that the nurse is personally responsible for his or her acts and omissions and that the nurse–patient relationship is not a derivative of other relationships. The case establishing the nurse–patient relationship precedent is a Texas case, *Lunsford v. Board of Nurse Examiners* (1983). In this case, a patient having chest and left arm pain was brought by a companion

---

**The Use of Unlicensed Personnel
in Dialysis Facilities
for Direct or Indirect Patient Care**

Unlicensed personnel should not perform any duties defined as "nursing practice" under the applicable state nurse practice act.

Unlicensed personnel must work under the direct supervision of a Registered Nurse.

A planned program of initial and ongoing training for unlicensed personnel must exist and be documented.

The competency of unlicensed personnel must be documented.

Figure 13-1. American Nephrology Nurses' Association: Position Statement. (*From American Nephrology Nurses' Association [1985]. ANNA position statement: The use of unlicensed personnel in dialysis facilities for direct or indirect patient care. ANNA Update, July/August 1985, with permission.*)

into a small hospital's emergency room. The patient's companion sought assistance from a physician in the hospital, who told her to see Nurse Lunsford, an R.N. The physician instructed Nurse Lunsford to send the patient to another hospital 24 miles away, since hospital policy was to send all patients to the area referral hospital unless they had a physician on the local hospital staff or it was a "life or death" situation. Nurse Lunsford saw the patient, obtained some history, and referred the patient as ordered.

The patient died on the way. The Board of Nurse Examiners (BNE) rescinded Nurse Lunsford's license for professional negligence. Nurse Lunsford sued, and appealed when the court decided in favor of the BNE. The Texas Court of Appeals upheld the decision of the court, stating that the nurse's duty to the patient is not derivative, and that the nurse's duty stems from the privilege granted by the state. The court of appeals also separated the nurse from any contractual agreement with her employer to act in a certain and prescribed manner.

This case is of extreme importance to nurses, because prior to this time the courts traditionally held that a nurse's professional relationship with a patient is derived from either the patient–physician relationship or the patient–health-care-facility relationship. As a result, damages resulting from a nurse's negligence have been imputed to the physician or health-care facility considered responsible for the patient. Lunsford versus the BNE puts the relationship, and the liability for negligence, squarely on the nurse's shoulders.

Negligence. Negligence measures a nurse's actions or omissions against what a reasonable and prudent nurse would have done in similar circumstances. There are four primary components of negligence upon which a finding of culpable liability is based: (1) a duty of some type owed from one individual to another, (2) a breach of that particular duty, (3) injury or damage suffered by an individual, and (4) a causal connection between the breach of duty owed and the damage suffered (Professor & Keeton, 1984).

Respondeat Superior. The employer can be found negligent in addition to the nurse. The concept of *respondeat superior* holds that the employer is liable for the negligent acts of an employee that are committed during the course and scope of the employee's employment. Numerous cases have relied on this premise for the finding of negligence and award of damages.

Premises Liability. Another area of negligence is premises liability, the responsibility of an institution open to the public to maintain the premises in a safe condition and to warn or guard against the risks and hazards located therein. This concept would apply to hospitals, dialysis facilities, and physicians' offices. Case law has further shown that health-care institutions are expected to assume that the public in their facilities will include the elderly and handicapped, and to make provisions accordingly.

Wrongful Discharge for Refusal to Give Care. Nurses often question whether or not they can refuse to care for certain patients if they have moral, ethical, or medical objections to the care they have been instructed to provide. In *Warthen v. Toms River Community Memorial Hospital* (1985), a discharged nurse sued the hospital for damages, alleging that the hospital had wrongfully discharged her for failure to administer dialysis to a terminally ill, double amputee patient. Nurse Warthen had worked for the hospital for 11 years, and in the dialysis unit for the 3 years prior to the incident. During the summer of 1982, she had dialyzed the patient several times, twice having to terminate dialysis when the patient suffered a cardiac arrest and severe internal hemorrhaging. The next time Nurse Warthen was scheduled to dialyze the patient, she informed the head nurse that she had moral, medical, and philosophical objections to dialyzing the patient. The head nurse reassigned her to another patient. Later that week, Nurse Warthen objected when she was again assigned to the patient, feeling that she had reached a prior agreement with the head nurse. Nurse Warthen then met with the patient's physician, who told her that the patient's family wanted the dialysis continued. The nurse continued to refuse to dialyze the patient, was terminated, and sued for wrongful discharge.

Nurse Warthen justified her refusal as adherence to the Code for Nurses developed by the American Nurses' Association (1981), which she believed constituted a public policy. The court disagreed, stating that the ANA Code of Ethics defined a standard of conduct beneficial to the individual nurse and not to the public at large; and that the nurse's conduct should not be at the expense of the patient's life or contrary to the family's wishes.

Protecting Yourself. In addition to providing the care that any reasonable and prudent nurse would provide in similar circumstances, the nurse must clearly document the care that is given. Most cases take years to come to trial, so the nurse is faced with defending actions long after they have occurred. It is virtually impossible to remember the specifics of a dialysis or a patient on a day that occurred several years ago. Without good documentation, you could be found negligent even if you were not.

ETHICAL ISSUES

The American Hospital Association's Special Committee on Biomedical Ethics defines ethics as the study of rational processes for determining the most morally desirable course of action in the face of conflicting value choices (American Hospital Association, 1985). The field of nephrology is overflowing with value choices. Who should be dialyzed? Who should receive the available kidney for a transplant? What should be sacrificed when budget cuts occur? When does assisting in the patient's decision process become coercive?

Ethics Principles

There are four major principles that form the basis for ethical decision-making. They are autonomy, beneficence, nonmaleficence, and justice.

Autonomy. Autonomy, the principle most familiar to nurses, is personal liberty of action. The only acceptable reason for removing an individual's autonomy is to prevent harm to others, yet one of the first things that occurs to a patient is a loss of autonomy. Home dialysis and in-center self-care dialysis promote patient autonomy. Nevertheless, the patient loses some freedom of action either because of the dialysis schedule or the lack of energy generally accompanying ESRD. Curtain (1986) has said that to deprive individuals of control of their lives is a most brutal rape of the ego.

In nephrology, the principle of autonomy demands that patients and staff be provided with complete and accurate information on which to base decisions, and that their decisions be respected and adhered to. The power of health-care professionals to influence the patient must be considered. Few things are as coercive as the threat of suffering and death. The statement "If your potassium intake gets too high, you could have a cardiac arrest and die" can be spoken in a manner that either provides information so that the patient can make a decision or in a manner that coerces the patient to do what the health-care professional wants. The choice to do certain things such as following a diet is psychologically distinct from compliance with the nurse's or doctor's orders. Hemodialysis patients are in an especially dependent position, in the worst of cases feeling as though they risk their lives if the staff doesn't like them or their actions.

Beneficence. Beneficence involves doing or contributing to good. Beauchamp and Childress (1983) divide beneficence into two components: provision of benefits and balance between benefits and harm. Health-care professionals are obligated to provide benefits, but not if those benefits produce equal or greater harm. The determination of how much harm the benefit is worth creates conflict.

Nonmaleficence. Nonmaleficence is the duty to do no harm. This principle forms the foundation of most codes of ethics. Harm can be mental as well as physical. Many medical and nursing procedures involve harm of one type or another. Generally, this is because the patient has made the decision that the benefit outweights the harm. The principle is violated when the patient is not consulted or is not provided with complete and adequate information.

Justice. Justice is generally seen to mean fairness. The problem arises in determining what is fair. Is it fair to use certain criteria to determine who receives a kidney transplant? Is it fair to deliver a lower quality of care to indigent patients than to those who pay full fare? Decisions of justice also occur daily when a nurse, having limited time, decides that the needs of one patient outweigh those of another.

Ethical Dilemmas

A number of ethical dilemmas face the health-care industry in general and specifically the field of nephrology.

Patient Competence. Whether or not the patient is competent to exercise his or her right to autonomy is an important consideration. The determination of competency crosses legal as well as ethical boundaries. It is not enough that the patient's family or the health-care professional does not believe the patient to be competent.

Consent. The patient, or guardian if the patient is deemed incompetent, has the right to give or withhold consent to any action upon the person. Inherent in consent is a view of the equality and dignity of all human beings. The legal minimum for consent requires full disclosure about the nature of the condition, all significant facts, and an explanation of the likely consequences resulting from treatment or nontreatment. Ethical considerations expand consent to include the maximal participation of the patient and the assurance that the disclosure, facts, and explanations are not skewed by the health professional's biases.

Confidentiality. Any unauthorized use of confidential information about the patient or organization is unethical. Too often, professional staff members discuss patients in hallways, elevators, and cafeterias, totally disregarding the people around them who may, in fact, know the patients. Nephrology nurses have an ethical responsibility to hold confidential all information about their patients, and to assure that all personnel working under their supervision do the same.

Resource Allocation. Resource allocation has always been a major ethical issue in the care of nephrology patients. It began once chronic dialysis became an accepted mode of therapy. There were too many patients for too few dialysis machines. Selection committees were formed to decide who should live and who should die. The advent of Medicare coverage for ESRD eliminated these committees, but created other ethical issues. Many people question whether it is fair or just to selectively spend federal tax dollars to care for ESRD patients. Subsequent ESRD Medicare cuts have created new resource allocation problems. The decision concerning which services to decrease or eliminate because of less revenue is often an ethical decision based on the principles previously described.

The resource allocation of organs for transplantation has become an ethical issue involving the entire country. The Organ Procurement and Transplantation Act described previously was a national attempt to mandate justice in the allocation of organs. Questions have also arisen concerning whether or not it is ethical for the donor (before death) or the donor family to direct an organ's destination. Ethical issues are prevalent with regard to deciding who will receive the kidney. Irwin (1986) notes that the two methods of selecting recipients are chance or the use of social worth criteria. In the chance method, all individuals are treated equally. If social worth criteria are used, principles of merit or utility are applied. Merit criteria give preference to individuals who have contributed the most to society, while utility criteria give preference to those who have the greatest potential of making a contribution. The problem, of course, is that the worth of contributions, either real or potential, is based on the value systems and ethics of those making the selections.

Conflict of Interest. A conflict of interest occurs when a person has two or more sets of obligations and duties that are in conflict with each other. This may occur, for example, when there are conflicts between the needs of the facility and the needs of the patients, or between the needs of the facility and the needs of the individual nurse, administrator, or physician.

Making Ethical Decisions
Nephrology nurses are continually faced with ethical decisions. To make these decisions effectively, it is first necessary for each nurse to assess his or her own value system—to determine what is important or valued—and to further determine the priorities of those things valued. For example, is life at any cost preferable to death? What is the nurse willing to compromise in the work setting before moving on to another job? Is it more important to maintain a good relationship with other nephrology professionals, or to assure that the patient receives adequate care? All of these questions and more must be answered in the mind of each individual nurse, before a state of values clarification has been reached. It is also important for organizations to work through the values clarification process.

Once the nurse has clarified his or her value system, he or she can proceed to making or contributing to ethical decisions. Many institutions have developed multidisciplinary ethics committees to assist in the decision-making process. One ESRD network, Network 3 in northern California, has created its own ethics committee with the objective of assisting in ethical decisions (Jones & Burrows-Hudson, 1986).

SUMMARY

Legal and ethical issues are critical to the practice of nephrology nursing. It behooves all nephrology nurses to become familiar with the legislative and case law affecting the profession, to clarify their own beliefs and values, and to understand the ethical principles involved in making decisions concerning themselves and their patients.

REFERENCES

American Hospital Association. (1985). *Report of the special committee on biomedical ethics. Values in conflict: Resolving ethical issues in hospital care.* Chicago: AHA.

American Nephrology Nurses' Association. (July/August 1985). ANNA position statement: The use of unlicensed personnel in dialysis facilities for direct or indirect patient care. *ANNA Update.*

American Nurses' Association. (1981). *Code for Nurses.* Kansas City, Mo. ANA.

Beauchamp, T. L., & Childress, J. F. (1983). *Principles of biomedical ethics* (2nd ed.). New York: Oxford.

Brennan, D. T. (1984). Impact of prospective payment regulations: Results of the head nurse survey. *ANNA Journal, 11,* 49–52.

Curtain, L. (1986). Autonomy, accountability and nursing practice. In P. L. Chinn (Ed.), *Ethical issues in nursing* (pp 95–102). Rockville, Md.: Aspen.

Davis, C. K. (1983). The federal role in changing health care financing. *Nurs Econ, 1,* 10–17.

Irwin, B. C. (1986). Ethical problems in organ procurement and transplantation. *ANNA Journal, 13,* 305–310.

Jones, V., & Burrows-Hudson, S. (1986). Ethics in nephrology: A regional approach. *ANNA Journal, 13,* 320.

Lunsford v. Board of Nurse Examiners. 648 SW2d (Tex Civ App 3 Dist 1983).

Professor & Keeton on the Law of Torts. (1984). Sec. 30, at 164–165.

Prospective Payment Assessment Commission (1986). *1987 adjustments to the Medicare prospective payment system: Report to Congress.* Washington, D.C.: Author.

Warthen v. Toms River Community Memorial Hospital. 199 N.J. Super. 18, 488 A.2d 229 (N.J. Super A.D. 1985).

14

Quality Assurance in Nephrology Nursing

Nancy Fredin

OBJECTIVES

After reading this chapter on quality assurance, the nurse will be able to:

1. Trace the development of nursing quality assurance activities in the past 150 years
2. Identify four factors affecting the continued evolution of nursing quality assurance activities
3. Define structure, process, and outcome criteria
4. Discuss five key points to consider when developing a quality assurance system
5. Discuss the relationships of nursing research and nursing quality assurance

The provision of quality patient care has long been a goal of the nursing profession. As nephrology nurses have become more comfortable with the roles of patient advocate and primary nurse, this interest in quality care has expanded. Shrouded in mystery and misunderstanding, quality assurance has traditionally been viewed with distrust and dislike. In reality, however, health-care professionals heartily agree with the need for objective patient care evaluation. *Quality assurance* (QA) may be described as the systematic approach to patient care evaluation. To ensure success, QA activities must involve not just one or two people, but all the professionals caring for a patient. The goal of QA activities is to assure provision of the best possible care for individual patients. Although the definition of QA activities is straightforward, the application of these ideas is more complex.

Patient care can generally be evaluated from three different perspectives: structure, process, or outcome. First used by Donabedian (1980) to describe medical care evaluation, these perspectives are generally used to construct criteria or standards for the evaluation of nursing care. The physical, financial, and organizational characteristics of a facility are addressed by *structure standards* or criteria. Fire codes, equipment availability, and staffing guidelines are monitored by structure standards. *Process standards* address how care is administered, focusing on methods rather than the end product. Examples of process standards include interventions to be included in standard postoperative nursing care or methods to be used for patient teaching. *Outcome standards* seek to define changes in health status, health knowledge, or behaviors as a direct result of nursing care. The focus here is on the end product rather than methods. Examples of outcome standards would be delineation of facts ESRD patients would be expected to repeat after successful patient teaching, or skills a home dialysis patient would demonstrate upon completion of home dialysis instruction.

HISTORICAL PERSPECTIVE

Florence Nightingale is generally credited as the first nurse to be concerned with evaluation and standards. *Notes on Nursing,* first published in 1859, presented basic care standards for patients and stressed the importance of meeting those standards whether care is provided by family members or a hired caregiver. The century following Florence Nightingale's first work was a period of dramatic growth and change. Rapid gains in the quality of nursing care were made, largely due to the emphasis on nursing education. Research conducted during this period concentrated on quality education as a means to quality care. World War II had a great impact on the nursing profession. A critical shortage of nurses during the war prompted studies of nurse staffing and nurse availability in the postwar years.

During the past three decades, much research effort has been directed towards the QA process as it applies to nursing practice, greatly contributing to the expansion of the QA knowledge base. These studies have approached QA from multiple perspectives and used various methodologies and data sources. Increasing sophistication in QA techniques should be one positive result of continued QA research.

FORCES INFLUENCING QUALITY ASSURANCE

As nursing practice continues to evolve, adjustments in practice evaluation must be made. While research activities continue, several other forces are influencing the expansion of monitoring and evaluation activities.

Economic Forces

The impact of economic concerns cannot be underestimated, particularly in the United States where health care is philosophically supported as a right for all people. However, the realities of growing concern for the cost of health care have forced the consideration of health care as a scarce resource that may need rationing.

Although many fear the advent of prospective payment will lead to decreasing quality of care, logic prompts a second look at this theory. Under a cost reimbursement system, institutions were reimbursed even if an error on the practitioner's part or a systems problem resulted in an increased length of stay. Under prospective payment, such as the current ESRD reimbursement system, reimbursement is predetermined, encouraging institutions to take new steps to ensure that costs are at or below reimbursement. Identification of factors impeding the delivery of quality care or causing increased patient resource use can directly impact the organization's bottom line.

Professional Factors

With the recognition of the nursing process as the scientific foundation for professional nursing practice, evaluation has become a more meaningful concept. Expansion of those concepts beyond evaluation of a single nursing intervention to patient care as a whole will make quality assurance activities more meaningful for nurses. As the nursing profession evolves, accountability for practice will continue to increase. The American Nurses Association (ANA) has played a central role in the promotion of QA activities. The first constitution of the ANA, in 1897, outlined goals for establishing ethical standards and improving nursing education. Continuing through recent history, the ANA has actively pursued establishment of standards for quality practice. In 1968, the ANA established the Congress for Nursing Practice, which published *Standards for Nursing Practice* (ANA, 1976). In 1974, Lang developed a model for quality assurance that was subsequently adopted as the ANA model for quality assurance. This model, which appeared in *A Plan for Implementation of the Standards of Nursing Practice* (1975), clearly indicates the dynamic nature of the quality assurance process. The ANA continues promotion and development of QA through several ongoing projects. The implementation plan was updated in 1980 by the American Nurses' Association. Other noteworthy activities include sponsorship of a conference on quality assurance as it relates to nursing, sponsored jointly with the American Hospital Association in 1963, and development of patient outcome criteria in the late 1970s. In 1982, the ANA published a series of quality assurance works outlining specific guidelines for monitoring and problem solving activities.

The American Nephrology Nurses Association (ANNA) has also been active in QA activities. In 1982, the ANNA first published the *Nephrology Nursing Standards of Clinical Practice*. As stated in the introduction, the ANNA firmly believes that "A profession's concern for the quality of its service constitutes the heart of its responsibility to the public" (p.1). These standards were revised in 1988. By recognizing and evaluating the unique contributions of all health-care team members to the care of the ESRD patient, excellent care may be assured.

Consumers
The advent of increasing consumer awareness and activism has also influenced the health-care industry. Gone are the days of investing health-care providers with unquestioning trust and the power to make decisions for the individual. While continuing to respect health-care providers for the knowledge and services provided, consumers are beginning to play a very active role in health care. Increased knowledge has led to close scrutiny of health-care services. More and more consumers expect options for meeting their health-care needs and the right to choose the option they perceive will best meet their own needs.

Accrediting Agencies
In 1918, the hospital standardization program was established by the American College of Surgeons. Hospital conditions at the time were deplorable, with initial surveys certifying only a small percentage of the hospitals surveyed. In 1952 a commission was established to assume surveying responsibilities from the College of Surgeons. This commission, now called the Joint Commission on Accreditation of Healthcare Organizations (JCAHO), has become a powerful influence in maintaining quality health care over the past several years (Roberts & Walczak, 1984). Although participation is voluntary, most hospitals across the country participate in JCAH surveys.

In 1986, the Health Care Financing Administration (HCFA), the federal agency charged with overseeing hospital participation in the Medicare and Medicaid programs, published revised guidelines for participation in the programs. Notably, a new standard requiring the establishment of a hospital-wide QA program was included. Specifically, these guidelines call for a comprehensive evaluation of care provided and actions and outcomes of those actions taken to correct identified problems. The standard has yet to be included in specific ESRD guidelines, but movement toward such a standard may be anticipated.

QUALITY ASSURANCE PROGRAM DEVELOPMENT

A successful quality assurance program begins with careful planning and a clear statement of the program goals. Although conceptualization is important to the planning process, careful operationalization of these concepts may also make the difference between success and failure. An assessment of patient needs and organizational needs will help clarify values and goals and provide insight into which methods might be most appropriate for your setting.

Goals

Goals of a QA program should address the needs of individual facilities and the patients commonly seen in the nephrology unit. Quality assurance program goals might include:

1. Assessing the current status of care administered or offered
2. Providing a system for problem identification and problem resolution
3. Assuring provision of the best possible care for the lowest resource consumption (cost:benefit ratio)

Roles

Once program goals are established, persons who will be involved in the QA system and their roles must be identified. Generally, it is wise to use as many existing lines of authority and communication channels as possible. Creation of new reporting procedures will only open the system to confusion and unnecessary complexity.

Final responsibility for the quality of care administered in any facility rests with the governing body. This may be a chief executive officer or president of the board of directors in a free-standing facility, or a board of trustees in a hospital setting. In constructing a quality assurance program, this body must be assured of regular, accurate reports summarizing QA activities in the facility.

The next level of accountability lies at the administrative level. By nature of their positions, administrators, including nurse-administrators, must actively support QA activities in their facility. Problems noted in patient care may at times require administrative intervention for problem resolution. Many times these types of problems center on resource use. Lack of equipment or supplies may have just as much impact on patient care as personnel availability. Administrators must take responsibility for acting quickly and prudently when the quality of patient care is threatened.

This administrative responsibility encompasses one or more administrative levels within an organizational hierarchy. Depending on the size of the facility, different administrative levels may have different scopes of responsibility.

The staff nurse is equally important to the QA program. All nurses must be involved in some manner, be it data collection, data evaluation, or planning problem resolution. Quality assurance cannot be delegated to one nurse or a small group of nurses. To obtain maximum benefit, everyone must be involved.

Education is frequently needed to achieve this level of effective involvement by all nursing personnel. Again, as demonstrated by the brief review of QA history, quality assurance has changed greatly over the past years. The knowledge base supporting QA activities has grown tremendously even in the past decade. Nurses generally do not possess a broad knowledge of QA concepts, let alone understand the application of those concepts. An initial overview during orientation to the facility, followed by ongoing in-service education programs, can meet the learning needs of staff nurses.

In addition to defining roles and lines of communication with nursing staff and administrators, consideration must be given to health-care team members. Although the care of most patients requires the skills of many disciplines, this is particularly true of the renal patient. A comprehensive QA program in the nephrology setting includes social workers, dietitians, physicians, and technical staff. Many facilities choose to design their QA program in a multidisciplinary format, while others choose to have each discipline conducting QA independently and merely interfacing at predetermined points. Regardless of the system used, the importance of sharing QA data with all health-care professionals cannot be underestimated.

Standards of Care

Before proceeding with further discussion of QA program development, consideration must be given to standards of care. A simple definition of "quality care" would be very difficult to construct. Quality care is not an absolute; rather, it must be defined in relation to a standard. As defined by Crow (1981), standards of care are some measure or measures by which nursing care can be judged or compared.

Standards are a common measure used in many different fields. In manufacturing industries, standards are generally concrete and easy to measure. For example, if a standard states that bolts manufactured by a certain company are to be within plus or minus 0.1 percent of the stated size, a quick measurement of bolts manufactured by this company will determine whether the standard has been met. In health care, while outlining a standard of care is difficult enough, the measurement of that standard is even more complex. For example, a patient care standard states that all newly diagnosed ESRD patients will be taught five specific points about their disease. Measurement difficulties arise when the patient is "taught" but 2 weeks later is unable to recall the points covered. In this instance, has the standard been met? Although standards may at times be difficult to measure, their importance to the nursing profession cannot be underestimated.

Standards come from a variety of sources including the ANA and specialty organizations such as ANNA, or may be developed within individual facilities. Regardless of the source, standards must be clearly identified and understood by all practitioners. Standards are the cornerstone of all QA programs.

QUALITY ASSURANCE TOOL DEVELOPMENT

The critical factor of any QA program is asking the right questions and using the right data sources. For this reason, tool development and methodologies of data collection must be given careful consideration.

Tool development focuses on asking the right question. In developing a QA tool, several factors deserve consideration. Validity refers to how well what is intended to be measured actually is measured. Criteria comprising a QA tool must be valid. Face validity addresses whether the tool is meaningful and reasonable. Face validity may be established by asking people familiar with what one is trying to measure (for example, patient care) if the tool is indeed reasonable. Content validity, on the other hand, may be obtained by asking a group of experts (such as professional nurses) to assess whether what is intended to be measured actually will be.

Reliability is another factor that is, at times, more difficult to establish. Reliability refers to the accuracy or precision of the tool. Is the tool stable and relatively predictable or is it inconsistent? Reliability may be tested by having two data collectors obtain data simultaneously and compare results.

As alluded to in the preceding paragraphs, before a tool can pass reliability and validity testing, it must be well written. Criteria must be written clearly and address only those things that can be objectively measured. Avoidance of jargon will decrease the possibility of misunderstanding and skewed results. Criteria must address only one behavior and should in fact be achievable. Testing the tool for validity will avoid setting goals that are unrealistic or unobtainable.

Using the appropriate data collection methods and data sources is also essential to a successful QA program. Although some systems may depend on only one methodology and one data source, more comprehensive systems will encompass combinations to yield a broader picture of the patient care being delivered. Common methodologies and data sources include medical record audits, patient and family interviews, nursing staff interviews, unit observations, and patient testing.

Prior to selecting a method and data source, consideration should be given to any requirements for use (such as special skills or equipment, ease of use, data compilation requirements, time commitments, and scope of data required (Schroeder & Maibusch, 1984). Although medical record audits are generally easy to conduct, the information obtained may not be as in depth as required for true assessment of the quality of care administered. Likewise, whereas some interviews may produce in-depth information, much attention must be given to interviewer training. Weighing the advantages and disadvantages of each methodology and consideration of the type of information required will make methodology selection somewhat easier.

The final consideration in this area is when to do data collection. Timing of data collection is generally referred to in relation to a patient receiving care. Retrospective data collection is conducted after a patient has received the care, generally after the patient has been discharged from the hospital or, has completed a treatment in the outpatient dialysis facility. Concurrent data collection is conducted while the patient is still receiving care in the hospital or during the course of a treatment. Consideration of the data collection time frame will also influence methodologies and data sources.

CASE STUDIES

As discussed earlier, care may be evaluated from a structure, process, or outcome perspective. To illustrate this point and describe actual QA programs, two hypothetical case studies are presented.

Inpatient Setting

Unit A is a 20-bed renal nursing unit, located within a large university hospital. Patients cared for on this unit are generally newly diagnosed ESRD patients, other ESRD patients with disease complications, or patients with dialysis access complications. As part of the entire hospital QA program, nurses take an active role in developing criteria specific to their unit or using generic evaluation criteria also used on other nursing units. Care in this unit is evaluated from structure, process, and outcome perspectives.

Organizationally, this unit is within a decentralized nursing department. A head nurse assumes 24-hour responsibility for unit operation as well as fiscal responsibility for the unit. As the unit manager, the head nurse also assumes responsibility for implementation of the unit QA plan. Each year a plan for QA monitoring is developed by the head nurse and his or her staff. The head nurse reports to a clinical director, who also reviews the QA plan and QA data collected. The director of nursing in this facility, responsible for all nursing units in the hospital, reviews plans for each unit's QA programs as well as all QA data. The director of nurses in turn reports nursing QA activities to the hospital QA officer for integration into the total hospital QA program. The QA officer then reports on all QA activities to the board of trustees.

As described previously, Unit A evaluates care from structure, process, and outcome perspectives. QA findings are reported to the unit medical director and to other disciplines as the data indicates. Data are collected while the patient is still receiving care on the unit. Data collection methodologies include medical record audit, patient and family interviews, nurse interviews, and visual observation.

The structure portion of the QA system uses a generic tool developed for use throughout the nursing department. After a thorough evaluation by the head nurse and staff, the tool was deemed valid in their clinical area. Sample criteria from this tool include the following:
1. Are all nurses currently licensed to practice in this state?
2. Are all nursing employees currently certified in CPR as required by hospital policy?
3. Are fire extinguishers inspected monthly?
4. Are internal and external medications stored separately?

The process and outcome tools developed for this unit rely heavily on this unit's standards of care. Patient care standards were developed by staff nurses working together in groups and approved by the staff as a whole prior to implementation. Criteria were then developed from identified patient outcomes and nursing actions. These criteria were also evaluated for content validity prior to use. Examples of process criteria to evaluate the care received by ESRD patients include these:

1. Are patient learning needs identified under the patient problem list?
2. Are physical assessments, including a complete review of systems, documented each shift?
3. Are patients asked how they wish to be addressed?
4. Are medications administered as ordered?

Examples of outcome criteria include the following:
1. The patient will maintain weight within 5 pounds (plus or minus) of his or her desired weight.
2. Patients will report a balanced dietary intake incorporating outlined restrictions.
3. Patients will describe signs and symptoms of dialysis access infection.

To facilitate data collection on this unit, the head nurse assigns all staff members data collection responsibilities. Upon completion of unit orientation, QA criteria and guidelines for data collection are reviewed with new employees. A brief review of the QA tool takes place quarterly in staff meetings.

Once collected, the QA data are compiled and presented to staff members in staff meetings. Using predetermined minimal compliance levels, the data are reviewed and potential problem areas identified. In addition to problem identification, positive feedback for practitioners is emphasized. Problem areas are further assessed for potential causes and priority identification. Plans are then made for problem resolution and follow-up evaluation. A summary of these activities is forwarded to the clinical director, the director of nursing, and eventually to the board of trustees.

Outpatient Setting

Unit B is a freestanding dialysis unit, owned and operated by three private physicians. Organizationally, management services are contracted to handle the financial side of the business, a board-certified nephrologist has been hired as the center's medical director, and a head nurse manages daily operations and personnel. Support services, such as those provided by dietitians and social workers, are also contracted.

This facility chose to approach QA through a multidisciplinary framework and to base evaluation on patient outcomes. Medical record audits and patient interviews are primary data sources. To facilitate this multidisciplinary approach, the head nurse and medical director hold joint responsibility for implementing the QA program. Quarterly reports are forwarded to the owners—the governing body.

A QA committee is established to oversee the QA activities in the facility. Committee members include the medical director, head nurse, a staff nurse, the dietitian, and the social worker. Annually, the committee reviews the data from the previous year and develops a plan for the upcoming year. Once the plan is developed, all health-care professionals employed by the facility participate in implementation. Data collection is assigned to personnel on a rotating basis. The services of a medical records reviewer are contracted on a semiannual basis to conduct an in-depth documentation analysis.

Once again, standards of care are central to this program. Standards outline not only patient outcomes but also speak to the process of delivering care. Outcome criteria were developed and reviewed by all disciplines before acceptance and use. Examples of outcome criteria include:

1. Patients will describe signs and symptoms of infected accesses.
2. Patients will verbalize plans to obtain treatment at alternate treatment facilities in case of emergency.
3. Documentation will reflect a complete dietary assessment by the clinical dietitian each 6 months.
4. Documentation will reflect monthly physician's progress notes.

Data collected are brought before the multidisciplinary QA committee for analysis and problem identification. Again, positive feedback and assessments of "quality" care delivered are stressed. Problems identified in the initial screening may result in more in-depth evaluation, and subsequent review or plans are made at that time for problem resolution. Follow-up monitoring is planned as part of the problem resolution step. Findings are shared with all other health-care professionals and the governing body.

RESEARCH AND QUALITY ASSURANCE

Although QA and research activities are related, there are some major differences. As indicated earlier, QA is a system of evaluation rather than a system of research. Research is generally concerned with uncovering new knowledge that may be generalized to other settings. Quality assurance, on the other hand, attempts to use information generated by clinical research. Gaps in present knowledge or contradictions in previously demonstrated relationships may be pointed out by QA activities.

SUMMARY

As the future of health care itself is unclear, the structure of future of QA activities is also unknown. Although actual systems and methodologies used may change, quality assurance as a concept will continue to be an increasingly important part of professional nursing practice. Attempting to quantify and evaluate the practice of nursing, with its many subtleties and multiple variables, is an overwhelming challenge. But the stakes are high. The provision of quality health care is a goal for all nephrology nurses.

REFERENCES

American Nephrology Nurses' Association. (1982). Standards of clinical practice. Pitman, N.J.: ANNA.

American Nurses' Association. (1975). *A plan for implementation of the standards of nursing practice.* Kansas City, Mo.: ANA.

American Nurses' Association. (1976). *Standards: Nursing practice.* Kansas City, Mo.: ANA.

American Nurses' Association. (1980). *A plan for implementation of the standards of nursing practice.* Kansas City, Mo.: ANA.

Crow, R. (1981). Research and the standards of nursing care: What is the relationship? *Journal of Advanced Nursing, 6,* 491–496.

Donabedian, A. (1980). *The definition of quality and approaches to its assessment.* Detroit, Mich.: Health Administration Press.

Roberts, J., & Walczak, R. (1984). Towards effective quality assurance: The evolution and current status of the JCAH QA standard. *Quality Review Bulletin, 10,* 11–15.

Schroeder, P., & Maibusch, R. (1984). *Nursing quality assurance.* Rockville, Md.: Aspen.

15

Research in Nephrology Nursing

Beth Tamplet Ulrich

OBJECTIVES

After reading this chapter on nursing research, the nurse will be able to:

1. Formulate a nephrology nursing research question
2. Perform an initial literature review
3. Begin the design of a nephrology nursing research project
4. Evaluate research endeavors of self and others

Nursing research is the process of validating and improving nursing practice—of systematically investigating new facts and relationships. It involves challenging tradition and asking "Why is this done in this manner?" More importantly, nursing research involves the search for objective data to demonstrate the worth of nursing activities.

The mention of "research" often brings to mind laboratories with beakers, Bunsen burners, and white rats. Although this may be accurate in the initial stages of the searching for a new cure or the development of a new diagnostic tool, research more often occurs in clinical settings such as nursing units and dialysis facilities. Nurses often believe erroneously that nurses do not do independent research, that research must be done by people with years of research training, that megabucks are required to fund any research endeavor, and—furthest from the truth—that research is boring. Nursing research has been compared to a mystery waiting to be solved, but nurses often make such a task out of research that the adventure is lost.

PERFORMING NURSING RESEARCH

The basic aspects of nursing research are performed by virtually every nurse every day as he or she uses the steps of the nursing process—problem identification, data collection, implementation of corrective measures, and evaluation. Only minimal change is required to convert the well-known nursing process into the less known research methodology.

Problem Identification

The best research is often done on what appear to be the simplest issues. A good research question is the next logical link beyond what is already known. There is a clear distinction, however, between what is known and what is thought. For example, patient and staff education is thought to be beneficial, but relatively few research studies have been done to prove this almost universal belief.

The simplest form of research is the *case study*, which describes one specific case. While better defined as an observation rather than actual research, case studies are the basis for descriptive studies (Fig. 15-1). Both case studies and descriptive studies involve determining what already exists. *Descriptive studies* include research questions such as: What is the current patient population? How much time do patients using different treatment modalities spend in the hospital? Why are they hospitalized? What is the peritonitis rate? What is the total cost of each treatment modality?

The results of descriptive research often give rise to more complex studies where conditions and variables are controlled. In the area of education, a researcher might use different teaching techniques and assess the success of each. The descriptive study on peritonitis could result in a study to determine which of several connection techniques is most successful. *Replication of studies* is necessary to validate the results and to show that the hypothesis or belief is applicable to a broad population, not just to that which was sampled.

In summary, anything that has not been objectively shown to be effective, anything that has been shown to work in other areas or patient populations but has not been studied in nephrology nursing, and anything that can be logically deduced or questioned, is a potential subject for nephrology nursing research.

Formulating the Research Question

Once the problem is identified, the research question must be formulated. The *research question* or statement is referred to as the *hypothesis*. It is a statement of the expected relationship among the variables being studied. Formulating the research question may involve narrowing the original scope of the project to a workable level. Rather than looking at overall adherence to the therapeutic regimen, a researcher might more successfully question one aspect of adherence, such as "What causes a patient to follow or not follow the prescribed diet?" Collaborating with peers during this phase of the research process is very beneficial. A peer critique can uncover missed variables and gaps in logic, and can lead to refinement of the study question. Small problems not identified at this stage can multiply and intensify as the research progresses.

Definitions

Operational definitions are series of words that clearly designate performable and observable acts. These definitions clarify terms used in the study for both the researcher and for future users of the research results. For example, the phrase "to heparinize the patient" can mean minimal or large dosages of heparin administered continuously or intermittently depending on the facility. A definition of "heparinization" would, therefore, be necessary in any study that involved its use. There is no such thing as a right or wrong operational definition. It must, however, convey exactly what is meant when a term is used.

Literature Review

The questions to be answered in a literature review are:

- What facts have already been studied?
- What relationships have already been found?
- At what level of confidence have those relationships been tested?

Computers have greatly facilitated literature reviews. Virtually all medical and university libraries can now easily access journal files. In some cases, the computer can provide the researcher with a copy of the article as well as the abstract. Searches should go beyond the nursing literature into related fields such as psychology, education, and medicine. Criteria for critiquing research are discussed later in the chapter.

The literature review, in addition to assisting in refinement of the study question, will help identify variables. *Variables* are characteristics that can have more than one value. The research question "Does adherence to the prescribed diet depend on the length of time on dialysis?" has many variables. The presumed cause, length of time on dialysis, is referred to as the treatment or *independent variable.* It can be measured by the researcher to determine a relationship to an observed phenomenon. The presumed effect, adherence to the diet, is termed the criterion or *dependent variable. Extraneous variables,* those that may also influence the study, would include such variables as age, sex, educational achievement, and presence of significant others. In many cases, these extraneous variables can be controlled through statistical analysis methods as long as the data are obtained from the subjects. The size of the sample is also important. In general, a small sample will yield results with low reliability. The more variables to be studied, the larger the sample required. Concerns about adequate sample size should be referred to a statistician.

The literature review assists in determining what data should be collected. At the end of the literature review, the research question is finalized.

Research Design

Research designs fall into two major categories, experimental and nonexperimental. In *experimental research,* all of the variables in the study are controlled by the researcher. *Nonexperimental research* generally occurs in a natural setting such as a nursing unit or dialysis facility. Between these two categories is the partially controlled nonexperimental study, in which the researcher exercises some limited control. This type of research is called *quasi-experimental.* Nonexperimental research can be retrospective or prospective. *Retrospective studies* make use of data already obtained, such as chart audits. *Prospective studies* use future data and are therefore more controllable.

Study Population and Sampling

The *study population* is the group that will actually be studied in the research effort. This may include, for example, all patients in a particular facility, network, or state. Since the *total population* can rarely be studied, sampling techniques are used to obtain a representative sample. Data gathered from this sample should then be able to be extrapolated to the larger population. As can be seen in Table 15–1, the methods of sampling vary in complexity and reliability.

TABLE 15-1. SAMPLING METHODS

Nonprobability sampling	No statistical generation can be made to a larger population
Purposive	Handpicked samples which the researcher believes will represent the total population
Convenience	Uses only subjects who are easily accessible
Quota	Convenience sample with controls to prevent overloading
Volunteer	Voluntary participation will influence results
Probability sampling	Provides a replica of the population so statistical techniques can be used and the probability of error computed
Random	Each subject has the same chance of being selected
Systematic	First subject is selected randomly, then every n^{th} subject is used
Stratified random	Ensures that each category is proportionally represented
Cluster	For geographically dispersed populations, it subdivides the population, then randomly selects subjects
Sequential	Includes all subjects from starting point to specified termination point
Matrix	Only some of the subjects complete some of the items. Provides group rather than individual data. Procedures and subjects are randomly identified.

Rights of Human Subjects

If human subjects are to be involved in the study, their rights must be protected. Three basic principles form the foundation of the ethical use of human subjects:

1. Each subject should be treated with respect, as an autonomous agent. The individual with diminished autonomy is entitled to protection.
2. The study should do no harm. Possible benefits should be maximized and possible harms minimized.
3. Benefits and burdens should be weighed judiciously. No group should benefit at the burden of another.

An informed consent should be given to each subject so that the individual can make an informed choice about his or her involvement. The consent must clearly outline the potential risks and benefits of the study. The subject must not be coerced in any way into participating. Nephrology nurses must be particularly alert to this issue. The lifeline dependency of the dialysis or potential transplant patient on the nephrology staff necessitates that the staff look carefully at any research requests from the perspective of the patient. If there is any chance that the patient may feel coerced, the study should be redesigned.

Collecting Data

The most popular methods of data collection include observation, document analysis, surveys, and simulations. Validity and reliability are the key issues in this aspect of the study. Both evaluate the quality of the data. *Validity* is the extent to which the data measures that which they purport to measure. *Reliability* is the accuracy and consistency of the data and measurement tools.

It is important to assure that data from each subject are collected in exactly the same way. If, for example, the study included weighing the patients, the researcher might specify that all weights be taken at the same time each treatment, on the same scale, and with the patients clothed alike.

Data Analysis

Data analysis techniques range from simple percentages to complex multiple regression models. In any health-care setting, there are people specializing in data analysis whose assistance can be and should be obtained. Although this may not be necessary in a descriptive study, it is virtually mandatory in studies of an experimental or quasi-experimental nature which require complex analysis. It is also useful to consult with a data analysis specialist or statistician prior to beginning the research, as these individuals are experts at designing data collection techniques that are both informative and efficient.

Presentation of Findings

Nursing research is of minimal use if results are not shared. Whether through oral or written forms, results must be communicated. This includes negative as well as positive results. If several researchers separately find that an intervention is unsuccessful, but don't report their results, there is sure to be another researcher who will try the same thing, oblivious to the pitfalls. It is more useful for the profession and the patient if the initial research is shared. Inventing a new cure is prestigious, but proving that a purported cure does more harm than good is equally necessary.

USING RESEARCH

As a consumer who wishes to use research findings to validate or alter practice, the nephrology nurse must be able to evaluate research endeavors. The following questions and criteria will assist in that evaluation (Fawcett, 1982).

- Is the theoretical framework explicit and logical? The overall framework should make sense to you.
- Has the problem been studied before? If so, the results should be compared.
- Is the study design appropriate to answer the research question?
- Are the tools reliable and valid? Data should be included as to how this was determined.
- Is the population described fully?
- How large is the sample? It should be large enough to produce reliable data and representative of the total population.
- Could the study be easily replicated based on the data presented? If not, some key facts have been omitted.

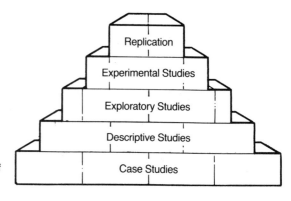

Figure 15-1. Building blocks of successful research.

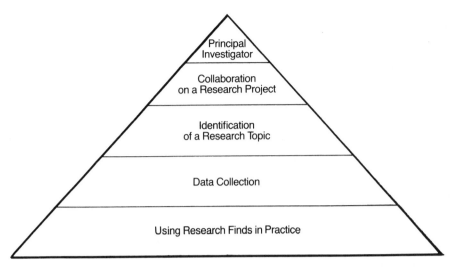

Figure 15-2. Levels of research involvement.

- Does the data analysis answer the original research question?
- Are the conclusions drawn by the researcher logical, based on the data presented?
- Can the results of the study be easily and cost-effectively applied to clinical practice? If not, additional study needs to be done.
- Finally, what overall contribution is made by this research? Does it advance the scientific practice of health care?

By subjecting a study to these questions and criteria, the nurse can determine the worth of the results and whether to incorporate this particular research into practice (Fig. 15-2).

SUMMARY

The nephrology nurse has many opportunities to become involved in nursing research. As a consumer, the nurse can use research findings to understand and validate the practice of nephrology nursing. As a participant, the nurse contributes to establishing the science of nursing. Through the use and performance of clinical research efforts, nephrology nursing can move from the tradition-based practice of the past to a scientific-based practice of the future.

REFERENCE

Fawcett, J. (1982). Utilization of nursing research findings. *Image, 14,* 57–58.

Index

Page numbers followed by *f* or *t* refer to figures or tables respectively.

Page numbers followed by *f* or *t* refer to figures or tables respectively.

Page numbers followed by *f* or *t* refer to figures or tables respectively.

Page numbers followed by *f* or *t* refer to figures or tables respectively.

Page numbers followed by *f* or *t* refer to figures or tables respectively.

Page numbers followed by *f* or *t* refer to figures or tables respectively.

Page numbers followed by *f* or *t* refer to figures or tables respectively.

Page numbers followed by *f* or *t* refer to figures or tables respectively.